The Dynamics
of Clinical Dietetics

The Dynamics of Clinical Dietetics

SECOND EDITION

Marion Mason, Ph.D., R.D.
Ruby Winslow Linn Professor of Nutrition
Simmons College
Boston, Massachusetts

Burness G. Wenberg, M.S., R.D.
Associate Professor and Coordinator
Undergraduate Dietetic Curriculum
Department of Food Science and Human Nutrition
College of Human Ecology
Michigan State University
East Lansing, Michigan

P. Kay Welsch, Ph.D.
Assistant Professor and Director
Center for Educational Services and Records
for Migratory Children in Missouri
College of Education
Southeast Missouri State University
Cape Girardeau, Missouri

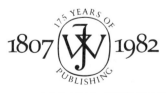

1807 1982

A WILEY MEDICAL PUBLICATION
JOHN WILEY & SONS
New York • Chichester • Brisbane • Toronto • Singapore

Cover design: Wanda Lubelska
Production Editor: Cheryl Howell

Library of Congress Cataloging in Publication Data:

Mason, Marion.
    The dynamics of clinical dietetics.

    (A Wiley medical publication)
    Includes index.
    1. Diet therapy. 2. Dietitians. I. Wenberg,
Burness G. II. Welsch, P. Kay. III. Title.
IV. Series: Wiley medical publication.

RM216.M435 1982   613.2   81-16160
ISBN 0-471-06088-7   AACR2

Printed in the United States of America

10 9 8 7 6 5 4 3

Preface
to the Second Edition

Times have changed since the first edition was written, and we have changed, too. As we have assumed some practitioner responsibilities, listened to our readers, and watched our students work with our ideas and organization, we decided to revise significantly the manner in which the text is organized and to present new tools and techniques where applicable.

Readers of the first edition will quickly note that only Part I, "The Practice of Clinical Dietetics," remains unaltered, with the exception of the addition of some new material and the movement of one chapter to a later section. Part II has been assigned a more appropriate title, and a new chapter on instructional resources has been added. In this section, *resources* for counseling are detailed, whereas Part III deals with *process*, a major change from the first edition. Each of the process chapters in Part III has been significantly revised, with major additions in the chapters on assessment and evaluation.

Part IV contains a new chapter, "Managing Client-Centered Care," which more truly reflects our philosophy that the client is the primary focus of professional attention while at the same time depicting the real world of clinical practice, that of multiple clients and responsibilities. The second of the chapters in Part IV presents some recent developments in evaluation of practice, including audit, peer review, and cost/benefit analysis. The last chapter retains the title from the first edition but is entirely new and deals with a futuristic look at the major responsibilities of all health care practitioners.

The second edition also contains 12 new figures, appearing primarily in the chapters devoted to assessment and to managing clinical practice. These figures graphically demonstrate clinical dietitians' relationships to and responsibilities for clients. We have also deleted some material, primarily in the appendices, to reflect more accurately that what we are about is philosophy and process of clinical dietetic practice, and *not* nutrition science content.

The last four years have witnessed significant changes in the profession, in the professional society, and in professional resources. In that time period, the numbers of practitioners, of those holding advanced degrees, of young members, and of members practicing full time have grown, reflecting the national economy.

Four years ago, the professional society put into operation a new set of bylaws that have already had significant impact on how the society and its members go about their business. Opportunities for leadership positions, once restricted to a relatively small group of people, are now abundant with the advent of special interest practice groups, both at the state and national levels. Thus, decision making is in the hands of more people—a time-consuming process, but one that is necessary for leadership development. The professional society has also, for the first time in its history, made significant strides towards examination of the profession. Studies of the mission of the profession, role delineation, manpower issues, staffing needs, and intervention costs and benefits are either in progress or completed. In this edition we have made a serious effort to record this era in our professional history.

We are also witnessing significant changes in our society, some of which are reflected in the publishing world. In this edition we have tried to use the masculine and feminine genders equally, both for clients and clinical dietitians.

We have been heartened by the reception that the text has received. We have made the discovery that there are literally hundreds of readers, practitioners and educators alike, who embrace our philosophy. New generations of practitioners are being initiated into the profession through the pages of this text. Knowing this makes our efforts worthwhile.

M.M.
B.G.W.
P.K.W.

Preface
to the First Edition

The increasingly visible role of nutrition as a component of comprehensive client care is an important force creating changes in the health care delivery system. Historical contributions to this increasing visibility include the U.S. Senate Select Committee on Nutrition and Human Needs; the 1969 White House Conference on Food, Nutrition and Health; the Ten State Nutrition Survey; and the Study Commission's Report on the Profession of Dietetics. Concurrently it has been ascertained that there is no available text that serves as a base for the preparation of the dietetic professional in those tasks related to meeting the nutritional needs of clients in comprehensive care. *The Dynamics of Clinical Dietetics* has been designed to respond to this need. In addition, the authors foresee that the text can serve to assist other decision makers in the health sciences. Health practitioners, administrators, and planners who participate in or contribute to comprehensive client care are provided an interpretation of the dietetic practitioner's unique role in this care.

The Dynamics of Clinical Dietetics proposes a theoretical base for the *practice* of Clinical Dietetics that has as its primary aim the provision of nutritional counseling and nutrient sources. The text utilizes a systems approach to identify assessment, planning, implementation, and evaluation tasks whereby the clinical dietitian can support the client in becoming an independent decision maker in selecting those foods that meet his nutritional needs. The conceptual framework for the text has evolved from the authors' practitioner, teaching, and research experiences, and thus is an outcome of many attempts to clarify for students the process of learning the behaviors incumbent on a clinical dietitian.

The genesis of *The Dynamics of Clinical Dietetics* may be found in Chapter 1, "The Clinical Dietitian at Work." This chapter defines the basic roles of the clinical dietitian in nutritional care. Subsequent chapters present definitive discussions of the processes necessary to fulfill those roles. All chapters, in one way or another, deal with the very heart of practice, the process of nutritional counseling.

The Dynamics of Clinical Dietetics provides learners in the profession of Dietetics with a comprehensive, timely view of the 'world of work.' It is expected that introductory course work in the biologic and behavioral sciences and, of course, in the disciplines of Food and Nutrition, will precede comprehension of the text's proposed model. Thus, the text is designed to serve dietetic students and/or interns in both the didactic and clinical components of the curriculum.

In addition to beginning learners, the authors believe that the text will assist advanced learners. As they become experienced in working with clients, advanced students can more readily conceptualize and thus act on the process of helping clients achieve independence in their nutritional care. It is also anticipated that the practicing dietitian will find the content useful in client-centered care, no matter the setting in which he finds himself.

The debt of the authors is without limit to those who have participated in either the conception or the completion of the manuscript. We gratefully acknowledge the contributions and support of our colleagues, our families, and our friends, but especially, our former and current students.

M.M.
B.G.W.
P.K.W.

Contents

PART II.
RESOURCES FOR NUTRITIONAL COUNSELING

J.   Preliminary Data Schedule   340

K.   Self-Evaluation Guide for Clinical Dietitians   342

GLOSSARY   345

INDEX   349

LIST OF TABLES

LIST OF FIGURES

LIST OF FIGURES, continued

PART
I

The Practice
of Clinical Dietetics

1
The Clinical Dietitian at Work

Most dietitians . . . are prone to think in terms of pathology and therapy. But, the bulk of Americans are healthy. To be effective, attention must be drawn to normal nutrition in its most positive aspects, to the preventive role of nutrition, to the changing life styles of a prosperous population.

Corrine H. Robinson, **Nutrition education— what comes next?** (*J. Am. Dietet. A.* 69:126, 1976).

One of the most common—and difficult—questions posed to dietitians by potential clients and by the public at large is, "What does a dietitian do?" As the reader will discover, there have been, and will continue to be, a host of responses, many of which are appropriate yet not mutually exclusive. To demonstrate this idea, one need only look at the summary report of the most exhaustive study ever undertaken of the profession of Dietetics.[2] In the words of the Study Commission on Dietetics:

It is clear that the answer to the question, Who and what are dietitians? is determined largely by the nature and purpose of the institution within which they work. In turn, the types of institutions which employ dietitians are those which have the resources to pay them.[2] (p. 17)

The Commission clearly emphasizes the point that the nature of the work of dietitians, including clinical practitioners, is determined largely by the professional environment in which they are practicing. In the ideas expressed in the lead quote above, Robinson[1] implies that dietitians are working primarily in acute care settings, thus leaving their important responsibilities in the vast areas of health promotion and maintenance unattended. Whether or not this is true remains to be seen.

In spite of myriad institutions and their reasons for existing, there are any number of responses to the query "What does a dietitian do?" that are common to all who practice in clinical environments. A first response may be that dietitians are health professionals[2] using their knowledge of foods, food composition, and nutrition to assist people, healthy or not, in developing patterns of food selection and consumption that will enable them to meet their physiologic, socioemotional, and intellectual needs. That particular answer implies, or should imply, that the *practice* of Dietetics is, in part, based on the *science* of Nutrition.[3]

NUTRITION AND DIETETICS DEFINED

The defining limits of the science of Nutrition have been enormously expanded in the last two decades as a result of the development of knowledge in a variety of technologies, and in the interests of a diversity of scientists. The definition of the science of Nutrition depends largely on the nature of the definer, whether he be cell biologist, physiologist, biochemist, anthropologist, psychologist, educator, internist, nutritionist, or dietitian. For the purpose of clarity in this text, nutrition is defined as:

> . . . the science of food, the nutrients and other substances therein, their action, interaction and balance in relation to health and disease, and the processes by which the organism ingests, digests, absorbs, transports, utilizes and excretes food substances. In addition, nutrition must be concerned with certain social, economic, cultural and psychological implications of food and eating.[4] (p. 955)

A universal definition such as this one encompasses both the biologic and behavioral aspects of the food consumption of humans and includes the premise that food *and* nutrition are not identical entities, but are to be considered as synergistic. Other definitions of the science of Nutrition include the hypothesis that the discipline is also a "social means" to achieve the goal of meeting health needs.

Earlier in these pages, we said that dietitians are health professionals who use their knowledge of foods and nutrition to meet particular needs of clients.* Thus, dietitians base their practice on the foundations of the science of Nutrition and the study of foods. But what is *Dietetics?* In 1969, the term "dietetics" was comprehensively defined by a committee of The American Dietetic Association as:

> . . . *a profession concerned with the science and art of human nutrition care, an essential component of the health sciences. It includes the extending and imparting of knowledge concerning foods which will provide nutrients sufficient for health and during disease throughout the life cycle and the management of group feeding for these purposes.*[5] (p. 92)

Dietetics, then, may be viewed as a very diverse profession concerned with virtually all human-oriented aspects of food and nutrition. Dietetics is basically a service profession, providing both tangible and intangible benefits to individuals, groups, and even whole populations! In this text, attention will be directed toward one particular aspect of Dietetics, the rendering of client-centered health care.

The definition of Dietetics that appears above incorporates a relatively new term, "nutrition care." In its broadest sense, nutritional care may be defined as the creative act of translating the bodies of knowledge of nutrition and other scientific disciplines to resolve the food problems and concerns of humans. From this global view, all aspects of dietetic practice are included, ranging from client counseling in private practice to the direction of large foodservice systems. For purposes of clarity, our definition of nutritional care is biased, in that we believe the *practice* of clinical dietetics and the provision of nutritional care are synonymous. Thus, we could title this first part "The Provision of Nutritional Care," since we believe that "The Practice of Clinical Dietetics" means the same thing!

We have now accepted a working definition of Nutrition, stated that the profession of Dietetics is anchored unequivocally to the disciplines of food and nutrition, and declared that the practice of clinical dietetics means the provision of nutritional care. It is now appropriate to examine further the term "clinical" and its meaning in these pages.

---

* The term "clients" has been chosen to designate all those persons benefiting from the practice of clinical dietetics. In these pages, the term "client" implies both apparently healthy *and* ill individuals. To many clinical dietitians, the term "patient" implies persons captive in acute care settings and, thus, is too restrictive for the principal theme of this text.

In the foregoing discussions, we have repeatedly used the term clinical to denote a particular aspect of dietetic practice. The phrase, clinical dietetics, describes a service aspect of the profession that results in both tangible and intangible benefits. That service was defined earlier as the rendering of client-centered health care. This view is in accordance with that of Johnson, who stated that ". . . clinical dietetics is a health service designed to aid people in maintaining or re-establishing a positive state of well-being"[6] (p. 219). In its brevity, Johnson's statement omits the idea that clinical dietetic practice is based on the disciplines of food and nutrition, but does emphasize the concept of health, and places no restrictions on environment or practice sites. The definition we shall accept in these pages is one that accounts for a more holistic view: *Clinical dietetics is nutritional care, offered in an environment where clients and their needs, physical, socioemotional, and intellectual, are the primary foci of professional effort.*

The practice sites of clinical dietitians have been the subject of debate because of the once conventional view that clinical dietitians restricted their activities to acute care environments. This belief is no longer viable, which is evidenced in part by the acceptance of the term "clinical dietitian" in place of the older phrase, "therapeutic dietitian." In this text, the term "clinical area" is used to denote any or all of those practice sites where dietitians are engaged in client-centered nutritional care. As such, the phrase "clinical area" may be used to describe institutional settings for acute or chronic health care; ambulatory care services located within the confines of an acute care setting or a community-based "open-door" clinic; an official or voluntary public health agency offering consultative services and morbidity care to individuals and families; the newer Health Maintenance Organizations (HMOs); or private practice in Dietetics.

"What does a dietitian do?" may be further answered by examining the roles and responsibilities of clinical practitioners in terms of their activities. An extensive review of the literature reveals, in almost every instance, that the clinical dietitian's work in primarily directed toward the interpretation of the disciplines of food and nutrition into the provision of a service designed to maintain or improve the health status of the clients she serves. In the global view, the clinical dietitian then:

1. Translates nutritional science and the study of foods into the skill of offering optimal nourishment to people
2. Assumes responsibility for supervision and facilitation of the nutritional care of individuals and groups

With the passage of time, especially since the 1972 Study Commission report, these ubiquitous role statements have been extensively refined. One such role refinement on the horizon is the assumption of the task of diet prescriptions. As this particular aspect of practice is the subject of considerable debate at the moment,[7-10] we shall look at the pros and cons of the issue later.

When clinical dietetics is viewed as a health profession, providing a unique service to individuals and groups with an enormous variety of needs, the role statements presented above seem inadequate to describe the everyday work of practitioners. In addition, the "rendering of client-centered nutritional care" is a phrase that itself is ubiquitous and demands further refinement. As clinical dietitians practice in a variety of health settings, they meet individuals who are totally unable to provide for themselves (e.g., acutely ill clients receiving nutients from nonfood sources). They also meet individuals, families, and groups who may be concerned about the safety of the food supply, the best ways to stretch food budgets, or the quality of meals offered in school lunch programs. The diversity of client interests and needs, therefore, is great and must be addressed by clinicians.

Clinical dietitians, then, attend to large numbers of clients and address themselves to diverse client needs. Therefore, in the view of the authors, the clinical dietitian:

Translates nutritional and behavioral sciences, and the study of foods, into the skills of nutritional care by:

1. Providing nutrient sources to clients who are incapable of both self-determination and self-sufficiency

2. Facilitating client participation, through nutritional counseling, in the selection of foods that provide nutrient sources. Captive in practitioner-managed settings, such clients are capable of self-determination, but are unable to be totally self-sufficient

3. Facilitating client independence in food selection and consumption, through nutritional counseling, for those who are capable of self-sufficiency and self-determination

A schematic presentation of these three statements is shown in Figure 1.1.

The first responsibility of clinical dietitians is concerned solely with the provision of nutrient sources to clients who are totally dependent, and therefore unable to be either self-determined or self-sufficient. Such persons may be hospitalized in acute care or even chronic care settings, and include those who are physically, mentally, or emotion-

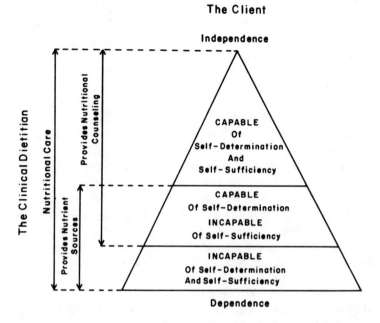

FIGURE 1.1   The Clinical Dietitian in Client-Centered Nutritional Care

ally unable to make decisions about food. In this segment, clinicians are responsible for the appropriateness of the nutrient sources provided each and every client,[11] but they are not primarily involved either in foodservice activities or the preparation of pharmaceutical products (e.g., intravenous feedings). In the figure, this statement occupies the small space on the bottom, to emphasize the premise that *clinical dietitians should be providing nutritional counseling as their primary professional role.* Such a view is supported by a recent federal government publication, *Disease Prevention & Health Promotion.*[12] The Task Force responsible for the preparation of this important document cited 12 categories of *behavior* (italics ours) that may be identified as important determinants of health status. Number two is Nutrition.

The second responsibility statement—that of facilitating client participation through nutritional counseling, in the selection of foods—is suggestive of the practitioner's responsibilities to individuals and groups who are able to make decisions, but who are not totally free to carry out those decisions. Such persons may be active residents of dormitories, retirement centers, or nursing homes. They may also be clients hospitalized in acute care settings, fully capable of self-determination, but consuming meals provided by the foodservice system. Other such individuals may be banded together in groups, such as children having lunch at school, older adults gathering at a Nutrition Center, or even individuals enrolled in a Meals-On-Wheels program. Thus, the second responsibility statement includes the two unique roles of the clinical practitioner: provision of nutritional counseling *and* provision of nutrient sources through food. Although the clinical dietitian is not primarily responsible for the foodservice aspect of feeding programs, she *is* responsible for the *appropriateness* of the foods offered each and every client. That statement implies that the clinician is responsible, through nutritional counseling, for helping clients make decisions when food choices are available. This is reflected in Figure 1.1 in the term "Capable of Self-Determination; Incapable of Self-Sufficiency."

The third responsibility statement—that of facilitating client independence through nutritional counseling—suggests the clinical dietitian's work with the greatest number of clients, and includes those activities suggested by Robinson.[1] In this responsibility, clinicians work with clients about to depart from practitioner-managed settings, ambulatory clients (as in the community open-door clinic), and both individuals and groups in the general population (as 4-H groups or church groups). Such persons are, by definition, capable of both self-determination and self-sufficiency. They are able to make decisions about food and carry out those decisions. Nutritional counseling, in this segment, is primarily directed towards the maintenance of health, although the achievement of health may be a goal as well.

In the triangle of Figure 1.1, this responsibility statement occupies the apex position as the authors believe that the work of clinical dietitians is most crucial here. The primary emphasis of practice should be health maintenance, through nutritional counseling, as ". . . the bulk of Americans are healthy"[1] (p. 128). Such a view is supported by Hirsch and co-workers in their design of a clinical training program for dietitians.[13] Dietetic learners in an ambulatory care unit are expected to adopt behaviors that support clients striving to achieve a greater state of self-determined actions.

The easiest way to watch the clinical dietitian at work, *fulfilling his two primary roles in the provision of nutritional counseling and the provision of nutrient sources,* is to examine those activities we will describe as "The Components of Clinical Practice." These components give specific direction to the activities described in the preceding sections, and provide some structure to the reply to "What does a dietitian do?"

THE COMPONENTS OF CLINICAL PRACTICE

Given many names by a variety of professionals in myriad disciplines, the components of clinical practice provide the structure within which the clinical dietitian functions. These basic and essential elements of nutritional care include four specific activities:

1. Assessment
2. Planning
3. Implementation
4. Evaluation

We shall examine each of these activities in this chapter and then later provide for the reader the beginning concepts and tools needed by the clinical dietitian in performance of his professional roles.

Assessment

Assessment is the term applied to the gathering of data for the client and from the client. The accumulated data are then analyzed and the results applied in the next stage of nutritional care, which is planning. In all cases, the assessment process involves the client, whether he is engaged by the clinical practitioner in a one-to-one conversation or the counselor uses secondary sources of data, or both. The assessment process includes the collection of information about the client's perceived needs, his attitudes and knowledge, and his food practices.

The methods by which assessment data are acquired may vary from clinician to clinician. The one common tool used by all practitioners is the diet history. This history may take many forms, but its primary objective is to obtain as complete a picture as possible of the client's food intake patterns. The tool includes not only a description of food intake, but a review of the many variables affecting food behavior. The diet history, then, provides the information necessary for the assessment of the adequacy of food intake and the parameters that affect that intake. The diet history is also a process. As such, the diet history represents the procedure for data collection, often using the skills of interviewing.

The effectiveness and reliability of the diet history depend greatly on the communication skills of the clinician. Inherent in these skills is the ability of the clinical dietitian to establish and maintain rapport with the client. The ability of a counselor to interact effectively with the client and his "significant others"* greatly affects the outcome of the communication process. In addition, the professional worker needs to be able to recognize his own strengths and weaknesses in working with clients. The way the counselor works, that is, *the performance of the role,* is an individual matter and significantly affects the diet history outcome as ". . . the manner in which he performs the functions . . . becomes a part of the role"[14] (p. 22).

It seems appropriate here to introduce to the reader another concept; that is "nutritional history." There has been abundant misuse of the terms "diet history," "nutritional history," "dietary status," and "nutritional status." As a tool, the *diet history* describes the food intake and food behaviors of a client. It includes information about food purchasing practices, food preparation facilities, special dietary supplement intake (e.g., vitamin preparations), and meal patterns. The diet history furnishes the information for statements about dietary status. Frequently the term nutrition history has been used interchangeably with diet history, but the two are not synonymous. *Nutrition history* is a broader concept, implying the incorporation of information obtained from the diet history *and* laboratory and clinical data.

Statements about status have also been inaccurately incorporated into the language of Dietetics. A clarification of the terms dietary status and nutritional status has been offered by Young:

> *"Dietary status" tells us only what the individual has been eating; it gives no direct indication of nutritional status—only presumptive evidence if his nutritional requirements are average and there are no conditioning factors present.*
>
> *"Nutritional status" refers to the actual nutritional condition of the patient as measured by physical examination, laboratory determinations, pathologic morphology, and therapeutic response under controlled conditions. Nutritional status is influenced not only by dietary intake, but also conditioning factors, such as increase in nutrient requirements, excretions, or destruction and interferences with nutrient intake, absorption, or utilization which may be operating either currently or in the past.*[15] *(p. 98)*

We therefore urge the reader to remember that the diet history, as an assessment tool, furnishes the foundation for statements about *dietary*

---

* "Significant others" is a sociologic term that denotes those important persons included in an individual's social systems; here the phrase is used to describe those persons with whom the client lives or shares food-centered activities, such as family and/or friends.

status. The diet history is just one of the many tools used for the assessment of *nutritional* status.[16]

In addition to the diet history, other data sources are available to the clinical dietitian for assessment purposes. One of these sources is the medical record, the primary communication tool used by all health professionals. The content of the medical record will vary according to the orientation of the care institution, but will usually contain a detailed explanation of the reasons for the client's admission to the system; the supporting evidence for his plan of treatment, including physical examination reports and results of diagnostic tests; notes about his progress with the treatment plan; and, eventually, a discharge summary with both statements of evaluation and plans for continuation of treatment, if necessary. In all sections of the medical record, valuable content may be obtained to be incorporated into the clinical dietitian's assessment. This is especially true of the sections devoted to reports of diagnostic tests.

Implied in the term "assessment" are also the analytic activities that follow the collection of pertinent data from a variety of sources. First, the adequacy of a client's food intake is evaluated, using appropriate sources of food composition data and nutrient intake guidelines. These professional tools will be discussed in a later chapter; suffice it to say here that knowledge of food composition and its application in designing nutritional care plans are two of the primary competencies that others expect of clinical dietitians.[17–19]

The impressions gained from both the client and his "significant others" are important contributions to understanding the client's needs, attitudes, and knowledge. In addition, the assessments of other health workers allow for a greater knowledge of the client, which provides the clinical dietitian further insight needed for the next step of planning.

There is one further obligation of the clinical dietitian in this phase and that is the responsibility for the interpretation, evaluation, and use of research related to nutritional care. The competent practitioner "Understands the significance of scientific inquiry and interpretation in advancing professional knowledge and improving standards of performance"[5] (p. 92). The wise utilization of new knowledge can only lead to assessment that serves ultimately to benefit the client.

Planning

In a health crisis. The second component of clinical practice, the process of planning, is achieved through the efforts of the practitioner alone or with other health workers during those periods of physiologic and/or psychologic stress that may occur in acute care settings. In such a situation, the client may be unable or unwilling to participate in the planning phase, or it may be that his participation is inappropriate *at this time*. The provision of nutrient sources, through foods or by other means, during a health crisis is the primary responsibility of the clinical dietitian.

The planning phase in a health crisis calls for a number of decision-making activities that are dependent on the clinical dietitian's knowledge of nutritional science and other related disciplines. The planning phase may be repeated a number of times as the nature of the crisis changes, or until some degree of health restoration is achieved. At the termination of a crisis, the nature of the client-practitioner relationship will change.

In preventive or maintenance care. In health maintenance and health improvement not of a crisis nature, the process of planning is achieved through the efforts of both the client *and* the clinical dietitian. After all, what is to be planned but a major portion of the client's life—his food? Johnson[6] has defined this orientation as client-managed care, in opposition to the plan manipulated primarily by the clinician (practitioner-managed care). The planning stage, then, is designed to meet the needs of the client, not the needs of the clinician. This hypothesis is in keeping with the view of the practice of clinical dietetics as a client-centered service.

Planning includes a variety of activities that should precede the stage of implementation and follow the steps of assessment. Planning begins with the formulation of goals with the client, based on hypothesized client needs arising from analyses of the assessment data. In this formulation, priorities should be organized and established in such a manner as to be acceptable to *both* the client and the counselor. The plan of treatment, derived from extensive study by all health professionals, should be acceptable to the client. The degree of acceptability is often determined by the degree to which the client was involved in the development of the plan.[20] Helping the client establish his priorities will create a climate for the acceptance of new behaviors. Self-determination is highly motivating and, conversely, authoritarian mandates usually engender passive resistance or active rebellion.

The clinical dietitian should not only assist the client with identifying goals to meet his needs, both perceived and real, but should also at this time confer with him on the appropriateness of the treatment plan. The design of learning experiences must be based not only on the expertise of the dietitian in behavioral and nutritional sciences, but also on the client's understanding and acceptance of the plan. An ill-conceived plan, regardless of the best of intentions on the part of the designers, will fail for any of a number of reasons. The statistical term "best of fit" is very applicable here. Everyone involved, clients and professionals alike, should have a vested interest in the achievement of desired goals.

The next facet of the planning stage is the selection of the appropriate strategies and tools to facilitate the implementation of the client-centered plan. Strategies may vary from self-instruction to individual to group instruction. There are also specific strategies recommended for the different thinking processes involved in learning. The term "tools" includes a variety of communication devices such as self-instructional booklets; interactive technology that requires a response on the part of the client (as in computer-assisted instruction); and printed texts and books. Learning experiences, however, need not be restricted to symbolic and semantic content. Audiovisual materials add sensory and behavioral content to encompass the breadth of informational data. Learning strategies and experiences must be carefully selected to meet the needs and abilities of the client.

Implementation

When the planning phase is completed, the next step in clinical practice is the implementation of the plan. Whether the plan is designed to meet long-term goals (as in the achievement and maintenance of health) or to meet short-term goals (as in the treatment of acute stress or as substeps to reaching long-term goals), there are numberous activities that take place in the implementation phase.

One activity that is a very basic responsibility of clinical dietitians is the documentation of all phases of the treatment plan. The keeping of records for his own use and the recording of specific notes in the medical record are two tasks of the clinician. The information recorded in the medical record serves as one channel of communication to all other health professionals.[21]

There is a relatively new system for the recording of information in medical records called the problem-oriented medical record (POMR). The POMR (or POR) is gaining steady acceptance in the health field as an improvement over the traditional source-oriented medical record (SOR). The effectiveness of the record as a communication tool is enhanced with the POR method since, by its systematic organization of data, it facilitates the ability of the clinician to evaluate rapidly the appropriateness of treatment. Indeed, Walters and DeMarco view the POR system as one in which the clinical dietitian is obliged to accept greater responsibility for client care.[22]

In health systems where foodservice is an integral part, the clinical dietitian works to achieve the plan implementation through the use of food and food combinations, or other sources of nutrients. The clinician is responsible not only for the accuracy of the food plan, but is alert and sensitive to the client's acceptance of the plan. Here, observation of clients' food consumption is a valuable "unobtrusive measure," which may not only serve the purpose of the implementation stage, but may serve also as assessment and evaluative devices.

In addition to the provision of food or nutrient sources for clients who are dependent on the health delivery system for their basic needs, the implementation phase includes the counseling of those clients who need or want to make changes in their food behavior. The learning scheme(s) derived from the planning phase now must be put into effect; that is, the client now needs to acquire from the clinical dietitian those new skills and knowledge that will allow him to achieve the mutually derived goals. In the process, the clinician must effectively interact not only with the client, but with his "significant others," in order to create the best possible learning environment for all who are involved. It is important to remember that the accepted definition of learning is a consistent change in behavior, not the storage of knowledge.

This facet of clinical practice has been labeled by a variety of terms, including patient teaching, diet or nutritional counseling, and nutrition education. Indeed, as we shall later see, nutritional counseling is in essence a microcosm of the components of clinical practice and is a much more comprehensive term than patient teaching.

In a 1975 report of the Diet Therapy Section Committee of The American Dietetic Association, diet counseling was described as a service:

> . . . providing individualized professional guidance to assist a person in adjusting his daily food consumption to meet his health needs. The process . . . actually involves three activities: interviewing, counseling, and consulting.[23] (p. 571)

In reality, diet or nutritional counseling is a concept that has not been as clearly defined as might be believed from the 1975 Committee's description. The activity conjures up a variety of images in the minds of educators and practitioners. Readers of this text require clarity, not variety; a more explicit definition of nutritional counseling is needed. *Nutritional counseling* is the total process of providing clients with the ability to self-manage their own nutritional care. Although there is no right way to counsel, there is a sequence of processes that almost always enhances the acquisition of new behaviors. These processes, in the order in which they should be carried out, are assessment, planning, implementation, and evaluation. The last component of nutritional counseling, that of evaluation, actually includes the activities of evaluation *and* revision, reimplementation and reevaluation, when needed. In contrast to the Diet Therapy Section Committee statement, the authors maintain that interviewing is a skill used in assessment as well as in the other three components of clinical practice.

That counseling is more than just simply providing professional guidance or information to clients is suggested by Danish.[24] He identifies counseling as a two-part process:

> *The first part involves the development of rapport, empathy, and a trusting relationship; the second, the implementation of specific behavior-change strategies and techniques directed at the client's problem.[24] (p. 107).*

Johnson[6] has alluded to the distinctions described by Danish by identifying two basic commitments of the clinical dietitian: "caring" and "helping." The authors would suggest that "helping" and "caring" are not separate but that successful "helping" is a series of behaviors contingent upon "caring" attitudes and a growing understanding of the human needs for self-direction, self-esteem, and integrity.

The term "nutrition education" is not synonymous with nutritional counseling, and, as such, should not be applied to client-counselor interactions. Nutrition education has been described by a variety of authors; one of the most complete definitions is that of Leverton:

> *Nutrition education is a multidisciplinary process that involves the transfer of information, the development of motivation, and the modification of food habits where needed. It must form the bridge that carries appropriate information from the research and development laboratories to the public, the ultimate user. During transport, nutrition educators and their counterparts in related professions must apply their skills and knowledge to adapt the information so it can be applied to a variety of everyday situations and then package it for distribution in a variety of ways, either directly or indirectly through intermediate agents.[25] (p. 17)*

As the reader can see, nutrition education is a broad concept, applicable to whole segments of society, as well as to individuals. In contrast, counseling is a very personalized process. It is this distinction that makes the interchanging of the two terms unacceptable in current dietetic terminology.

Upon completion of the implementation phase, the practitioner moves next to measure the quality of his work in the evaluation period. For some, the last component is the most difficult and, as such, is frequently avoided. The competent practitioner, however, *always* evaluates his work.

Evaluation

For the client in a health crisis, as indicated earlier in the section on planning, the evaluation process may be repeated a number of times as the nature of the crisis changes, or until some degree of health restoration is achieved. The primary activity of the evaluative process for such clients is the continual monitoring of the treatment process in order to ensure a steady progression towards reestablishment of health. Once some degree of restoration is achieved, the client's needs will probably change. Thus beginning again with assessment is essential.

In the nutritional counseling process, evaluation is the means by which the clinician judges whether or not her activities on behalf of the client have been successful in terms of the client's acceptance and incorporation of new behaviors. The client's acquisition of knowledge and skills may be measured by paper-and-pencil quizzes; question-and-answer sessions; or other more technically innovative (and usually expensive) techniques. Evaluation differs from assessment in that it looks at the outcome value of intervention. More important, however, is the follow-up evaluation that checks to see if the client is both able and motivated to apply the skills in his normal environment after a trial period. The evaluation process implies that the clinician is involved in follow-up activities for continuity of care; that she does not dismiss the client from her surveillance upon the client's departure from the health care site. This also suggests the use of different evaluation techniques than are typically employed.

Was the client successful at the conclusion of the evaluative process? We hope so, since client success is the goal. In the event that the client has not achieved the goals of the plan, there is a need for the clinical dietitian to consider revision of the care plans, based on the collection of additional data. In other words, why has the *plan* failed? Note that we do not talk about client failure, but failure of the plan. The reader will recall that the client and the clinical dietitian are partners in the ordering of priorities and the formulation of the plan; thus, if failure occurs, some part or parts of the plan were inappropriate for the client. The evaluation process should include an analysis of the elements of assessment, planning, and implementation in order to determine the inappropriate elements of the total process, and to facilitate an effective revision.

With a revised nutritional care plan, the next step for the clinician and the client is reimplementation of instruction, directed toward the objectives that have not been met. Learning from failure is a valuable experience. Achieving success on top of an earlier failure is an even more savory event.

In this phase of clinical practice, the clinician continues to apprise others of the progress of the client, through the use of records as well as clinical conferences with other health professionals.

Recapitulation

The answer to the query, "What does a dietitian do?" will vary according to the interests and orientation of the respondent. A comprehensive reply, applicable in *all* clinical settings, is that the clinical dietitian:

Translates nutritional and behavioral sciences, and the study of foods, into the skills of nutritional care by:

1. Providing nutrient sources to clients who are incapable of both self-determination and self-sufficiency
2. Facilitating client participation, through nutritional counseling, in the selection of foods that provide nutrient sources. Captive in practitioner-managed settings, such clients are capable of self-determination, but are unable to be totally self-sufficient
3. Facilitating client independence in food selection and consumption, through nutritional counseling, for those who are capable of self-sufficiency and self-determination

The processes with which the clinical dietitian works are the four basic components of clinical practice: assessment, planning, implementation, and evaluation. But is this all? A negative answer is the proper response here, as the competent practitioner will be simultaneously engaged in a number of supportive activities. We shall continue to remind the reader that the primary reason for all such professional activities is the provision of quality client-centered health services.

OTHER FACETS OF THE CLINICAL DIETITIAN'S WORK

Management of Resources

The clinician who delivers quality care is also the effective manager of the resources available to him. Every reader knows that one resource, time, is a very scarce commodity that can never be replaced. Therefore, the clinical dietitian manages the resource of time in many ways, one of which is through the delegation of authority and responsibility to others. In a number of clinical settings there are supportive personnel who are capable of assuming many tasks of the clinical dietitian. A great challenge to many clinicians is the release of certain traditional tasks, thereby freeing them to assume the responsibility for more complex endeavors. The competent practitioner will seek ways to delegate selected tasks in order to release his time for these challenging activities. In this manner, the clinical dietitian uses human resources both effectively and efficiently.

Clinical dietitians also have a responsibility for the evaluation of their own programs and, in some cases, the total program in which they are working. This type of evaluation may be accomplished in a number of ways, such as examining the functions of the dietetic unit, collecting and entering certain kinds of information into data analysis systems, or simply participating in departmental planning. The basic principles of management in clinical practice will be examined in an ensuing chapter.

Interactions with Other Health Workers

Everywhere one looks in the literature, the concept of the clinical dietitian serving as a member of the "health care team" arises as a major role. Service on a team may be expressed as contributing to team care plans, sharing knowledge of the client with other health professionals, assisting primary health care providers to make appropriate decisions, or participating in team conferences. The responsibility of team membership was not one assumed early in the development of the profession, as dietitians once worked autonomously.[26] However, as the directions of health care have changed, so has the manner in which the clinical dietitian functions.[14]

A health care team is usually a small group of people working together for a common purpose: the provision of quality health services.[27]

More specifically:

> *A health team is a group of health professionals with a variety of skills, knowledge, values, and attitudes, who work together to solve health problems. What makes this group of people working together a team is that each member of the team needs the other team member to provide . . . services. Because of the complexity of patients' problems, no one person has all of the skills and knowledge to manage these problems.*[28] *(p. 342)*

The clinical dietitian's participation in team management of client care is a natural one that follows his acceptance of the responsibility of the nutritional care of individuals and groups. Whether or not clinicians are truly effective "team members" is a matter of speculation,[26] but the fact remains that they are expected, at least by peers, to participate in interdisciplinary teamwork.

Practitioners also have a responsibility for the dissemination of nutritional information to other health professionals, either formally in such structured situations as teaching rounds and inhouse publications, or informally, as the exchange of information during walking rounds. Others working in care units *expect* that clinical dietitians will serve as the resource persons for queries on foods and nutrition. Part of the success of the clinician in the dissemination of information is the establishment *and* maintenance of effective channels of communication.

Interactions with the Community-at-Large

The literature devoted to delineation of the responsibilities of dietitians is replete with references to the fact that members of the profession communicate as a public service. Such communication may take the form of writing a newspaper column; serving as a telephone consultant for local dial-a-dietitian projects; developing and distributing topical material for consumers on nutrition education concerns or food purchasing practices; appearing as a guest speaker with local groups of varied interests. In each of these settings, clinical dietitians participate because they are the acknowledged experts and, as such, meet a special need of their communities. They may also serve as consultants to the food industry in the development of new products or modification of existing products.

Clinical dietitians have a special responsibility for communicating with their elected representatives about pending food and health care legislation; they may take the initiative in identifying a need for particular programs or legislation.[29] Clinicians may also use the fruits of such legislation in their practice by referring clients to food assistance programs that are available in their community.

THE CLINICAL DIETITIAN AS A PROFESSIONAL

Inherent in every profession* is a set of guidelines or "norms" that state, either implicitly or explicitly, how an individual should conduct himself in a given set of circumstances. This is as true for the health fields as it is for the practice of law or architecture, or other "service" professions.

One basic characteristic of practitioners of clinical dietetics is a respect and concern for people and their value systems.[31] Clinicians who do not respect the rights of others violate a basic tenet of "professionalism." Therefore, the clinical practioner, at all times, respects and maintains the confidentiality of the medical and social information documented in the medical record. The record is not only a legal document, but is also, to a degree, an unveiling of an individual; as such, the client has the right to expect that information about him will be treated with the utmost confidentiality. A concern for people is expressed in many ways, not the least of which is the conveyance of a sense of respect for the dignity of others.

In the professional role, the clinician also separates personal and professional responsibilities and problems. Such a division of attention is sometimes difficult to achieve, but is vital to the performance of the professional role. The clinician who is sensitive to his own needs will seek out experiences that will provide continued growth and opportunity to deal with personal problems.

The clinician also has a strong sense of commitment to his profession; that is, he believes that the area of expertise defined by his practice or profession possesses dignity and credibility, and that his work affects the quality of life for others. In this context, the clinical dietitian has a sense of commitment to the growth of his profession, both as a field of intellectual endeavor, and as a society where people of similar purpose band together.

In a health discipline, there is one last responsibility placed on each and every practitioner, and that is the responsibility for "continuing

---

* A ". . . profession is a body of persons engaged in (a) . . . common mission . . . bound together by a common discipline in a spirit of fraternity, learning, and public service. The profession is synonymous with its membership."[30] (p. 281)

learning":

> *Perhaps the noblest element in the life of a professional person is his or her commitment to programmes of continuing renewal. When one thinks of it, the whole professional world of practitioner and client or patient is one of commitment and trust. . . .*
>
> *. . . the patient or client of the dietitian has a right to assume and usually will assume that this important health professional is operating in therapy and in prevention not only from the heartland of her or his knowledge, but from the frontiers of medical and natural science wherever episodes of discovery enrich dietetic knowledge and give new strategies for healing and prevention.*[32] *(p. 279)*

Thus, the professional is expected by both peers and clients to assume accountability for his own ongoing learning.[33,34] This learning may take the form of "keeping up with the literature" (reading journals and texts); attending and participating in local, state, or national meetings; or enrolling in courses pertinent to the discipline at a local college or university. In each of these circumstances, the clinical dietitian seeks to enhance his capacity to act responsibly toward the ultimate consumer of his services, the client. Galbraith said it best: "The practice of a profession means continual growth, and *that* is the challenge and the reward!"[35] (p. 169).

SUMMARY

It is clear that nutritional counseling is the clinical dietitian's primary role. The manner of acting on this premise varies with the practitioner and the setting. The following pages of this text propose one approach for this crucial role in a client-centered setting.

CITED REFERENCES

1. Robinson, C. H. Nutrition education—what comes next? *J. Am. Dietet. A.* 69:126, 1976.
2. Study Commission on Dietetics. *The Profession of Dietetics.* Chicago: The American Dietetic Association, 1972.
3. The dietitian in primary health care. *J. Am. Dietet. A.* 70:587, 1977.
4. Council on Foods and Nutrition. Report of the Council on Foods and Nutrition. *J. Am. Med. A.* 183:955, 1963.

5. Committee on Goals of Education for Dietetics, Dietetic Internship Council, The American Dietetic Association. Goals of the lifetime education of the dietitian. *J. Am. Dietet. A.* 54:91, 1969.

6. Johnson, C. A. The need for better nutritional care. Who's responsible? *J. Am. Dietet. A.* 67:219, 1975.

7. Forcier, J. I., Kight, M. A., and Sheehan, E. T. Point of view: Acculturation in clinical dietetics. *J. Am. Dietet. A.* 70:181, 1977.

8. Krause, T. O., and Fox, H. M. Nutritional knowledge and attitudes of physicians. *J. Am. Dietet. A.* 70:607, 1977.

9. Hasson, W. E. Legal issues facing dietetic practice. *J. Am. Dietet. A.* 70:355, 1977.

10. Schiller, M. R., and Vivian, V. M. Role of the clinical dietitian. II. Ideal vs. actual. *J. Am. Dietet. A.* 65:287, 1974.

11. The American Dietetic Association position paper on recommended salaries and employment practices for members of The American Dietetic Association. *J. Am. Dietet. A.* 78:62, 1981.

12. The Departmental Task Force on Prevention. *Disease Prevention & Health Promotion: Federal Programs and Prospects.* DHEW (PHS) Publ. No. 79-55071B. Washington: Publ. Health Service, 1979.

13. Hirsch, E. Z., Benassi, R., Liddle, L., and Rogers, P. An interdisciplinary clinical training program for dietitians. New primary care functions. *J. Am. Dietet. A.* 70:149, 1977.

14. Cason, D., and Wagner, M. G. The changing role of the service professional within the ghetto. *J. Am. Dietet. A.* 60:21, 1972.

15. Young, C. M. The therapeutic dietitian—a challenge for cooperation. *J. Am. Dietet. A.* 47:96, 1965.

16. Obert, J. C. *Community Nutrition.* New York: John Wiley & Sons, Inc., 1978.

17. Spangler, A. A., Cederquist, D. C., and Blackman, C. A. Physicians' attitudes on dietitians' contributions to health team care. *J. Am. Dietet. A.* 65:646, 1974.

18. Schiller, M. R., and Vivian, V. M. Role of the clinical dietitian. I. Ideal role perceived by dietitians and physicians. *J. Am. Dietet. A.* 65:284, 1974.

19. Johnson, C. A. Entry-level clinical dietetic practice as viewed by clients and allied professionals. A pilot study. *J. Am. Dietet. A.* 66:261, 1975.

20. Zifferblatt, S. M., and Wilbur, C. S. Dietary counseling: Some realistic expectations and guidelines. *J. Am. Dietet. A.* 70:591, 1977.

21. Joint Committee of The American Hospital Association and The American Dietetic Association. *Recording Nutritional Information in Medical Records.* Chicago: Am. Hosp. Assoc., 1976.

22. Walters, F. M., and DeMarco, M. The dietitian/nutritionist and the problem-oriented medical record. II. The role of the dietitian. *J. Am. Dietet. A.* 63:641, 1973.

23. Diet Therapy Section Committee, The American Dietetic Association. Guidelines for diet counseling. *J. Am. Dietet. A.* 66:571, 1975.

24. Danish, S. J. Developing helping relationships in dietetic counseling. *J. Am. Dietet. A.* 67:107, 1975.

25. Leverton, R. M. What is nutrition education? *J. Am. Dietet. A.* 64:17, 1974.

26. Schiller, M. R. The dietitian's changing role. Increased responsibilities place dietitian on health care team. *Hosp.* 47:23:97, 1973.

27. Frankle, R. T., and Owen, A. Y. *Nutrition in the Community. The Art of Delivering Services.* St. Louis: C. V. Mosby Co., 1978.

28. Seigel, B. Organization of the primary care team. *Pedia. Clin. N. Am.* 21:341, 1974.

29. Cross, A. T. Nutrition legislation: Strategy for success. *J. Am. Dietet. A.* 76:50, 1980.

30. Report of the Task Force on Competencies, Council on Educational Preparation, The American Dietetic Association. *J. Am. Dietet. A.* 73:281, 1978.

31. Thomasma, D. C. Human values and ethics: Professional responsibility. *J. Am. Dietet. A.* 75:533, 1979.

32. McLeish, J. A. B. The challenge of professional and personal renewal. *J. Canad. Dietet. A.* 39:274, 1978.

33. Boissoneau, R. Point of view: The importance of continuing education for dietitians. *J. Am. Dietet. A.* 71:49, 1977.

34. The American Dietetic Association position paper on continuing education. *J. Am. Dietet. A.* 64:289, 1974.

35. Galbraith, A. L. The President's Page. *J. Am. Dietet. A.* 69:168, 1976.

SUGGESTED REFERENCES

A.D.A. statement to federal government regarding major gaps in nutritional knowledge. *J. Am. Dietet. A.* 70:294, 1977.

Andrew, B. J. Interviewing and counseling skills. Techniques for their evaluation. *J. Am. Dietet. A.* 66:576, 1975.

Bennedict, J., Sortome, E., and Watson, B. Continuing education concerns of the practicing dietitian. *J. Canad. Dietet. A.* 39:281, 1978.

Broski, D. C., and Upp, S. C. What allied health professionals want from continuing education programs: A study of five disciplines. *J. All. Health* 8:24, 1979.

Chapman, N. Incorporating nutrition into family planning services. *J. Nutr. Ed.* 10:129, 1978.

Committee for a Report on Health Promotion and Disease Prevention for the U.S. Surgeon General. *Healthy People: The Surgeon General's Report on Health Promotion and Disease Prevention.* Background Papers, 1979. DHEW (PHS) Publ. No. 79-55071A. Washington: Nat'l. Aca. Sci., 1979.

Fruin, M. F., and Campbell, J. D. Developing behaviorally anchored scales for rating dietitians' performance. *J. Am. Dietet. A.* 71:111, 1977.

Galbraith, A. L. Excellence defined. *J. Am. Dietet. A.* 67:211, 1975.

Gifft, H. H., Washbon, M. B., and Harrison, G. G. *Nutrition, Behavior and Change.* Englewood Cliffs, NJ: Prentice-Hall, Inc., 1972.

Houle, C. O. *Continuing Learning in the Professions.* San Francisco: Jossey-Bass, Inc., Publ., 1980.

Johnson, C. A., and Hurley, R. S. Design and use of an instrument to evaluate students' clinical performance. *J. Am. Dietet. A.* 68:450, 1976.

Karkeck, J. M. Continuing education: To be useful, a thing must be used. *J. Am. Dietet. A.* 74:566, 1979.

Kunis, B. S. Family nutritionist on the primary health care team. *J. Nutr. Ed.* 8:77, 1976.

Owen, A. L., and Owen, G. M. Training public health nutritionists: Competencies for complacency or future concerns. *Am. J. Pub. Health* 69:1096, 1979.

Schwartz, N. E., and Gobert, R. C. Continuing education in nutrition and dietetics: A working model. *J. Canad. Dietet. A.* 39:288, 1978.

Scialabba, M. A. Functions of dietetic personnel in ambulatory care. *J. Am. Dietet. A.* 67:545, 1975.

Sims, L. S. Identification and evaluation of competencies of public health nutritionists. *Am. J. Pub. Health* 69:1099, 1979.

The American Dietetic Association position paper on child nutrition programs. *J. Am. Dietet. A.* 64:520, 1974.

The American Dietetic Association position paper on nutrition education for the public. *J. Am. Dietet. A.* 62:429, 1973.

The American Dietetic Association position paper on the role of the registered dietitian in consultative service to group care facilities. *J. Am. Dietet. A.* 67:579, 1975.

The American Dietetic Association position paper on nutrition services in health maintenance organizations. *J. Am. Dietet. A.* 60:317, 1972.

The colors of Dietetics are raised on a medical flagship. *Nutr. Today* 14:5:30, 1979.

Traylor, M. N., and Lincoln, G. H. Experiences of a dietitian in a Health Systems Agency (HSA). *J. Am. Dietet. A.* 71:638, 1977.

Wade, J. E. Role of a clinical dietitian specialist in a nutrition support service. *J. Am. Dietet. A.* 70:185, 1977.

Weigley, E. S. Professionalization and the dietitian. *J. Am. Dietet. A.* 74:317, 1979.

White, P. L., and Mondeika, T. Somewhere under the iceberg. *J. Am. Med. A.* 235:1873, 1976.

2
Health Teams in
Client-Centered Care*

> . . . it should be remembered that the interdisciplinary team in human service organizations owes its existence to the need for coordinated care of the client. The team, therefore, should always be focused on the central issue of client care.
>
> Alex J. Ducanis and Anne K. Golin, **The Interdisciplinary Health Care Team**. (Germantown, MD: Aspen Systems Corp., 1979).

THE TEAM CONCEPT

Teamwork is an experience familiar to all of us. On many occasions in our lives we find it necessary to associate with others in a cooperative effort to achieve a particular goal. Whether in the form of cooperative games, family growth and development, voluntary associations and clubs, or participation in the institutions of our society, we are asked to make our own particular contribution to a shared goal. Our participation may range from such simple and straightforward activities as casting a ballot or collecting money in a fund drive to a more complex set of activities that describe our participation in a particular *role*, such as father, senator, or dietitian. That particular role (set of activ-

---

* This chapter was written by Madeline H. Schmitt, R.N., Ph.D., Associate Professor of Nursing and Sociology, University of Rochester, Rochester, New York.

ities) is coordinated with other roles (other sets of activities) so that when all the activities are performed in a coordinated and cooperative fashion, a desired goal is achieved. Thus, it takes not only the efforts of a father, but also those of a mother, children, and, perhaps, an extended family to achieve family goals. It takes voters, senators, congressmen, and a president to achieve democratic government goals. And it takes clients, dietitians, nurses, physicians, and many others in roles to achieve health care goals. Teamwork, thus, has three major aspects:

1. Shared goals
2. Individuals acting in roles that encompass a diversity of skills and experiences
3. A plan for coordinated effort

In some teams, the shared goals are few in number and specific, team membership is stable, the role of each member (his particular set of activities) is well-defined, and the plan for coordinated effort is spelled out. A football team, for example, is an association of persons who work together to make touchdowns or field goals (while preventing the other team from doing the same) in order to win games. Each person brings specialized skills to the team, such as running, passing, or blocking skills. These skills are organized into particular roles (sets of activities) such as halfback, end, or linebacker. The various roles are coordinated through a variety of plays that are the football team's coordinated effort to achieve their goal of winning games.

In other teams, the shared goals are greater in number or diffuse, team membership may fluctuate, the role of each member (his particular set of activities) may be less clearly defined, and the way to reach the goals through coordinated effort may consist of actions involving many alternative choices with many possible outcomes. For example, a family is an association of persons who work together around multiple and generally identified goals such as childrearing, provision of shelter, food and other basic necessities for survival, and emotional and physical growth for all family members. Family size may fluctuate and affect goals, roles, and plan of coordination. Family members' roles (sets of activities) are only generally defined in relation to the goals. Thus, provision of food involves a set of activities: generating resources for, obtaining, and preparing the food. Such activities may be the responsibility of one family member or the set of activities may be divided among several family members. Finally, no one *particular* set of activities provides the way to reach the goal. For example, food may be provided by farming and harvesting one's own, by using money to buy it at a retail store, or by organizing a "co-op" among a group of families to obtain foods without preservatives, organic foods, or to buy food in bulk quantities at less than retail price. The accomplishment of multiple goals may contribute to achievement of an even broader one, defined by some "ideal" created that focuses the team's or the family's goals, roles, and plan of coordination. In the absence of fixed membership, clear roles, and plans (such as the football team has), the team may be encouraged to move toward a "collegial" ideal and the family toward an "egalitarian" one.

Other factors affect team goals, roles, and organization. A particular team may exist only briefly, organized around a short-term goal. In such cases, there is usually a clear set of role activities for each member and relations are clearly spelled out. Little of the person-in-the-role (individuality) is expressed. An example of such a team, in addition to the football team presented previously, is a flight team. The pilot, copilot, attendants, and flight assistant are organized around a particular airplane flight, have clear activities in relation to one another, and a particular plan of coordination that moves them toward their short-term goal. A team may also exist for a long period of time organized around a set of continuing goals. In such cases, people know each other and their individual capabilities more completely; consequently, there may be more individual variation in roles and coordination. A family is a good example of such a team organized around long-term maintenance of its members, where changing characteristics of individual members (ages, physical capabilities, cognitive developmental abilities, and so forth) contribute to a flexibility in goals, roles, and coordination.

HEALTH CARE TEAMS

Development

The provision of health care has not always been, and still frequently is not, a team endeavor. Physicians have traditionally been solo practitioners or have been engaged in group practice with other physicians in providing medical care. Other health care professionals have been affiliated with institutions for the purpose of providing institutional support services—food, laboratory service, nursing care, and so on—which allowed the physician to provide medical care to clients in those institutional settings.[2] Often there is still not good articulation between institutional medical care and these "support" services. The initial idea of providing team care grew out of the need for physician-extending and physician-supporting services.[3] The early teams in health care were organized for joint action around medical goals for clients. The phrase "allied medical personnel" brought to mind clearly defined roles in relation to the physician's goal of treating the client's disease. The physician was the leader and ultimate authority in such teams. Typically, in such teams, allied medical personnel might contribute information to the assessment of the medical problem, the physician would make the diagnosis and give the orders, and then the allied medical personnel would implement the orders and report the results. This model is still advocated,[2,4] and as a pattern of interaction, fits many existing health care teams, according to those who have studied team functioning.[5–10] Silver sums up this point of view in discussing the model of care for his demonstration project for family health maintenance:

A family-oriented health team introduced into group medical practice will help carry out the social function of medicine along with the scientific, creating a family medical service.[4] (p. 145).

Treatment of disabled veterans following World War II required a type of health care that went beyond the traditional medical approach of "doing to" the client in order to cure. It required a focus on "returning the client to the community as a socially and economically useful citizen" and on maintenance therapy.[3] This shift in focus created more of an emphasis on the person than the disease, on a broader range of needs, and on a broader range of treatment variables as contributing to a desired outcome. It also became clearer that the client's own motivation and active cooperation were central factors in providing successful care. The change in emphasis created an awareness of the lack of preparation of physicians for assessing and providing treatment for the client in many aspects of care having to do with rehabilitation. The effect was to create a team whose added membership had the qualifications to define, organize, and implement these broader goals in a more collegial* relationship with the physician member. This type of team is receiving increasing attention as a result of changing ideas about what health care is (that it is much broader than the provision of medical care), increasing appreciation of the complex problems of etiology and treatment of chronic illness, and increasing profession-

* "Collegiality is defined as a relationship characterized by equivalent status and complementary skills"[11] (p. 213).

alization of a wide variety of health services, including dietetics. There is modest evidence that such an approach may improve outcomes of care.[9]

In the newest forms of health teams, additional, nonprofessional team members have been added to represent areas of expertise unfamiliar to more traditionally prepared professional members. An example is the family health worker or family aide, who has become an integral part of many care teams working in community settings, as so many of the health problems encountered in the community are tied to social, economic, and cultural issues. The family health worker, selected from the community and given some additional health care skills, becomes a communication link between the client and family and the health professionals, and is the specialist on the team in dealing with social, economic, and cultural barriers to families in receiving health care.[8,12,13]

Another example is the expansion of the role of the basic care attendant who provides long-term care in institutions serving patients with a variety of problems. Through supplementing their knowledge of client needs in areas such as basic developmental patterns, physical and occupational therapy, and nutrition, a pattern of team delivery of health care that capitalizes on professional knowledge while conserving scarce professional resources can be created. For some institutionalized individuals, concentrating services through one nonprofessional "primary deliverer of services" also seems to be easier for the patient to accept.[14]

Phrases such as "health care team," "multidisciplinary team," "interdisciplinary team," and "health team" are commonly used to describe comprehensive care teams. Generally these teams are organized around a client's health goal that (a) is broader than the medical care problem, (b) is understood through the separate assessments by all the team members in their special areas of expertise, and (c) results in an overall assessment together with a plan that includes the contribution each team member is expected to make in implementing the plan to achieve the stated goal. Leadership may depend on the expertise required to solve the problem. The relationship among members is that of colleagues rather than a central person and assistants. Such teams may or may not actively incorporate the client or the client's perspective into the assessment and planning for care.

Most recently, health care professionals have become interested in helping clients assume more responsibility for their own ongoing health care. It has become clear, with enhanced knowledge of the etiology of chronic illnesses, that only long-term changes in client behaviors will curb many endemic diseases of civilized countries (e.g., obesity, heart disease, and pulmonary disease). To encourage commitment to self-care, some teams have actively incorporated clients or the clients' points of view in assessment and planning for care. Such teams often use the terms "individualized," "patient-centered," or "client-centered" in describing the emphasis of joint action with the aim of facilitating the client's independence in the provision of his own health care.[11,15] "Individualizing" or "centering" the assessment and planning process on the client means inclusion in the assessment of (a) how the health problem is perceived by the client and his significant others, (b) what they would like to do about it and why, and (c) the plan of action that incorporates everyone's (including the client's) assessment and priorities for health care services.

The organization of such care requires some effective means of association among the team members and the client. It cannot be emphasized enough that awareness of the client's perspective is attained through time spent with him in listening and effective interviewing.

Goals, Roles, and Coordination of Plans

As with other kinds of teams, health care teams have three major aspects: shared goals, individuals acting in a diversity of roles, and a plan for coordinated effort. As noted in Chapter 1,

A health team is a group of health professionals with a variety of skills, knowledge, values, and attitudes, who work together to solve health problems. What makes this group of people working together a team is that each member of the team needs the other team member to provide . . . services. Because of the complexity of patients' problems, no one person has all of the skills and knowledge to manage these problems.[12] *(p. 342)*

Beyond this broad definition, however, health care teams (as can be assumed from the discussion of team development) encompass a wide variety of orientations to specific goals, roles, and methods of coordination.

Goals. Health care teams may be a very transitory association of persons around a few short-term goals, such as a team organized at the scene of an automobile accident to direct traffic, get the injured first aid and medical care, and so forth. Another example might be a health team conference in an acute care setting, where because of his short stay, the client is discussed in conference on only one occasion.

The health care team may also be an association of persons organized around many short- and long-term goals, such as a primary health care team* that assumes responsibility for the coordination and integration of health care for a particular group of clients for an indefinite period of time. The shared goals range from specialized medical ones to comprehensive health goals.

Roles.   Health team membership may be decided by some "ideal" set of standards or goals and, hence, the identification of the team members follows. Seigel[12] lists eight such "ideals" from a literature review on primary health care teams. A differing belief is that health teams should be organized around the health assessment and intervention needs of the particular clients to be served, and the professional resources available.[12] Most health teams encompass both perspectives. Generally, there is some overall health team organized and ready to provide the kind of health care potentially needed. Yet, only those members who have the skills required by particular clients at any given point in time will be involved with them.

Team membership may be differentiated between "core" members and "consultants." Some members of the team provide health care services that are needed by most clients. These members are termed "core" members and develop the closest ongoing relationship with each other.[10] An example of a "core" member is the speech therapist when the client is a child with cleft palate. "Consultants" may include a variety of persons. Examples are a medical specialist as consultant to the physician member of the team;[4] others, such as the psychiatrist, social worker, clinical dietitian, health educator, sociologist, or psychologist, may be consultants to individual members or the team as a whole.[4,13]

The specialized preparation that is the basis for membership in the health team creates numerous difficulties for meeting together as a team. Specialized preparation is often of a form that does not fit team delivery of care. For example, the physician is traditionally trained in a university medical center so that he can function as a solo or phy-

* A primary health care team, defined as follows by Seigel, provides:
  1. *First contact* care, where a majority of personal health services are provided and ready access to specialty services is facilitated, for a specified population of clients
  2. *Continuous* care, which implies a long-term relationship between client and professionals
  3. *Family-based* care, which recognizes the importance of significant others in the therapeutic process
  4. *Coordination* and *integration* of health care by continuous support and education to the client and significant others[12] (p. 343).

sician-group practitioner. The physician is prepared to diagnose and treat, rather than deal with patient management and health maintenance; to respond to acute problems rather than problems of a chronic or psychosocial nature.[7,8] She is used to practicing with an array of assistants. Similarly, the professional education of the dietitian has traditionally occurred in the large acute care setting with emphasis on dietetic skills, which more often than not results in minimal contact with professionals of other disciplines. When individual care is provided to the client by the clinical dietitian, it is usually on the physician's specific order to meet a nutritional care prescription. The contact may not involve communication with the other professionals involved in the care at all. Thus the educational setting, the nature of the problems attended, and the lack of relationships developed with other professionals mitigate against successful team sharing experiences. Typically, then, when such professionals try to meet as a health team to deliver "team" care, there is often little real collaboration.[3] At best, in the absence of familiarity with each other, stereotypical expectation for roles (sets of activities) and relationships may operate. Thus, in the absence of familiarity with a particular dietitian, a health care team might basically expect the dietitian to have knowledge of food composition and be able to apply it in designing nutritional care plans. There would be a general lack of awareness of other elements of the role of clinical dietitians. This lack of awareness is likely to continue and to limit useful contributions of team members unless team members can meet together over time, get to know each other, and learn about one another's particular capabilities and potential contributions to client care.

Other factors contribute to the role held and relationships experienced by any particular professional member in a health care team. Occupational status outside the team is a powerful influence on one's role and relationship. Most health professions have not attained an occupational status equivalent to the physician, and this influences the association and actions of team members, regardless of the particular client situation. The general effect of the physician's higher status on the team's interaction is that the other professionals supply information to the physician while the physician seeks information, makes the decisions, gives the opinions, and sets the direction. The physician receives most attention compared to other team members. This pattern of interaction typifies teams organized around medical care goals. Sex and age differences among team members may also influence team members' roles and relationships—women deferring to men, and younger professionals deferring to older ones—in ways not productive of effective patient care delivery. In any given situation an extensive familiarity with a particular client or differences in prior experience may outweigh the various status factors. However, expertise per se has counted surprisingly little as influencing interaction in the few experimental studies designed to look at this question in small group situations.[16]

The education of professionals for team practice is still novel and not widely available.* There is a major task of effecting association between specialized professionals to accomplish team care. Team members need to redefine and clarify to other team members the stereotyped roles they are given upon first entering a health team, so as to be consistent with ideas of their own professional responsibilities. The best way to do this is through demonstrating their capabilities.

As team members' capabilities are demonstrated, it is not unlikely that they will discover their roles contain overlap as well as specialization. The overlapping may be related to similarities in the education and skills of the professionals, such as in psychiatric interdisciplinary teams where psychiatrists, clinical psychologists, social workers, and psychiatric nurses have many similar repertoires of knowledge and skills. Another example is that nurses have historically overlapped with dietitians in assuming considerable responsibility for the nutritional care of clients, though their preparation in nutritional care is not at the same level as that of clinical dietitians. Such overlapping requires role negotiation so that where more than one individual on the health team is capable of engaging in a particular activity with a client, it is clear who has the responsibility to do so. Horowitz has indicated that:

> *In an employment setting, a worker must anticipate a settling in stage in which he discovers (usually over a period of time) exactly what is expected of him and what he can reliably expect of others. In interdisciplinary team practice, the newcomer commonly finds that his job is rather undefined and that his colleagues have differing conceptions of the division of labor and the part he should play. Each member of the group sizes up the situation and indicates . . . what he believes he can and should do, among the things he determines must be done. . . . Team operations almost invariably*

---

* The Institute for Health Team Development[15] is the only organization specifically committed to experiments in educating a variety of health professionals for team practice. It has been sponsoring a variety of experimental educational endeavors around the United States.

engender a continuing process of role clarification and redefinition.[17] (p. 16)

Depending on how a health care team views such overlap, it can provide the team with some flexibility or with the basis for a territorial dispute. In the former case, the client benefits, and in the latter he loses!

Coordination (Plans).   The plan for coordinated effort may be clear or uncertain. If the health care team has a small number of clearly delineated goals, the plan of coordinated effort (how and what each team member is to do related to the total effort to reach the shared goal) is also likely to be reasonably clear. If they have a large number of ambiguous goals organized around a generally stated goal, such as "total patient care," "comprehensive health care," "individualized health care," "primary health care," and so forth, the plan of coordinated effort (how and what each team member is to do related to each of the goals and how these are related to the overall goal) is also likely to be ambiguous. Focusing the goal(s) of the team's effort is critical to the team's success or failure. Following some general goal identification like comprehensive health care, or primary health care, or client-oriented care, the team must specify in more detail the client(s)' desired health status and activities to be engaged in which will produce this desired outcome. Without consensus on these divisions, the team will have no focus for organizing the work, for role negotiation, or for evaluation of successes; and it will flounder, creating high dissatisfaction among team members. It becomes much easier for the team members to assign responsibilities for assessment of current status and intervention responsibilities once they have made decisions about the end points of client health status to be attained.

Examples of Two Extremes of Health Teams

A surgical team is a good example of a health care team with delineated goals, clear roles (sets of activities) for each team member, and a clearly stated plan for coordination of effort towards the goals.[12] The goal of the team is defined by the surgeon's identification of the needed surgical intervention. The membership of surgical teams is clear: surgeon, assisting surgeon (one or more), anesthesiologist, scrub nurse (or technician), and circulating nurse. The coordinated plan is contained in the details of the specific surgical procedure, as is the role each member of the surgical team carries out in completion of that procedure. The leader of the team is the surgeon; the other members assist him in accomplishing the surgical goal.*

The primary care team is a good example of a health care team that is opposite to the one described above. The goals of the primary care team—first-contact care, continuous care, family-based care, and coordination and integration of health care—are very general ones. They are not focused exclusively on implementing medical goals (ideally!). No clearly accepted set of detailed goals relates to the general goals. For example, there is no sequence of specific goals usually identified for "family-based" care. No particular set of members has been defined as the "core"—or "best" combination—of members for achieving any of these goals. No clear responsibility for leadership rests with any particular role. Roles (sets of activities) in relation to goals have many alternative arrangements. There is no clearly accepted "procedure" (or steps in intervention) to assist clients in moving toward identified goals, but rather there are many alternative choices with many possible outcomes. Seigel has noted that:

> In the community, where primary care is being delivered, the goals (what is medical, what is social, what is nursing, what is really the problem) are not so clear. Thus, there is considerable and necessary overlapping of roles, and a multiplicity of alternative approaches to any one health problem.[12] (p. 342)

The consequence of this lack of focus is that many reports of primary health team efforts contain references to serious problems relating to goal achievements, role satisfaction, and interprofessional coordination.[7,12,13]

HEALTH TEAMS IN CLIENT-CENTERED CARE

Goals

An example of a client-centered care team is the primary care team previously described. Two characteristics in particular, its family-centered focus and its broad health goals, contribute to making it a client-centered health care team. "Family-centered" infers that the team incorporates the client and his family (or significant others) as the central members of the team. The planned care is directed toward goals

---

* This is a simplification of surgical teams who engage in complex goals. However, even in these cases, the team is an expanded version of an accepted *core* team. Thus, *more* physicians or nurses may be added, but it is unlikely that a health educator or dietitian will be.

that are likely to increase the client's desire and capacity to assume responsibility for his own ongoing care. "Broad health goals" implies a concern for enhancing the many factors that contribute toward a client's health or, conversely, decreasing the factors which contribute toward ill health. Such goals range from changes in physical environment (e.g., removal of lead-based paint from surfaces on which children are likely to chew), to social environment (decreasing overcrowding that spreads disease, or supplementation of economic resources for adequate health), to cultural environment (changing cultural practices that are known to contribute to development of disease), to psychologic environment (reducing isolation and loneliness that result in poor motivation to maintain health), to biologic environment (correction of physical problems that impair ability to ingest and absorb vital resources such as food and oxygen and impair the ability to ward off disease). The major difference between primary care teams and client-centered care teams is that primary care teams operate at a specific location in the health care system, i.e., first-contact care, whereas a client-centered care team can be found any place where various disciplines, together with the client, are actively planning his care in a broad range of needs for health.

Roles

Teams attempting to provide client-centered care may encounter difficulties in integrating their priorities for health with the client's priorities. This is because professionals have often identified health goals in terms that reflect requirements for their own behaviors. An example of this from clinical dietetics might be to instruct a client to reduce his sodium intake. A better statement is made in terms of the desired client goals (e.g., reduce the amount of fluid retention). Even when stated in client-focused terms, such professional goals for client outcomes may need to be linked to client priorities in order to obtain commitment and participation. For example, reducing fatigue and increasing energy as a client priority may be linked to the professional goal of reducing fluid retention. Means by which the goal can be accomplished are then planned, such as reducing daily sodium intake to 2 grams. After adequate assessment of the client's food behaviors, the clinical dietitian can assist the client to alter those behaviors in ways most acceptable to him while achieving the goal of limiting sodium intake. The client-centered approach recognizes that such a change in food intake may not be accepted unless there is assistance in altering established food behaviors in ways that accomplish the goal, but are still consistent with the importance of food and usual eating patterns and preferences in a client's daily living.

Simultaneously, in terms of the broad health care goals for the same client, a social worker on the team may be sensitive to the client's lack of economic resources for obtaining adequate food, medications, and shelter. In addition, the social worker may be aware of a lack of social contact that decreases any motivation to work toward health. The physician may be aware of multiple biologic reasons for the fluid retention and be planning therapy that takes into account complicated biologic interrelationships. The nurse may be aware of the client's concern that his illness will impair his ability to continue to live alone, or create a burden for his significant others. In each case, the professional will be more successful in helping the client cope with these difficulties if the care takes into account his priorities and preferences. What kind of social contact does the client prefer? Do the medical therapies cause side effects that the client finds difficult to tolerate? How can the client be taught to manage necessary limitations so that he maintains a feeling of independence?

In such client-centered teams, the roles are not necessarily neatly defined by the individual professional's sphere of responsibility. Managing the problem of fluid retention requires more than the action of the physician in prescribing medication and a limited sodium intake. It requires that the clinical dietitian help the client work out a nutritional care plan consistent with the sodium restriction. It requires that the social worker explore social isolation, and so forth. One client problem generates many different role responsibilities. Furthermore, the nature of the problems and role responsibilities reflects a team situation where members relate to each other as colleagues with independent spheres of responsibility and with no one member's role more important than the others. The physician's prescription will not be effective over time if other team members do not recognize and respond to needs for social contact, economic resources, and ability to function in "normal" adult tasks in an independent manner.

Coordination of Plans

The efforts of the various professionals in client-centered care, as in the example described, require planning by the total team. What aspects must be initiated first? Perhaps the problem is severe enough to require hospitalization and an immediate, strict regimen of medications and sodium restriction. The financial difficulties may also need immediate attention. Other plans can be made as the client is ready to attend to other aspects of the problem. Or perhaps the problem of fluid retention is not serious now, but has the potential for becoming so. Other aspects of client need may then be attended to first (e.g., education about the potential difficulties and suggestions for altering daily living that would decrease the chances of the fluid retention becoming a serious problem). Such decisions require information sharing, priority setting, and distribution of role responsibilities at the level of the total team. The ideal outcome of such effort is described by Seigel:

> *From the notion of interdependence and bilateral influence of behavior develops the hoped for outcome of any team function: the idea of synergy. Thus the outcome of the care process, with more than one health professional working in a team, produces an effect which is greater than the effect produced by individual efforts.*[12] *(p. 342)*

THE CLINICAL DIETITIAN'S ROLE IN CLIENT-CENTERED CARE TEAMS

Core Member vs. Consultant

Most descriptions of health teams do not identify the clinical dietitian as a member of the team. Serious deficits in the nutritional management of a wide variety of acute and chronic disorders may accompany institutional medical care that does not utilize the expertise of the clinical dietitian.[18] Occasionally, if the clinical dietitian's role is mentioned, a consultant role is identified. The major reason for other health professionals not identifying the clinical dietitian as a core member of the team has to do with a narrow perception of the clinical dietitian's role by the dietitian and other health team members. In one study of four interdisciplinary teams' attempts to provide client-centered care, the dietitian, who had considerable personal and professional knowledge of the clients involved, had such a low rate of participation it could not be reliably analyzed.[9] It would seem necessary for clinical dietitians to educate team members about their ability to provide client-centered care in conjunction with others. Such education will require the clinical dietitian to engage in the processes of role redefinition and role clarification in teams in which they participate, as described earlier in this chapter, and to write about their experiences.

Core Team Membership

In most client-centered health teams, there are clear potential roles for the clinical dietitian in the area of nutritional care. In some instances, clinical dietitians are beginning to describe such roles organized around specific disease entities.[19] Many diseases, in both the acute and chronic phases, require temporary or permanent modifications in usual food intake patterns so that complications may be prevented in the acute illness, and may be minimized in chronic illness. Such modifications (contributing to secondary and tertiary prevention*) can best be implemented by the client with assistance from the professional who knows in detail the nutritional value and composition of the food to be eaten, yet is sympathetic with the client in helping him to make modifications in such a way as to meet his needs and maintain his satisfaction. Even more crucial is the role of the clinical dietitian in the client-centered care team, as she assists the client in the primary prevention of illness through nutritional counseling. Thus, clinical dietitians have a role in contributing to all three kinds of prevention. Further, if a client is institutionalized for a long or short period of time for treatment of his illness, institutional eating routines and kinds of food served may place great strain on the client's ability to achieve the desired goals in relation to nutritional care. A clinical dietitian working as a member of a client-centered health team can assist the client by reducing the inconsistencies between the client's personal care requirements and the institution's policies and procedures.

SUMMARY

The team approach to providing health care has become increasingly popular because it is thought to provide an effective way of dealing with the fragmentation of care, as well as providing the client with a broader range of health care services. Attributes of the team are: shared goals, individuals assuming roles that imply a diversity of skills and experiences, and a plan for coordinated efforts. Beyond these general commonalities, the specific nature of the team goals, membership, and responsibilities, and plans for organization and operation can vary

---

* For purposes of clarity in these pages, primary prevention is defined as that directed towards the prevention of illness; secondary prevention is the prevention or limitation of disability concurrent with or following an acute, critical illness; tertiary prevention is the restoration of ability through rehabilitation after bodily damage becomes irreversible[20]

widely from rather simple and clear ones, to complex, multiple, and unclearly defined goals, membership, and responsibilities, and plans for coordination and operation.

Client-centered care teams are complex, emphasizing provision of a broad range of health care services by multiple professionals in co-operation with the client. The latter's stated priorities are actively incorporated into the care plan with an aim of enhancing the client's sense of knowledge and responsibility for his own health care. This form of health care delivery is a very new one, and is beginning to emerge as a component of health professionals' education.

Essential first steps in participation in such teams include role re-definition and clarification in order to deal with stereotyped images among team members. A second task is to define the areas of shared goals in concrete terms so that the team will have an opportunity to assess its own progress toward the goals. Role redefinition and clari-fication, plus clear team goal setting, have been identified as serious problems to be addressed by teams.

Clinical dietitians have not often been viewed as core members of teams, but have been more frequently perceived as specialized con-sultants. If they wish to assume the role of core members of teams, they will need to demonstrate their interest in and capabilities for such participation. This demonstration should include a client-cen-tered approach to nutritional care which illustrates the application of the clinical dietitian's special skills and knowledge at all levels of prevention.

CITED REFERENCES

1. Ducanis, A. J., and Golin, A. K. *The Interdiscriplinary Health Care Team.* Germantown, MD: Aspen Systems Corp., 1979.
2. Magraw, R. M. Interdisciplinary teamwork for medical care and health services. *Ann. Int. Med.* 69:827, 1968.
3. Margolin, R. J. Rationale for teamwork. *Rehab. Rec.* 10:32, 1969.
4. Silver, G. A. *Family Health Care: A Design for Health Maintenance.* Cam-bridge: Ballinger Publ. Co., 1974.
5. Caudill, W. A. *The Psychiatric Hospital as a Small Society.* Cambridge: Harvard Univ. Press, 1958.
6. Wessen, A. F. Hospital ideology and communication between ward per-sonnel. *In* Scott, W. R., and Volkhart, E., Eds. *Medical Care.* New York: John Wiley and Sons, Inc., 1966.
7. Wise, H. The primary-care health team. *Arch. Int. Med.* 130:438, 1972.

8. Wise, H. Making health teams work. *Am. J. Dis. Child.* 127:537, 1974.

9. Feiger, S., and Schmitt, M. H. Collegiality in interdisciplinary health teams: Its measurement and its effects. *Soc. Sci. and Med.* 13a:217, 1979.

10. Parker, A. W. *The Team Approach to Primary Health Care. Neighborhood Center Seminar Program.* Monograph Series No. 3. Berkeley: Univ. Extension, Univ. Calif., 1972.

11. Aradine, C. R., and Hansen, M. F. Interdisciplinary teamwork in family health care. *Nurs. Clin. N. Am.* 5:211, 1970.

12. Seigel, B. Organization of the primary care team. *Pedia. Clin. N. Am.* 21:341, 1974.

13. Beloff, J. S., and Willet, M. Yale studies in family health care III. *J. Am. Med. A.* 205:73, 1968.

14. Modrow, C. L., and Darnell, R. E. Cross-modality: Delivery of health services through non-professionals. *J. Am. Dietet. A.* 74:337, 1979.

15. *Health Team News.* The Institute for Health Team Development, Montifiore Hospital and Medical Center, Bronx, New York. 1:1974.

16. Richardson, J. T., Dugan, J. R., Gray, L. N., and Mayhew, B. H. Expert power: A behavioral interpretation. *Sociom.* 36:302, 1973.

17. Horowitz, J. J. *Team Practice and the Specialist.* Springfield, IL: Charles C Thomas, 1970.

18. Tobias, A. L., and VanItallie, T. B. Nutritional problems of hospitalized patients. *J. Am. Dietet. A.* 71:253, 1977.

19. Carson, J. S. Nutrition in a team approach to rehabilitation of the patient with cancer. *J. Am. Dietet. A.* 72:407, 1978.

20. Shamansky, S. L., and Clausen, C. L. Levels of prevention: Examination of the concept. *Nsg. Outl.* 28:104, 1980.

SUGGESTED REFERENCES

Andreopoulos, S. *Primary Care. Where Medicine Fails.* New York: John Wiley & Sons, Inc., 1974.

Banta, H. D., and Fox, R. C. Role strains of a health care team in a poverty community: The Columbia Point experience. *Soc. Sci. Med.* 6:697, 1972.

Beckhard, R. Organizational issues in the team delivery of comprehensive health care. *Milb. Memor. Fund Quart.* 50: Part 1:287, 1972.

Beloff, J. S., and Korper, J. The health team model and medical care utilization. *J. Am. Med. A.* 219:359, 1972.

Brill, N. I. *Teamwork: Working Together in the Human Services.* Philadelphia: J. B. Lippincott Co., 1976.

Christensen, K., and Lingle, J. Evaluation of effectiveness of team and non-team public health nurses in health outcomes of patients with strokes or fractures. *Am. J. Publ. Health.* 62:483, 1972.

Drew, A. L. Teamwork and total patient care. *J. Psy. Soc. Work.* 23:25, 1953.

Folta, J., and Deck, E., Eds. *A Sociological Framework for Patient Care.* New York: John Wiley and Sons, Inc., 1966.

Golden, A. S., Carlson, D. G., and Harris, B. Non-physician family health teams for health maintenance organizations. *Am. J. Publ. Health.* 63:732, 1973.

Goldstein, S., Birnbom, F., and Miller, B. The team approach in a psychogeriatric unit. *J. Am. Geria. Soc.* 23:370, 1975.

Lewis, J. M. The organizational structure of the therapeutic team. *Hosp. Comm. Psy.* 20:36, 1969.

Rubin, I. M., and Beckhard, R. Factors influencing the effectiveness of health teams. *Milb. Mem. Fund Quart.* 50: Part 1:317, 1972.

Rubin, I. M., Plovnick, M. S., and Fry, R. E. *Improving the Coordination of Care: A Program for Health Team Development.* Cambridge: Ballinger Publ. Co., 1975.

Schiller, M. R., and Vivian, V. M. Role of the clinical dietitian. *J. Am. Dietet. A.* 65:284, 1974.

Spangler, A. A., Cederquist, D. C., and Blackman, C. A. Physicians' attitudes on dietitians' contributions to health care team. *J. Am. Dietet. A.* 65:646, 1974.

Tichy, M. K. *Health Care Teams: An Annotated Bibliography.* New York: Praeger, 1974.

Wise, H. Beckhard, R., Rubin, I., and Kyte, A. L. *Making Health Teams Work.* Cambridge: Ballinger Publ. Co., 1975.

3
Nutritional Counseling in Client-Centered Care

Counseling is less a profession than a technique or art which is to be employed as part of a more inclusive responsibility in those professions whose chief business is with persons. . . .

Rollo May, **The Art of Counseling** (New
York: Abingdon Press, 1967).

The authors have assumed the position that the provision of nutritional counseling is the primary professional role of clinical dietitians in client-centered nutritional care. It is recognized that nutritional care is only one of the components of total health care for the individual, but a more significant one than has traditionally been accepted.[2] Combs and coworkers[3] describe dietitians' contributions to caring for people as a qualification for their inclusion as members of the "helping" professions. Though professionals in medicine, nursing, and social work have long been recognized as helpers, a large number of other professionals have recently acquired this characterization. Though each profession has its own philosophy, emphasis, tools, and techniques, they all subscribe to the same basic aim, the optimal well-being of people. To achieve this goal, effective helpers need to be guided by the best that is known of the dynamics of human behavior offered by the discipline of psychology. These helpers include the clinical dietitian.

WHAT IS NUTRITIONAL COUNSELING?

The term counseling is generally, but not always, used by professionals to denote the practice of providing to people who seek their help, the needed resources, instruction, support, and guidance for the purpose of enabling them to achieve a given level of functioning.[4] A relatively new word, counseling has naturally assumed a variety of connotations, most often that of helping emotionally troubled people. Although this is one aspect of counseling, it is much too limiting. In reality, there are financial counselors, pastoral counselors, academic counselors, marriage and family counselors, and a number of others with specified problem orientations. In other words, counseling is the process of helping people learn improved ways of dealing with their everyday or very complex and deeply ingrained problems. Thus, counseling may lead to better ways of coping with life situations.[5]

Counseling is exactly what the practice of clinical dietetics is about: helping people with present or potential nutritional problems, whether they exist because of lack of knowledge, or motivation, or both. The goal or *purpose* of the process the authors have labeled *nutritional counseling* is to help the client select and implement more desirable nutritional behaviors by using a variety of skills that are elements of the process.

The primary outcome of nutritional counseling is to acquire or *learn* new behaviors, and the essence of nutritional counseling is the process of personalized *teaching*. These terms need to be clarified. In today's educational vocabulary, *learning* is defined as a process that is directed toward a relatively persistent *change in behavior*.[6] This is in contrast to the rather traditional view of learning as acquisition of facts and information. At the same time, *teaching* is defined as the manipulation of system variables to produce behavior change (learning).[7] This means that teaching is not equivalent to "telling," since experience has taught us that providing information to a client is less than adequate in helping him change his behavior. To quote Guthrie:

We need only to look at the food habits of professionally educated nutritionists and food scientists to demonstrate that food choices are not made on the basis of nutrition information alone. For them, as for the less informed public, food choices are the result of a host of social, psychological, economic and emotional variables. . . . The challenge to educators and nutritionists is to discover the mechanisms by which information is processed and translated into be-

havioral change and the social reinforcements necessary to initiate and maintain it.[8] *(p. 89)*

Providing information, therefore, is only a small component of the teaching process. As teaching is defined here, there is, for all practical purposes, no difference in the process of teaching and the process of counseling.

May[1] suggests that there is an artificial distinction between education (teaching) and reeducation (counseling). Teaching is evolving today toward a more personalized approach to meeting students' cognitive, affective, and psychomotor needs.[9] Counseling has also moved toward integrating the client-centered approach of Rogers[10] with the action-oriented approach of the behaviorists[11,12] into a more holistic model.[13] Counselors seek to deal with changing behaviors, not only by working with attitudes, but also by teaching skills, such as communication, assertiveness, and problem-solving. Consequently, the differences have become blurred. The authors have elected to use the word counseling, because the clinician and the client will infer that counseling is a more personalized, individualized approach to working with people, based on common usage. Such a belief on the part of the client is a critical prerequisite to successful behavior change. The success of counseling is also enhanced by an eclectic selection of change strategies exemplified by Kanfer and Goldstein.[14]

Because the outcomes of counseling are so far-reaching, there is a wide spectrum of skills and knowledge needed by the clinical dietitian for the provision of nutritional counseling. According to White and Mondeika,[15] it should be the responsibility of the dietitian to plan the client's nutritional care with the client and the health team, implement and evaluate that care, and then communicate the outcome to the team. Such a description is obviously that of a clinical dietitian functioning on a team of health specialists whose primary goal is optimal care for the client. This description is supportive of the team concepts presented in Chapter 2.

CONCEPTS BASIC TO NUTRITIONAL COUNSELING

Two basic components are prerequisite to the clinical dietitian's effectiveness in nutritional counseling. He should be knowledgeable about nutrition, and about human behavior. Figure 3.1 illustrates these components at the core of nutritional counseling.

A definition of nutrition to serve the purposes of this text was presented in Chapter 1. A simplistic restatement of the definition is that

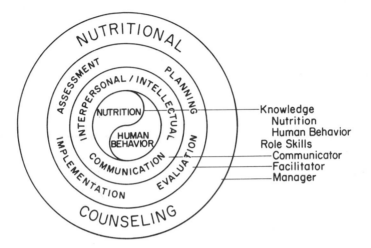

FIGURE 3.1   Relationship of knowledge and role skills to nutritional counseling.

nutrition knowledge encompasses the complex interdependence of food and nutrients for clients in their environments. Stone described Dietetics as the profession that ". . . involves the translation of . . . current, spectacular knowledge of nutrition . . ."[16] (p. 27). We earlier declared that it is not the purpose of this text to include what is known about nutritional science as there is already an abundance of such texts. Nonetheless, the authors are cognizant that it is essential for clinical dietitians to be knowledgeable in the discipline. That knowledge base continues to change and carries with it an aura of excitement; it follows that one responsibility of the practitioner is to assess new data, compare them with what is known, and determine whether or not the new data are applicable to current practice.

Understanding human behavior is also at the core of the clinical dietitian's effectiveness in nutritional counseling. The ability to facilitate behavior change derives from an understanding of the dynamics of behavior. The depth of understanding required for counseling can come only from the experience of self-understanding.[17] This point is underscored by Brill:

The worker who aspires to utilize himself in a disciplined and knowledgeable way in relationships with other people must have a personal objectivity based on: (1) awareness of himself and his own needs, (2) ability to deal with personality patterns within himself, and (3) resultant relative freedom from the limitations they may place on his ability to perceive with clarity and relate with honesty.[18] *(p. 1)*

Thus, at the core of nutritional counseling is the clinical dietitian's understanding of his own behavior, and success in implementing necessary changes in that behavior. The skills involved in achieving this are extensive and beyond the scope of this text. As a resource for the reader, there is included at the end of this chapter a list of suggested references for the topic. In addition, conferences and workshops related to the topic are frequently offered by professional societies and educational institutions in various parts of North America.

ROLE SKILLS OF THE CLINICAL DIETITIAN IN NUTRITIONAL COUNSELING

The clinical dietitian's success is dependent upon both a wide variety of skills and a client-centered value system.[19] Stone's remarks also contain a description of what he believes is the relationship between the science of nutrition and the practice of clinical dietetics. The relationship:

. . . involves the translation of our current, spectacular knowledge of nutrition and the interpretation and distribution of this knowledge to the individual; . . . the function of the . . . dietitian is the conversion of theory into practice, of science into art.[16] *(p. 27)*

Once the clinician becomes secure in his knowledge of nutrition, the next step is to meaningfully apply the knowledge. The avenue of application includes interpreting nutritional knowledge in terms of *food* as an individual's nutritional needs are reflected as food to be consumed. A client's food behavior (selection, preparation, and consumption of food) is the primary focus of nutritional counseling for the clinical dietitian. Consequently, knowledge of foods and their composition is also a basic prerequisite to practice.

The clinical dietitian's successful conversion of theory into practice and science into art (thus achieving the goals of nutritional counseling) requires a number of skills. The skills are behavioral and intellectual, as opposed to mechanical ones, and require a solid knowledge base to be utilized appropriately. This wide array of skills evolves from the many tasks that constitute the complexity of counseling. Lack of expertise in any one area hinders the progress toward the desired outcomes of counseling. We shall examine these areas as they relate to the process of nutritional counseling.

Figure 3.1 illustrates a composite of the role skills of the clinical dietitian in client-centered nutritional counseling. The perceived role skills are communication, facilitation, and management. Related to these role skills are the nutrition knowledge base and an understanding of human behavior. We shall examine the interrelationships of these skills and processes in the following paragraphs.

Communication Skills

Effective communication is primary to pursuing the goal of nutritional counseling with clients, clients' significant others, and other members of the health care team. Communication skills are viewed as being composed of two basic types: intellectual and interpersonal communication. Effective intellectual communication[21,22] is an indispensable skill as it is the ability to speak and write in a clear, concise, organized manner, so that the "receivers" can understand intellectually what has been said. Instructions, information relayed via the medical record, and knowledge shared with both colleagues and clients require expertise in this area. In addition to being a competent "sender," it is important to acquire the skill of being a proficient "receiver." "Receiving" implies reading and listening for comprehension. The magnitude of knowledge in nutrition and dietetics is such that no one can possibly learn all there is to know—ever! The implication is that the dietetic practitioner is a lifelong learner and, as such, is continually dependent on the literature and other professionals to keep abreast of constant change.

Although intellectual communication is extremely important, it is not the only kind of communication. In recent years, much has been learned about the process of interpersonal communication.[3,4,13] This type of communication extends the sharing of knowledge to a sharing of meanings for people. If a client says, "I don't eat meat," and the counselor notes, "client doesn't eat meat," intellectual communication has been established. Human beings, however, have motives for their behavior and unless the clinician has an awareness of these motives, behavior change may be difficult. Investigation of the meaning of the client's statement may produce a variety of motives: that he is vegetarian as a result of religious commitment or social mores, that he has no teeth, that meat is too expensive, or that he detests meat. As people are often unwilling to share personal meanings and feelings with those they don't trust, interpersonal communication requires an additional set of skills that are, for most people, not a part of their regular communication repertoire. These skills are often referred to as empathic listening skills.[23] They are particularly important in the interviewing and instruction segments of nutritional counseling.

Facilitation Skills

The facilitation skills encompass a great many activities and behaviors (see Figure 3.1). The model for nutritional counseling to be presented in this text includes the components of Assessment, Planning, Implementation, and Evaluation. The successful facilitation of these components is incumbent on the clinical dietitian. This implies that the clinician provides a support system for the achievement of client independence. That is, the clinician shows the client how to remove the obstacles that render a behavior difficult to change; she does not coerce or do for the client anything the client can do for himself. Other synonyms most often substituted for facilitator are counselor and helper. The best counselor or helper works herself out of a job with each client by facilitating client independence.

Contingent on successful facilitation are a number of related activities. Included are interviewing, investigation, observation, analysis, design, instruction, innovation, and evaluation.

A skill for the assessment component of counseling is that of *observation*, as it is a data-gathering skill. There is an overwhelming tendency on the part of human beings to be subjective, selectively "seeing" only what they prefer to see. Consequently, there is a need to acquire the skill of objective observation, recording that which actually occurred without observer interpretation. For example, a subjective observer might describe a client as a chain-smoker. An objective observer would describe the client as having lit and smoked, by inhaling, eight king-sized filter-tipped cigarettes to the end of the filter in a one-hour session, removed from the mouth only to exhale. Total objectivity is the preferred means of observation.[24] Depending on the purpose of the data collection, however, some subjectivity can be tolerated. In another situation, it might be adequate to say that the client smoked eight cigarettes in an hour. They could have been king or regular, smoked half way or all the way, in the mouth constantly, or mostly held in the hand. If the decisionmaker needs to know only approximately how many cartons the smoker will consume in a week, the latter is adequate. If there is a need to know the amount of exposure to smoke tars, the most objective observation is preferable. In any event, the skill of objective observation is invaluable to the dietitian who works with a concrete entity such as food.

Another skill is that of *investigation*. There are myriad facts that must be gleaned from a variety of sources. The clinical dietitian must know how to obtain them and then know which are most reliable. This includes learning to discriminate between subjective and objective data provided by others.[25,26]

In the first phase of counseling, assessment, the clinician gathers and analyzes client data from a variety of sources. One of the basic skills needed in the gathering of data is that of *interviewing*. The very heart of interviewing is the use of both intellectual and interpersonal communication, primarily the latter. Interpersonal communication is also used as a means of establishing a relationship between client and clinician that is necessary for many people to deal with the complexities of their own food behaviors. The interviewer skills are also appropriate in certain aspects of implementation and evaluation.

The clinical dietitian must also be a systems *analyst*. As such he examines the biologic, food intake, environmental, and behavioral elements of a client's system of food practices in order to describe the components and their interrelationships. The practitioner analyzes those components of the system to determine which components are appropriate and functioning optimally, and to present recommendations for improvements.

Following assessment, the client's care must be planned. The practitioner is then a planner/systems *designer*. That which he designs is termed a learning system. Such a system will include[7,27]:

1. Clearly stated behavioral objectives based on client need
2. Learning experiences, based on tested educational theory, to help the learner reach the objective
3. A method of evaluating whether or not the client met the objective, and if not, why not

At this point, it is also of tremendous value for the clinical dietitian to be an *innovator*. The skills of creative problem solving are very beneficial in developing learning experiences and support services, particularly in circumstances where the solution is not readily evident.[28] Creativity, the production of novel ideas, can be fostered by structured experiences and continued practice.[29] It is also nurtured in an environment where it is all right to take a risk and fail, and where human beings feel accepted rather than judged.[30] Creativity, as defined here, is not limited to the production of artistic works, but describes a broader process of freeing the mind to do "what can't be done."

The skill of *instruction* is descriptive of the clinical dietitian's participation in providing the client with appropriate learning experiences and resources. Instructing involves providing information, practice, and feedback to the client *vis à vis*, or guiding the client to self-instructional learning materials. This new technology in education provides a wide variety of instructional tools and techniques that can challenge the instructor's imagination and accommodate various learning styles of clients.

The failure of nutritional counselors to evaluate the results of their efforts is comparable to running the football to the 1-yard line and then dropping it. There is, in both instances, no evidence of the goal being achieved. Therefore, nutrition counselors must be *evaluators*.[26] An evaluator determines the value of the components and outcomes of a system in order to make decisions about change. In other words, he decides not only whether something worked, but if it was appropriate. The evaluator is concerned with success in a given milieu and is always judging each unique system once it is put into operation.

The evaluator continually monitors his learners, not just when they exit the learning system. Early and continual feedback* is called *formative* evaluation. It permits the system designer to make alterations that increase the probability of the learner meeting the established criteria. At the termination of a learning experience, *summative* evaluation is used both to evaluate the system and define the learner's achievement. Both forms of evaluation are integral and indispensable parts of nutritional counseling.

Management Skills

The clinical dietitian must be prepared to apply management skills. Figure 3.1 illustrates that the role of nutritional counseling is executed using such skills. In essence, then, the clinician is viewed as a manager when providing nutritional care to clients. An efficient management system is indispensable for clinical dietitians whose goal is to provide optimal nutritional care for their clients.

Management is frequently viewed as the province of the foodservice systems dietitian. Though the environment is different, the tools by which management is implemented are the same. The clinical dietitian as a *manager* is discussed in Chapter 14. In the view of the authors, management of clinical practice is deserving of a chapter of its own. Unless the clinical dietitian has an operative system and can serve as

---

* We shall use the term "feedback" to indicate the process of providing information to the learner about his progress in meeting an objective, describing to him that progress in terms enabling him to more readily achieve that objective.

an effective manager, less than optimum nutritional counseling will be provided to clients.

THE RECIPIENTS OF NUTRITIONAL COUNSELING

The Client

Concurrent with acquiring the skills necessary for successful nutritional counseling, it is essential that clinical dietitians begin to develop an objective, theoretical base regarding their attitudes and beliefs about the nature of being human.[31] These beliefs and attitudes will significantly affect the approach used with clients, as there is some evidence to support a hypothesis termed the "self-fulfilling prophecy".[32] This hypothesis suggests that what a significant other believes about a person will often materialize. A testing of the hypothesis was reported in 1968 in a classroom situation. Teachers were assigned randomly selected students but were told some were overachievers and some underachievers. In actual fact, there was no significant difference between groups. After a period of time during which the teachers worked with the students, it was ascertained that those students deliberately mislabeled "overachievers" actually did significantly better than those deliberately mislabeled "underachievers." In some manner, the teachers seemed to place more emphasis on helping those they felt could succeed. If they had viewed all students as achievers, perhaps many more would have done well. This description should give clinical dietitians pause in examining their attitudes toward those whom they may label in such ways that imply *inferior*, e.g., retarded, illiterate, unmotivated, disorganized. Larson, for example, found that some nurses stereotyped lower-class patients as dependent, passive, unintelligent, lazy, forgetful, ignorant failures.[33] If a clinician feels this way about a client it seems likely, following the hypothesis described, that he will unconsciously make less effort and perhaps convey a sense of hopelessness in counseling, thus dooming the client to failure.

The client in the counseling process can be anyone who exhibits food behaviors detrimental to his health and/or one who desires a change in his food behaviors. In one study, Rae found that the reasons for referral to nutritional counseling included excessive weight (61%), Diabetes Mellitus (14%), other problems of nutritional pathology (10%), pregnancy (10%), and a variety of general problems (5%), such as food budgeting.[34] The client may also be a person who actually has desirable food behaviors, but needs to receive acknowledgment that reinforces his behavior. Initially, the client does not need to request counseling, nor does he need to have medical evidence of a nutrition-related problem. If he either wants or needs counseling, anyone can be a client.

Utilization of levels of needs awareness may be helpful in understanding the vast audience of potential clients and their counseling needs (Table 3.1). Such a grouping attempts to state clearly the various circumstances in which a client might seek and enter counseling. There are many potential clients who are unknown to clinical dietitians because they fail to seek counseling. Others fail to continue once begun; the clients in Rae's study are an example.[34] Of the referrals made, 12 percent never came to a first appointment and, of the ones who did come, 30 percent did not return for a second visit. Clients may not enter counseling because they are either unaware of their need or do not know where to turn for help. Many probably do not know that dietitians are available to provide services. Other potential clients may not want to change their behavior. The ones who try counseling once may find the counselor or the experience threatening and choose not to continue. This will be true particularly when clients perceive that

TABLE 3.1   Levels of Needs Awareness

Level	The Client:
1	Doesn't know whether his behavior is detrimental or beneficial.
2	Knows his behavior is detrimental but doesn't know a preferable behavior or how to get the assistance needed.
3	Knows his behavior is detrimental and knows what he should do, but doesn't know how to do it.
4	Know his behavior is detrimental, what to do, and how to do it, but says he doesn't want to change.
5	Knows his behavior is detrimental, what to do and how to do it, says he wants to change, but fails when he tries.
6	Knows his behavior is detrimental, what to do, how to do it, and can maintain desired behavior.

the clinician is judgmental and unaccepting of them or their behaviors. Furthermore, clinical dietitians may tend to overlook those clients who are represented by Levels 4 and 5 because motivation is considered to be a magical quality that the client either does or does not have. Thus, dietitians tend to concentrate on clients who, once they know what to do and how to do it, will follow through on their own. Helping clients to develop their own motivational strategies and a desire to continue counseling can be an extraordinarily difficult task for many practitioners, but not an impossible one.

Significant Others

Obviously, when others besides the practitioner and the client become involved in the counseling, the dynamics quickly assume a greater complexity. If, however, we look at human beings as functioning in their own ecosystems in which they both act and react, it is apparent that the clinician must be in touch with those significant others who stimulate client behavior. Therefore, the immediate family is a very crucial contact. As family therapy is becoming an increasingly preferred in-depth method of working with people with emotional problems,[35] some nutritional problems may be treated by a professional family therapist in conjunction with the clinical dietitian. In this situation, the family therapist has the primary responsibility and thus is the team leader. Family counseling, the inclusion of family members in assessment, planning, implementation, and evaluation, is a valid method of nutritional counseling that may be employed by clinical dietitians. For example, even though a husband doesn't prepare meals, he may knowingly or inadvertently be encouraging his wife's undesirable eating patterns or meal-planning choices. Interactions between parents and children have tremendous influence on developing food behaviors in the child, as well as some influence on the meal preparation patterns of the mother.

Health team members often have insights from additional contact they have had with clients. A social worker might suggest that a family is not ready for nutritional counseling until they have resolved some marital problems. In this instance, the social worker functions as the family therapist and takes the lead in providing counseling. Frequently there are indications that the clinical dietitian can most effectively provide nutritional care for the client when working in cooperation with other health care providers. The history compiled by the health team can be of value to the clinical dietitian; simultaneously, the clinical dietitian contributes to the health and social history of the client. Optimal nutritional care is a component of the team's goal of health for the client.

THE COUNSELING ENVIRONMENT

An overview of nutritional counseling would not be complete without an examination of the environment in which it occurs. Too often the first site that comes to the minds of many is that of an acute care setting, where the majority of clinical dietitians historically have practiced. Limiting counseling to that environment assumes that nutritional care is basically a component of secondary and tertiary prevention programs. That is, the client has a pathologic problem that includes a nutritional facet and the dietitian instructs him on the basis of the prescribed care plan. Nutritional care is rightfully a significant component of primary prevention as well. In an examination of the diseases that rank highest in mortality rates, a wide array of cardiovascular diseases and cancer are found to rank first and second in numbers of nonaccidental deaths.[36] These are the diseases that are of complex etiology, are relatively irreversible, and are more than likely the result of less than adequate concern for, or ignorance of, desirable health care by the individual. Proper nutritional behavior has been demonstrated to be of value in the prophylaxis of some of these diseases and hypothesized as important in others.[37]

What does this mean to the clinical dietitian? It should demonstrate that there is a tremendous need for a nutritional component in primary prevention programs, programs directed toward the prevention of illness. It means clinical dietitians must work with clients in and out of formalized institutions to help them become aware of discrepant nutritional behaviors, and to encourage them to accept counseling as a means of helping them select and put into action nutritional behaviors that will promote health.

Where Clients are Found

If the preceding assumptions about primary prevention are acceptable, consideration of the various places in which such programs can occur is now appropriate. Nutritional counseling will be practiced in diverse facilities such as walk-in clinics, family practice centers, nutrition sites for senior citizens, schools, offices of dietitians in private practice, clients' homes, facilities that provide space and/or activities for special groups (e.g., weight-control groups at YMCAs), community education program sites, and in almost any other imaginable place where people gather to learn. The opportunities are limited only by our perceptions of the purpose and process of nutritional counseling.

The most obvious place, next to acute or chronic care sites, is undoubtedly an ambulatory care facility, such as a clinic or physician's office. Of particular interest are the clinical sites of the evolving Health Maintenance Organizations (HMOs). These are prepaid health plans to which clients subscribe and pay a monthly fee in return for health care. Such organizations are built on the assumption that it is economically beneficial for the health care team to keep its subscribers healthy. As more physicians consider group practice, particularly in the form of health care teams, nurse clinicians, social workers, dietitians, counselors, and dentists will be functioning members of the team.

Clinical dietitians in private practice provide individual and group nutritional counseling, as well as consultant services.* The privately employed dietitian may take referrals from both health professionals and from clients.[38,39] In private practice, the dietitian needs to develop a format and facilities for provision of individual and group counseling,† and consultant services. Rooms designed for individual and group counseling must be available, as well as time allotted in some cases to visit clients' homes and institutionalized clients for consulting purposes.

Beyond the conventional health care sites, nutritional counseling should be available in places where individuals and groups of people in need of a better understanding of nutrition can be found. As the importance of nutrition is being acknowledged to a greater degree than ever before, public school systems are beginning to include nutrition units in the comprehensive curriculum, often at the mandate of the state.[40] More recently, the federal government has identified the provision of nutrition education in public schools as a major priority in health promotion services.[41] It follows that there is a tremendous need for clinical dietitians to participate as consultants in the development

---

* The term consulting is used here in the context of providing information and recommendations to a secondary client where there will be others (the primary clients) affected by that secondary client's decisions and actions. An example is the dietitian employed by a public health agency whose responsibilities include client nutritional care and staff education. When providing client nutritional care, the practitioner is counseling a primary client. In staff education, the practitioner is a consultant to other health care providers (secondary clients), who will in turn be counseling their clients (primary clients).

† As stated in the preface, course work in the behavioral sciences is prerequisite to the provision of nutritional counseling.

of public school programs and as instructors for in-service workshops for teachers.[42]

In conjunction with public schools, there are often adult education programs where dietitians need not be certified as teachers by the state.[43] The response to these programs has been quite significant. Many adults are eager for new learning experiences; the vehicle is now there for clinical dietitians to participate as instructors and be remunerated for their efforts, as they should be.

There are also increasing numbers of government-funded nutrition programs where potential clients can be identified and counseled.[44,45] Examples of these are programs for older adults, children in day-care centers, and migrant workers. Client contacts can and should take place in many and diverse circumstances, thus broadening the scope of dietetic practice.

The Actual Counseling Site

We have considered the four major types of counseling settings where clients are found: institutions, ambulatory care settings, offices, and community sites. There are, of course, other considerations related to the specific environment in which counseling may occur. It is often useful to leave a formal office environment and enter the client's own world. The office formality may serve to confer an aura of authority on the clinical dietitian and thus establish a communication barrier unless the counselor takes great care to avoid it. Going to the client may communicate that the dietitian doesn't need the "trappings" to be effective. Certainly clinicians can go the other way and be so informal as to suggest that their role is not important. The key is an awareness of what is being communicated nonverbally by the selection of the environment, and that will vary with the client.

Within an acute or chronic care setting, counseling may take place in a client's room, lounge, classroom, or, preferably, a room designed for nutritional counseling. Clinical dietitians should be cognizant of the special value to be derived from learning about the client's home situation, which can be achieved through seeing the client in his own environment.

SUMMARY

Nutritional counseling is the process by which clients can be most effectively helped to acquire more healthful nutritional behaviors.

Clinical dietitians, therefore, must acquire a number of role skills related to client-centered care. It is important to understand the diverse concerns and problems of the clients who seek or need counseling, and to consider not only the individual client, but all of the significant others who interact with the client, including family, peers, colleagues, and the health team. In counseling, it is probably most beneficial to use family counseling when possible. There are also advantages to providing group counseling with participants who have similar concerns.

For successful counseling, attention should be given to the counseling environment, which need not be limited to traditional sites. The potential sites in which counseling can occur are much broader than is usually perceived. Within these sites, the actual surroundings should be conducive to counseling as they send nonverbal messages to the client just as the counselor communicates his view of himself, his role, and his attitude toward the client. Conscious attention to all these factors and the implementation of a systems approach, as exemplified by the model presented in Chapter 9, can help the clinical dietitian provide the best nutritional care of which he is capable, and increase his ability to help the client achieve desired change.

CITED REFERENCES

1. May, R. *The Art of Counseling*. New York: Abingdon Press, 1967.
2. Wylie, J., and Singer, J. Growth process in nutrition counseling. *J. Am. Dietet. A.* 69:505, 1976.
3. Combs, A., Avila, D., and Purkey, W. *Helping Relationships: Basic Concepts for the Helping Professions*. 2nd Ed. Boston: Allyn and Bacon, Inc., 1978.
4. Carkhuff, R. R. *Helping and Human Relations: A Primer for Lay and Professional Helpers. Vol. II. Practice and Research*. New York: Holt, Rinehart and Winston, Inc., 1969.
5. Brammer, L. M., and Shostrom, E. L. *Therapeutic Psychology: Fundamentals of Actualization Counseling and Psychotherapy*. 3rd Ed. Englewood Cliffs, NJ: Prentice-Hall, Inc., 1977.
6. Gagné, R. M. *The Conditions of Learning*. 3rd Ed. New York: Holt, Rinehart and Winston, Inc., 1977.
7. Davis, R. H., Alexander, L. T., and Yelon, S. L. *Learning System Design: An Approach to the Improvement of Instruction*. New York: McGraw-Hill Book Co., 1974.
8. Guthrie, H. A. The role of nutrition education in dietary improvement. *Food Tech.* 32:9:89, 1978.

9. Schalock, H., and Garrison, J. The personalization of teacher education programs. *In* Anderson, D., Cooper, J., DeVault, M., Dickson, G., Johnson, C., and Weber, W., Eds. *Competency-Based Teacher Education.* Berkeley: McCutchan Publ. Corp., 1973.

10. Rogers, C. R. *Client-Centered Therapy: Its Current Practice, Implications, and Theory.* Boston: Houghton-Mifflin Co., 1951.

11. Krumboltz, J., and Thoresen, C. *Behavioral Counseling: Cases and Techniques.* New York: Holt, Rinehart and Winston, Inc., 1969.

12. Bandura, A. *Principles of Behavior Modification.* New York: Holt, Rinehart and Winston, Inc., 1969.

13. Gazda, G. M. *Human Relations Development: A Manual for Educators.* 2nd Ed. Boston: Allyn and Bacon, Inc., 1977.

14. Kanfer, F. H., and Goldstein, A. P., Eds. *Helping People Change: A Textbook of Methods.* New York: Pergamon Press, Inc., 1975.

15. White, P. L., and Mondeika, T. Somewhere under the iceberg. *J. Am. Med. A.* 235:1873, 1976.

16. Stone, D. B. A true role for the dietitian: A scholar in nutrition. *J. Am. Dietet. A.* 49:26, 1966.

17. Hamachek, D. E. *Encounters with the Self.* 2nd Ed. New York: Holt, Rinehart and Winston, Inc., 1978.

18. Brill, N. I. *Working with People: The Helping Process.* 2nd Ed. Philadelphia: J. B. Lippincott Co., 1978.

19. Brammer, L. M. *The Helping Relationship: Process and Skills.* 2nd Ed. Englewood Cliffs, NJ: Prentice-Hall, Inc., 1979.

20. Thiele, M. C., and Hankin, J. H. Training nutritionists for comprehensive health delivery systems. *J. Am. Dietet. A.* 70:189, 1977.

21. Purtilo, R. *The Allied Health Professional and the Patient: Techniques of Effective Interaction.* Philadelphia: W. B. Saunders Co., 1973.

22. Howard, J. C., Tracz, R. F., and Thomas, C. *Contact: A Textbook in Applied Communications.* 2nd Ed. Englewood Cliffs, NJ: Prentice-Hall, Inc., 1974.

23. Sydnor, G., Akridge, R., and Parkhill, N. *Human Relations Training: A Programmed Manual.* Minden, LA: Human Relations Development Training Institute, 1973.

24. Watson, D. L., and Tharp, R. G. *Self-Directed Behavior: Self-Modification for Personal Adjustment.* 2nd Ed. Monterey, CA: Brooks Cole Publ., 1977.

25. Hurst, J. W., and Walker, H. K., Eds. *The Problem-Oriented System.* New York: Medcom Press, 1972.

26. Owen, A. L., and Owen, G. M. Training public health nutritionists: Competencies for complacency or future concerns. *Am. J. Pub. Health.* 69:1096, 1979.

27. Kaufman, R. *Educational System Planning.* Englewood Cliffs, NJ: Prentice-Hall, Inc., 1972.

28. Carkhuff, R. R. *The Art of Problem-Solving.* Amherst, MA: Human Resource Devel. Press, 1974.
29. Welsch, P. K. *The Nurturance of Creative Behavior in Educational Environments: A Comprehensive Curriculum Approach.* Unpublished Ph.D. dissertation, Michigan State University, 1980.
30. May, R. *The Courage to Create.* New York: Norton, 1975.
31. Stefflre, B., and Matheny, K. *The Function of Counseling Theory.* Boston: Houghton-Mifflin Co., 1968.
32. Rosenthal, R., and Jacobson, L. F. Teacher expectations for the disadvantaged. *Sci. Am.* 218:4:19, 1968.
33. Larson, P. A. Nurse perceptions of patient characteristics. *Nurs. Res.* 26:416, 1977.
34. Rae, J. Evaluation of demonstration models for delivery of nutrition services: Effects upon health of clients. *J. Canad. Dietet. A.* 38:201, 1977.
35. Satir, V. *Conjoint Family Therapy: A Guide of Theory and Technique.* Rev. Ed. Palo Alto: Science and Behavior Books, Inc., 1967.
36. Gori, G. "Introductory Remarks and Historical Perspective of the Relationship of Diet to Cancer." Symposium: Cancer and Nutrition, Presented at the 59th Annual Meeting of the American Dietetic Association, Boston, October 13, 1976.
37. Wynder, E. "Relationship of Diet to Cancer Epidemiology." Symposium: Cancer and Nutrition, Presented at the 59th Annual Meeting of the American Dietetic Association, Boston, October 13, 1976.
38. Trithart, E. S., and Noel, M. B. New dimensions: The dietitian in private practice. *J. Am. Dietet. A.* 73:60, 1978.
39. Kunis, B. S. Entering private practice in dietetics. *J. Am. Dietet. A.* 73:165, 1978.
40. The Nutrition Education Task Force. *Food—What's in It for You?: Teacher Reference Guide.* Lansing, Mich.: Mich. Dietet. Assoc. and Mich. Publ. Health Assoc., 1976.
41. The Departmental Task Force on Prevention. *Disease Prevention & Health Promotion: Federal Program and Prospects.* DHEW (PHS) Publ. No. 79-55071B. Washington: Publ. Health Serv., 1979.
42. Significant issues in nutrition. *J. Am. Dietet. A.* 70:13, 1977.
43. The American Dietetic Association position paper on the scope and thrust of nutrition education. *J. Am. Dietet. A.* 72:302, 1978.
44. Owen, A. Y. *Community Nutrition in Preventive Health Care Services. A Critical Review of the Literature.* Health Res. Admin. Publ. No. HRP-0300701. Washington: U.S. Dept. Health, Educ., and Welfare, 1978.
45. Owen, A. L., Owen, G. M., and Lanna, G. Health and nutritional benefits of federal food assistance programs. *In* Mason, M., et al. *Costs and Benefits of Nutritional Care: Phase 1.* Chicago: The American Dietetic Association, 1979.

SUGGESTED REFERENCES

Biondi, A. *The Creative Process*. Buffalo: DOK Publishers, Inc., 1972.

Bloom, B. S., Hastings, J., and Madaus, G. *Handbook on Formative and Summative Evaluation of Student Learning*. New York: McGraw-Hill Book Co., 1971.

Bullough, B., and Bullough, V. L. *Poverty, Ethnic Identity, and Health Care*. New York: Appleton-Century-Crofts, 1972.

Carruth, B. R., Mangel, M., and Anderson, H. L. Assessing change-proneness and nutrition-related behaviors. *J. Am. Dietet. A.* 70:47, 1977.

Ellis, A. *Growth Through Reason. Verbatim Cases in Rational-Emotive Therapy*. No. Hollywood, CA: Wilshire Book Co., 1975.

Ellis, A., and Harper, R. A. *A New Guide to Rational Living*. No. Hollywood, CA: Wilshire Book Co., 1976.

Hamachek, D. E., Ed. *Human Dynamics in Psychology and Education. Selected Readings*. 3rd Ed. Boston: Allyn and Bacon, Inc., 1977.

Harris, T. A. *I'm OK—You're OK. A Practical Guide to Transactional Analysis*. New York: Harper and Row, 1969.

Jourard, S. M. *The Transparent Self: Self Disclosure and Well-Being*. 2nd Ed. New York: Van Nostrand Reinhold Co., 1971.

Maslow, A. H. *Toward a Psychology of Being*. 2nd Ed. Princeton, NJ: D. Van Nostrand Co., Inc., 1968.

Powell, J. *Why am i afaid to tell you who i am?* Niles, IL: Argus Communications, 1969.

Rogers, C. R. *On Becoming a Person. A Therapist's View of Psychotherapy*. Boston: Houghton-Mifflin Co., 1970.

Saulnier, L., and Simard, T. *Personal Growth and Interpersonal Relations*. Englewood Cliffs, NJ: Prentice-Hall, Inc., 1973.

Shostrom, E. L. *Man, the Manipulator: The Inner Journey from Manipulation to Actualization*. New York: Abingdon Press, 1967.

PART

II

Resources for Nutritional Counseling

4
The Medical Record

Most dietitians . . . are prone to think in terms of pathology and therapy. But, the bulk of Americans are healthy. To be effective, attention must be drawn to normal nutrition in its most positive aspects, to the preventive role of nutrition, to the changing life styles of a prosperous population.

Corrine H. Robinson, **Nutrition education— what comes next?** (*J. Am. Dietet. A.* 69: 126. 1976).

In the first stages of the assessment process, the clinical dietitian turns to the medical record* of the client she is counseling. The record is the most valuable communication device existing in health care settings, and serves as the reservoir or depository of information concerning an individual. Thus, the medical record is a historical document, vividly summarizing over time a description of the course of care. Unfortunately, there is no one well-defined pattern of organization for medical records, as institutions rendering health care differ considerably in their function and structure. Some commonalities do exist, however, and these will be examined in this chapter. The clinician is again reminded that the medical record *is* a legal document, representing the course of an individual's health care, and thus is treated with the

* For once the authors accept for their own the terminology in common usage. In our opinion, however, "medical record" is a misleading label, incompatible with Robinson's and our philosophy. The correct terminology is "health record," thereby placing emphasis on wellness and *not* on pathology. Stay tuned for the third edition.

utmost confidentiality.[2] Since the record is a legal document, it is often submitted for examination in a court of law when some aspect of health care is being contested.

The clinical dietitian in private practice or in certain ambulatory settings is in a unique situation, in that she does not usually have ready access to the medical record of a client who presents himself with a nutritional care problem. In such circumstances, the practitioner should request the record from the referral source during the assessment phase of the counseling process. This may require that the clinician go to the site of record storage or that the record be copied and sent to her office.*

Every client's medical record is maintained and stored for future use usually by the Medical Records Department of the health facility. The medical record administrator is not only responsible for the completeness and safety of this vital document, but is often called upon to "audit" records. An audit of a medical record is an evaluation of the quality of care and is based upon criteria established by those health professionals rendering the care. Involvement of clinical dietitians in health care audit will be discussed in Chapter 15.

In summary, the medical record is:

1. A communication tool
2. A legal document
3. A confidential document

THE SOURCE-ORIENTED MEDICAL RECORD

The traditional medical record format has been used in American health care institutions for more than half a century.[3] In view of recent changes in the organization of medical records, the traditional record is now referred to as the source-oriented record (SOR), to distinguish it from the newer problem-oriented record (POR).[4,5] The format of the SOR is governed by the principle that similar records are filed together; that is, all x-rays appear in one section, all laboratory reports in another, and so on. The organization, then, is based on the *source* of information obtained during the course of health care—hence the name, source-oriented record.

The SOR contains a number of documents that are independently inserted into the record in separate sections, usually in chronologic

---

* Written permission of the client may be required.

order. Presented in random order, the sections include:

The problem list (optional)	Consents
Patient identification information	Consultations
	Laboratory reports
Physicians' orders	Medication records
Graphic sheets	Operating room records
Progress notes	

The following paragraphs are devoted to an examination of these sections. The first to be discussed, the problem list, is not always included in this record; the listing of problems has been "borrowed" from the POR system by many institutions still using the SOR, as they have found such a listing to be valuable in client-centered health care.

Problem List

The page called "The Master Problem List" is based on the principles of the POR, and serves to highlight those active and inactive "problems" that represent the client's need for diagnostic, therapeutic, or educational health care. The problem list asks for the date the problem was found to exist and its resolution (if any). Pertinent inactive problems are listed in the event that they may relate, either directly or indirectly, to the defined active problems. Each problem is numbered in sequence and appropriately titled.

Identification Data

The next section of the record is the form for recording information pertaining to the identification of the client in a variety of ways. This page is often referred to as the "front sheet" or the "face sheet." The following information about the client is recorded, usually by the admitting officer, on the front sheet:

PATIENT IDENTIFICATION INFORMATION

Section A (for admission to health care facility):

Name	Institution unit number
Address	Reentry: yes or no
Home telephone	Age
Birthdate	Birthplace
Sex	Marital status

Religion	Occupation
Place of work	Social security number
Father's name	Mother's name
Spouse's name	Spouse's occupation
Spouse's place of work	
Admission date	Patient care unit
Admission diagnosis	
Attending physician	Family physician
Insurance carrier	
Medicare number	Medicaid number
Notify in emergency:	
Address:	Telephone:
	Home:
	Work:

Section B (for discharge from health care facility):

Discharge date	
Primary diagnosis	Other diagnoses
Complications (including drug reactions)	
Operations or treatments	Reportable diseases
Discharge status	
Alive	Date of return to ambulatory unit
Deceased	
Treatment and orders	
Date of return to work	Activity restriction

As the reader will no doubt realize, the face sheet contains a wealth of information useful to the practitioner in her assessment of the client. Much of the socioeconomic status (SES) information, useful in compiling the initial data, is available here.

Physicians' Orders

Usually following the patient identification information is the section devoted to the physicians' orders. These pages will contain the specific orders for all forms of treatment, including those directly involving the clinical dietitian (the plan for the client's nutritional care). In those institutions where there are primary care providers other than physicians recording directions for specific treatments, the written orders will be countersigned by the attending physician.

Graphic Sheets

The next section of the medical record is usually that called "graphic sheets," and contains information recorded by the nursing staff. The graphic sheets demonstrate visually the following information about the client:

> Heart rate
>
> Temperature (F or C)
>
> Respiration rate
>
> Height
>
> Weight
>
> Fluid intake: Mouth   Output: Urine
>   Parenteral   Emesis
>   Blood   Other
>   Stools

All of the information is recorded according to date and time so that an ongoing record of the physical descriptions is available for quick inspection. Of particular significance to the clinical dietitian are the records of height, weight, body temperature, fluid intake and output, and defecation.

Progress Notes

Those pages marked "progress notes" may follow next in the SOR. In some respects, the term "progress" is misleading, as this section usually contains not only chronologic notes entered by members of the health team, but also includes a retrospective review of the events leading up to the client's admission to the health care facility. Nonetheless, the progress notes *do* provide an ongoing description of the care of the client.

To follow along with the time sequence of events, the first entry in the progress notes will be a report of the findings of the complete admission examination of the client, usually performed by the attending physician. In care facilities that are also teaching institutions, it is highly likely that there will be two or more complete admission examinations, each of which is recorded by the person conducting the review. The basic elements of the physician's admitting notes are as follows:[2]

Source and reliability of
information (optional)
Present illness and chief
complaints
History: physical, social,
emotional, and family health
Review of systems: a
systematic listing of
symptoms, past and present
Physical examination
Initial laboratory data:
comments on the reported
values of admission
diagnostic tests

Preliminary prognosis:
including the severity of
illness and the expected
results of treatment
Plan of study: the manner in
which the diagnosis is to be
established (radiologic
examinations, laboratory
studies, etc.)
Plan of management: the
manner in which the client is
to be treated (including the
overall plans for nutritional
care)

Following these pages in the progress notes, the practitioner will usually find a multitude of remarks recorded by a variety of professionals, including core members of the health care team and consultants. The great bulk of these notes will be written by two groups of persons: nurses and physicians. As the nursing staff is usually the group most intimately involved with the direct care of the client, nursing progress notes will be of vital importance in the temporal evaluation of client progress. The physicians, of course, monitor progress as well, but from a different orientation than that of the nursing staff.

In many clinical practice settings, clinical dietitians use the progress notes section to record the ongoing relationship of the client and his nutritional care plan. In some settings, special forms are used for the recording of such information; these will be discussed in the next major section of this chapter. The notes recorded by the clinical dietitian should be clearly labeled, concisely written, and signed appropriately, using the initials R.D. (Registered Dietitian) when applicable. For a partial listing of the common abbreviations found in this and other sections of the medical record, see Appendix A.

Consents

Since "informed consent" is a major issue in health care today, the practitioner may expect to find a section of the medical record devoted to "consents." This section includes the forms for consent of the client for a variety of procedures, including surgical operations, certain types of radiologic treatments, and the like. This section will also include all forms signed by the client permitting his inclusion in any type of experimental procedure.

Consultations

Primary care providers frequently have need to request assistance in a particular aspect of client care. Such assistance, referred to as "consultation," is an everyday event that serves the purpose of enhancing care by providing expert attention. Any health professional may serve in the role of consultant, including the clinical dietitian.

A request for consultation is frequently recorded on a special sheet, which states the nature of the problem and any other pertinent information that may assist the consultant. The consultant's report back to the initiator of the request may appear on the original request-for-consultation sheet, on another sheet, or in the progress notes.

Laboratory Reports

A significant part of the objective data collected in the assessment phase will consist of the results of procedures, which may be used initially to establish a diagnosis and then employed to monitor progress. Laboratory results may also be used as screening procedures for apparently healthy individuals enrolled in a health maintenance program.

The clinical dietitian has two opportunities to use this section of the medical record. The first, of course, is in the assessment stage, when the practitioner is collecting the data necessary for the development of treatment and/or counseling plans, and again in the evaluation phase when he is measuring the value of intervention. The second, less obvious to many clinicians, is in the activity of screening. Very often when he is reviewing the record of a client new to the health care facility, the clinical dietitian may examine the results of laboratory tests and find values reported that are incompatible with adequate nutritional health. He may find, for example, hemoglobin values that are lower than the accepted norms, or elevated blood levels of glucose. In such an event, it is the responsibility of the clinician to intervene on behalf of the client if plans are not already underway for the provision of corrective measures, especially in the area of nutritional care. The primary care provider should be notified of the clinical dietitian's observations, and together they may take further action on behalf of the client.

The *general* types of laboratory and other diagnostic procedures employed in modern health care facilities are shown in Table 4.1.[2,6] The word "general" is emphasized, as such procedures may not be all-inclusive for every type of institution. The results of diagnostic proce-

TABLE 4.1   General Classes of Laboratory Tests and Other Diagnostic Procedures

---

Laboratory Tests (classified according to biologic specimen):

Blood, serum, or plasma determinations: e.g., ascorbic acid, blood volume, calcium, serum enzymes, pH, total protein, urea nitrogen, lipoprotein profiles

Urine tests: e.g., acetone and acetoacetate, creatinine, lead, glucose, pH, osmolarity

Special endocrinology tests (primarily using serum or plasma): e.g., calcitonin, insulin, thyroid-stimulating hormone (TSH)

Hematologic determinations: e.g., coagulation factors, hematocrit, hemoglobin, folic acid, vitamin B_{12}

Cerebrospinal fluid tests: e.g., pressure, glucose, protein

Miscellaneous determinations: e.g., fecal fat or nitrogen; microbiologic cultures of blood, urine, or other body fluids; renal or liver function tests; analyses of gastric and duodenal contents

Other Diagnostic Procedures:

Cytology and pathology tests: e.g., biopsy reports of specialized tissue (as liver), cytologic examinations

Endoscopic studies: e.g., sigmoidoscopy

Electrographic studies: e.g., electrocardiogram (EKG), electroencephalogram (EEG)

Roentgenographic and isotopic studies: e.g., chest films, gastrointestinal series, radioactive iodine uptake

Anthropometric measures: e.g., estimations of body fat and weight of lean body mass

---

dures may not be found in this section of the medical record; often they are placed with the progress notes or inserted in a section called "other reports." The ranges of "normal" values of the common laboratory tests are often printed on the forms used for reporting test results.

It is an enormous and questionably profitable task to list in these pages all of the laboratory determinations that are pertinent to the practice of clinical dietetics. The values of interest to the practitioner are dependent on the nature of the client's needs, both in health and in illness. Those practitioners interested in laboratory diagnoses in disease states are referred to other sources.[6-8]* In the interests of the

---

* The degree to which laboratory test results are employed by a dietetic learner is dependent on where the learner is in his sequential educational program. That is, beginning students are encouraged (and advised!) to think in terms of primary prevention, and not in terms of morbidity.

healthy client, and for intervention purposes, the clinician should pay particular heed to reported values for determinations involving nutrients.[8] In general, the values of interest include those shown in Table 4.2.

Many of the nutrients listed in Table 4.2 are routinely assessed in health care settings. Others, such as the fat-soluble vitamins and most of the water-soluble vitamins, are not ordinarily measured. Some of the nutrients are measured directly and reported quantitatively (as mg ascorbic acid/dl serum or mEq sodium/l serum). Others may be measured indirectly and then reported in units of enzyme activity (as thiamin, riboflavin, or B_6). Still other nutrients may be evaluated by the use of "load" tests and the results reported in quantitative units of intermediates or endproducts of specific metabolic pathways (as folic acid or B_6). There is usually more than one evaluative method available for nutrient assessment in biologic specimens; the method chosen for analysis will depend on the degree of accuracy required and the availability of laboratory equipment and trained personnel.[10,11] Guidelines for evaluation of nutrient concentration in biologic fluids are given in Appendix B.

A relatively simple pragmatic indicator of obesity may be calculated from the measurement of triceps skinfold thickness with a skinfold caliper.[12] A guide to determining obesity from such skinfold measurements is given in Appendix C. A method for approximating ideal body weight is shown in Appendix D.

Earlier in this section, the phrase "normal" value was used. The quotation marks were deliberately placed around the word normal to indicate that some degree of variation is expected for any individual in a given population. That is, *there is no such thing as "normal,"* only a range of values into which a specific determination made at a given

---

TABLE 4.2 Listing of Nutrient Assessments

Blood-forming nutrients:
  Iron, folic acid, vitamins B_6 and B_{12} (as an adjunct to iron, hemoglobin, and hematocrit values)
Vitamins:
  Water-soluble: thiamin, riboflavin, niacin, and ascorbic acid
  Fat-soluble: A, D, E, and K
Minerals:
  Sodium, potassium, calcium, phosphorus, iron, iodine, and other trace elements
Serum protein and serum albumin

---

point in time may be expected to fall. When evaluating laboratory determinations, it is pertinent to consider that:

> . . . *normal ranges have been obtained for measurements made on large groups of apparently healthy people using the statistical approach which equates the normal range to two standard deviations above and below the mean. By definition five per cent of the population will be outside these limits. . . .*[13] *(p. 80)*

It is the accepted practice, therefore, to consider that reported values falling above or below the "normal" range represent the probability of "at-risk" (vulnerable) situations.

There is considerably less stock placed in the reported values of nutrient determinations for the simple reason that the ranges are too great, a result of the smaller number of determinations made on healthy individuals. In both types of laboratory determinations (standard biologic tests and nutrient analyses), there are any number of factors that influence the outcome. How the samples are collected, stored, and transported; the method of analysis; and the experience of the laboratory personnel, all cause variations in results. Another variable, often overlooked, is the individual himself. Individual variations can be attributed to such diverse events as pregnancy, the time and content of the individual's last meal, and the time of day the sample is collected.[13-15]

Medication Records

Often at the back of the medical record, may be found the forms used to list the medications administered to the client. In addition to the name of the drug, the list will show the dose, frequency, and route of administration. The medication list includes those drugs administered over time, drugs given as needed, and single-order medications.

In this section, the clinical dietitian should be alert to four general classes of drugs and their relationship to nutrition:

1. Medications that are sources of nutrients (e.g., multivitamin preparations, IV solutions)

2. Drugs that in some way interfere with nutrient metabolism (e.g., isoniazid, a therapy used in the treatment of tuberculosis, acts as a B_6 antagonist)

3. Drugs whose effectiveness is in some way altered by the ingestion of certain nutrients (e.g., tetracycline absorption is diminished when ingested with calcium-containing foods)

4. Medications that have an effect on taste sensation or appetite (e.g., potassium chloride liquids, used in electrolyte replacement therapy, may cause nausea and/or depressed appetite)[16]

Operating Room Records

In most health care facilities, the last section of the SOR will contain the records of surgical procedures, if any were performed. The operating room record will show, among other things, the type of anesthesia administered and the name of the surgical procedure. This information is useful to the practitioner making plans for the initiation of oral feedings to the client in the immediate postoperative period.

The SOR in Summary

The source-oriented record will usually contain nine or ten sections, each of which contains specific kinds of information relevant to the nutritional care of the client. These sections may occur in the following order:

The problem list	Consents
Patient identification information	Consultations
	Laboratory reports
Physicians' orders	Medication records
Graphic sheets	Operating room records
Progress notes	

Enelow and Swisher[3] have commented that the most serious criticism of the SOR is of its rather arbitrary separation of the chronology of a disease process from the current physical and laboratory findings. Taken together, past and present events and findings form the basis of clinical diagnosis; the format of the SOR tends to confuse readers by the separation process.

OTHER DOCUMENTS OF IMPORTANCE

A great many other documents or record forms are used in health care settings. The exact nature and quantity of such records is dependent, of course, on the institution and its purposes. Some of these documents will be maintained and preserved along with the basic elements of the traditional medical record, while others are used only on a temporary basis and then discarded when the original purpose no longer exists.

Records maintained for the nutritional care of clients vary greatly. In most settings, however, clinicians will use a version of a *diet cardex card*. On this card is listed basic information about the client, often obtainable from the face sheet of the medical record. In addition, the card will show the specifics of the nutritional care plan and will include a section for recording notes about the client's progress with the plan. Unless the clinician is in solo practice, it is probable that a number of practitioners will interact with the client; some communication device, such as a diet cardex card, must be available for use by all those working with a particular client. Such a card may be preserved for future use (in the event of reentry to the setting), or all or some of the information entered and preserved in computerized data banks. If a computerized data bank is available and utilized, the practitioner may have individual printout sheets for each client instead of a card. Whatever the format, the information and its implication for care are the same.

Actions taken on behalf of the client will usually be based on the orders of the primary care provider and often recorded on a form called "Diet Orders." *Diet order records* will indicate the type of nutritional care desired, the effective date and time of the order, and so on.

Other records of importance to the clinical dietitian include the forms used to document nutrient intakes of selected clients. In certain types of stress situations, both psychologic and biologic, it is of prime importance to know just what the client is actually ingesting every day. In general, *nutrient intake records* include summary calculations for kilocalories, and carbohydrate, protein, and fat (all in grams). Other nutrients may be included in such intake records (e.g., sodium, potassium, ascorbic acid), depending on the nature of the client's needs. Such calculations are made by determining the exact quantity of the food ingested by the client and then calculating the nutrient content of that intake. This may be done by one of two ways: entering the consumption data into a computer terminal programmed to do nutrient analyses, or using handbooks of food composition. The latter method, still the most widely used in this country, is by far the more time-consuming and error-filled way of computing intake totals.

Another document of importance, the *diet history*, will be discussed in a subsequent chapter. Occasionally the diet history will be contained in the medical record; the history or its lucid summary should be placed there with greater frequency because of its significance in terms of both past events and planning for the future.

The nursing staff more likely than not will keep many detailed records of clients' care. Many of these records will contain information useful to the clinical dietitian, especially the nursing history, which may include such details as the client's physical and emotional needs, and her response to care.

Finally, one of the most important records to the clinical dietitian is that which is sent to another health care organization on behalf of the client. In the event that she no longer needs the type or intensity of care she is currently receiving, a client may often be referred to a second health service for continuation of care on a different level. The role of the practitioner in assisting the client in making her nutritional needs known to the personnel of the new agency is an important one. The clinical dietitian, therefore, has a responsibility for participating in the preparation of the *referral*. Most referral forms call for two kinds of information: statements about the client's physical ability to feed himself, and specifics about the nutritional care plan. An exchange of information between professionals in the same or different health disciplines is the one way in which some degree of continuity of care is achieved.[17]

THE PROBLEM-ORIENTED MEDICAL RECORD*

The health professional considered by most to be the originator of the POR system is a physician, Dr. Lawrence Weed. In 1970, in the preface of his text, Weed wrote:

> *There is in existence at the present time no body of literature on how to structure the medical record, particularly progress notes on long-term problems, and so there is no framework within which discipline can develop.*[18] *(p. 6)*

Since the time of publication of Weed's work, the POR system has been gaining in its acceptance in a variety of health care settings. According to Caserta,[19] some advantages of the system include allowing the practitioner to plan client care in a logical manner, and providing a disciplined framework that allows an infinite variety of care situations to be created.

In contrast to the SOR, the basic premise of organization of the POR is that all information must be associated with the client's health problem to which it relates, regardless of the source of that information.[20] Thus, the distinctive feature of the POR is that it is problem

* The terms, problem-oriented medical record and problem-oriented record, are used interchangeably to designate the same system. Preference is given to POR in these pages.

structured; the information contained in the POR is organized according to a series of problems, which are identified through the process of data collection. The progress notes are chronologically recorded as in the SOR, but as new data are recorded for each problem, the persons obtaining the information (e.g., the clinical dietitian) record their data according to the number and title of that problem.

There are four basic elements to the POR system:[18]

1. The defined data base
2. The complete problem list
3. The initial plans
4. The progress notes

An examination of these sections follows.

The Data Base

The data base ordinarily incorporates the information found in the admission notes of the SOR. In most health care settings using the POR, the data base will contain the following information:[20]

Patient profile—a description of the client, including relevant social, family, and environmental data

Present illness (PI) and chief complaints (CC)

Past medical history (PH) and family (medical) history (FH)

Review of systems (ROS)

Physical examination (PE)

Reports of laboratory work

Reports of other initial diagnostic procedures

In some settings, the data base will also contain nursing assessments.[21] According to Yarnall and Atwood,[22] the defined data base should contain the routine, explicitly defined information that pertains to a particular client in a specific setting.

The Complete Problem List

In this context, a problem denotes ". . . some aspect of the patient's health or environment that produces, or threatens to produce, functional disability, morbidity, or increased rate of mortality"[22] (p. 219). Therefore, the complete problem list is a carefully constructed list of all of the client's problems, which have been identified through the compilation of the defined data base.[23] The problems may be diagnostic, therapeutic, or educational in nature.

Each problem is identified by name and number, with new problems added as they become known. Past and present problems, active or inactive, are recorded in this section. In the event of resolution, the problem is so marked on the list with the date of resolution. Even though the list is developed after the data base is defined, this section of the POR appears as the first page.

The Initial Plans

The initial plans are the overall planning strategies and evaluations of the client's problems. Each area of concern on the problem list is examined in light of the others appearing on the list, and then a plan is developed for each one.[22] Each plan is titled and numbered to coincide with the problem with which it deals.

There is a general scheme for developing every plan according to the needs of the client. Thus, each problem plan is divided into three sections:[18]

1. Diagnostic
2. Therapeutic
3. Client education

The diagnostic section is designed to increase the data base where needed; that is, to provide for further information when the defined data base is insufficient. The therapeutic portion indicates management procedures to be used in treating the problem, including the overall plan for nutritional care. The last section is usually a brief statement indicating the involvement of the client in the plan of management and to ensure, when possible, that he is an active participant in the care process.

As the data base and problem list change, so will the ensuing plans. If there is no plan for a particular problem, the reasons are usually given in this section. In essence, the third section of the POR should specifically outline those actions related to diagnostic studies, therapy procedures, and client activity and education.

The Progress Notes

As in the SOR, the progress notes section of the POR is organized chronologically, and is the place in the medical record where various health team members and consultants record their observations and plans for client-centered care. In the POR, however, the progress notes serve a variety of functions that incorporate many sections of the SOR.

There are three major elements to the progress notes section:

1. Narrative notes
2. Flowsheets
3. Discharge summary

Narrative notes. The narrative notes are written in a unique fashion, in that they follow the acronym SOAP (**S**ubjective, **O**bjective, **A**ssessment, and **P**lan). In this manner, each narrative note is written according to a defined format, regardless of the orientation of the note's author. The elements of the narrative progress notes are as follows:[20]

Subjective data: describe the client's perception of the problem and outline his expression of his symptoms, changes experienced, or thoughts related to the outcome of the problem. Food intake and subjective expressions made by the family or significant others are recorded here

Objective data: contains verifiable information such as laboratory test results, physical findings, or clinical evaluations by the health professional

Assessment: devoted to an analysis of the problem based on the recorded subjective and objective data

Plan: contains the formulation for diagnostic and therapeutic procedures, and plans for client education relating to the specific problem. When the plan represents a change in a strategy listed in the initial plans section, a note to this effect is made

Each narrative note is related directly to the problem recorded on the problem list, and is titled and numbered accordingly. Often operative notes are included in this section. In the pages to follow, a case study demonstrating the use of SOAP notes in an ambulatory health care setting will show more clearly the uniqueness of this section of the POR.

Flowsheets. The second element of the progress notes is the "flowsheets." These are records of all continuing measurements (or parameters), which are kept over time as part of the follow-up activities once an initial plan is established. Parameters that may be recorded on flowsheets include the cardinal signs (temperature, pulse, and respiration); records of medications administered; reports of laboratory tests; and the client's daily consumption of selected nutrients. Since flowsheets are considered to be the "dynamic center" of the POR, it is essential that they be maintained consistently so long as the problem under treatment exists.[4,18] In this manner, the interaction between the recorded data and therapy plan can be reviewed.

Discharge summary   The discharge summary is the final section of the progress notes. In this summary, there should be a complete retrospective note on each numbered problem on the problem list.[18] Each note is written according to the SOAP format, and outlines the level of resolution of each problem.

The POR in Summary

Proponents of the POR format write vigorously about the advantages of the system. The POR is viewed by one user as ". . . . providing a means whereby the medical record will better reflect the health problems of patients and the professional responses to them on the part of physicians, nurses, and other major participants in care"[24] (p. 8). The key phrase in the quotation above is "professional responses," as the POR is almost unanimously seen as facilitating the work of health *teams* by promoting trust between practitioners and reducing confusion about plans.[25] In addition, the format of the SOAP notes is designed in such a manner that documentation of the process of clinical judgment is inevitable.[26]

For purposes of review, the four basic elements of the POR and their major sections are outlined below:

1. The data base:
   Patient profile
   PI, CC
   PH, FH
   ROS
   PE
   Laboratory reports
   Other initial Dx procedures

2. The complete problem list

3. The initial plans:
   Dx
   Rx
   Client education

4. The progress notes
   Narrative notes (SOAP format)
   Flowsheets
   Discharge summary

A CASE STUDY

Clinical dietitians are one group of health professionals who are expected to participate in the diagnostic, therapeutic, and client education functions delineated by the POR. By recording in the progress notes, practitioners have the opportunity not only to participate more fully in client-centered care, but may demonstrate their particular skill and abilities to others.[27,28] The following case study serves to illustrate not only some of the processes of the problem-oriented medical record, but focuses attention on the responsibilities of clinical dietitians in diagnosis, treatment, and client education.

Case Study: SOAP in Action

Mrs. S. R. is a 19-year-old Caucasian woman who first visited the obstetric ambulatory clinic at the Medical Center on May 5th. On that date, her EDC was calculated to be about December 13th.*

The client's initial physical examination and interview revealed the following information, recorded in the data base of her POR:

Mrs. S. R. is a primigravida, and presents with a gestational age of 8 weeks. Client denies any history of hypertension, heart murmurs, Diabetes Mellitus, or other major medical problems. Menarche occurred at age 11. Prior to this pregnancy, client took birth-control pills for 3 years. Presently she smokes a half-package of filtered cigarettes daily. She is 5 feet, 7 inches tall and weighs 115 lb. Present lab data include hematocrit of 30% and hemoglobin of 10.3 gm/dl; all other values are within normal limits. The client's major concern on this visit is relief for daily nausea and vomiting, and occasional headaches.

PROBLEM LIST

Date	Problem	Resolved
5/5	#1 Pregnancy	
5/5	#2 Nausea and vomiting	

* Refer to Appendix A for record abbreviation meanings.

According to clinic procedure, Mrs. S. R. is referred to the clinical dietitian, Ms. Dawson. Following the visit, Ms. Dawson decides which problem is appropriate for her remarks, and records the pertinent information about this interview in the progress notes.

PROGRESS NOTES

5/5 Problem #2: Nausea and vomiting

S: *Mrs. S. R. states that she had had nausea and vomiting for at least 5 weeks. Last week the problem became worse, so she resigned her job. During this time, Mrs. S. R. relates that she has not been eating much and thinks she has lost 2 or 3 lb. She has not taken vitamins. One day's diet recall indicates that Mrs. S. R. skips breakfast, eats lunch at 11 AM, prepares supper at 5:30 PM, and snacks on pretzels and coke in the evening. She drinks 1 cup of milk per day and omits fruit altogether.*

O: *Eighth week of pregnancy; body weight = 115 lb (ideal = 135 lb); hematocrit—30%; hemoglobin—10.5 gm/dl.*

A: *Client's weight is less than the calculated ideal body weight for a nonpregnant adult female. Mrs. S. R. has reduced food intake because of nausea and vomiting. This could precipitate nutritional anemia in light of her borderline hemoglobin value and decreased weight. Protein, kilocaloric, and calcium intake must be increased to meet the fetal requirements.*

P: *Dx: Will check with the nurse-midwife (CNM) to recommend iron and folic acid supplements. Weight gain must be monitored at each visit.*

   Rx: Showed Mrs. S. R. how to incorporate more milk, and breads and cereals in her diet. Stressed the value of protein for the developing fetus. Suggested consuming toast with jelly in the morning, drinking liquids between meals, and avoiding the use of fat for cooking to overcome the nausea difficulty. Gave client pamphlet of Nutritional Guidelines for Pregnancy.

Client Education: Requested client to bring a 2-day food record when she returns in 2 months.

R. Dawson, R.D.

Mrs. S. R. came for her second visit to the clinic on July 5th. Physical examination is satisfactory. Gestational age is now 17 weeks. Weight is 119 lb. Blood chemistries show that hematocrit is 29% and hemoglobin is 9.3 gm/dl. Client told CNM that she has been taking her iron and folate supplements daily. Nausea and vomitng have subsided. Chief complaints now are tiredness and constipation. The CNM recommended a stool softener for the latter problem.

A quick review of Mrs. S. R.'s medical record provides the clinical dietitian with a basis to guide her interview. Ms. Dawson notes the new problem and writes her comments as follows:

PROBLEM LIST

Date	Problem	Resolved
5/5	#1 Pregnancy	
5/5	#2 Nausea and vomiting	7/5
7/5	#3 Constipation	

PROGRESS NOTES

7/5 Problem #3: Constipation

   S: *"I have been trying to drink more milk, but can only stand 2 cups per day. Something is keeping me from having bowel movements, and I'm afraid it is the milk. Besides, I'm so tired I can't seem to even move." Mrs. S. R. brought a very brief 2-day food record. Three small meals with a few between-meal snacks of cookies and Koolaid are the general pattern. During these 2 days, the client ate no fresh fruits or vegetables, and only one serving of canned pears and one of cooked green beans.*

   O: *Pregnant—seventeenth week; body weight = 119 lb.*

   A: *Weight gain = 4 lb. Still below recommended body weight. Mrs. S. R. is not eating enough of the proper kinds of foods, as evidenced by her small weight gain in 2 months and her persistent constipation. The constipation could be caused by a decrease in exercise or more probably a lack of roughage in her diet.*

   P: *Dx: Will check with the CNM about increasing exercise.*

   Rx: Encouraged the substitution of fresh fruit for snacks as a way of providing necessary nutrients and promoting elimination. In addition to the 2 cups of milk, suggested that she drink at least an additional quart of liquid for better elimination.

   Client Education: Client will state alternative methods of incorporating additional fluids into daily intake.

R. Dawson, R.D.

The clinical dietitian decided after this interview that another distinct problem had arisen. Accordingly, she entered "7/5 Problem #4,

low hemoglobin and hematocrit values" on the problem list and recorded the following narrative in the progress notes:

PROGRESS NOTES

7/5 Problem #4: Low hemoglobin and hematocrit values

S: *"I don't eat that much meat. Liver? Can't stand the smell or
taste of that stuff." Client also remarked that she might like
food stamps because all her neighbors use them. Mrs. S. R.'s
food record indicated that her daily sources of high biologic
value protein are 2 cups of whole milk and about 2 ounces
of meat. No leafy greens, egg yolk, or legumes are included.*

O: *Lab values of hematocrit—29% and hemoglobin—9.3 gm/dl.*

A: *Lab values show that the client's hemoglobin in 2 months
has dropped from 10.3 to 9.3 gm/dl; hematocrit has also fallen
from 30% to 29%. Mrs. S. R. has limited sources of ingested
iron. Perhaps the prescribed ferrous sulfate, with its consti-
pating effect and bad taste, has been frequently omitted. The
client also exhibits poor calcium and protein consumption.*

P: Dx: *Will contact CNM about change in iron supplement
and consult with community health nurse about a
home visit.*

Rx: *Reviewed with client important nutritional principles
in pregnancy by using the models of a developing fetus,
along with the printed food guidelines. Suggested the
use of dried peas and beans, and enriched breads for
increasing dietary iron; encouraged greater calcium
and protein consumption by eating cheese, custards,
puddings, or ice cream. Gave Mrs. S. R. phone number
of county social service office to determine if she is
eligible for food stamps.*

Client Education: *Client will state alternative methods of
incorporating two additional calcium-rich foods into
daily food intake, e.g., cottage cheese, milk puddings,
yogurt.*

R. Dawson, R.D.

*On Tuesday, August 3rd, Mrs. S. R. returned to the clinic for
another physical examination and follow-up hematology tests. The
CNM reports that the client is progressing normally at a gestational
age of 21 weeks. No edema present; weight is 123.5 lb. Laboratory
chemistries show an iron-binding capacity of 350μ/dl, hematocrit
of 30.2%, and hemoglobin of 9.8 gm/dl. Mrs. S. R. stated that her*

new pills taste much better than the old ones. Her only complaint now is of low back pain after a day of work about the house.

The clinical dietitian, encouraged by the laboratory report, was anxious to see Mrs. S. R. Her progress note follows:

PROGRESS NOTES

8/3 Problem #4: Low hemoglobin and hematocrit values

S: *Mrs. S. R. states that the new iron pills taste like candy, and occasionally she has taken two a day. Client relates that meat still does not hold much appeal, but that she did like pork and beans 1 night a week. Client reported that she has been determined eligible for food stamps.*

O: *Body weight—123.5 lb; hematocrit—30.2%; hemoglobin— 9.8 gm/dl; iron-binding capacity—350μ/dl.*

A: *Hematocrit has increased 1.2% and hemoglobin 0.5 gm/dl in 4 weeks. At a gestational age of 21 weeks, Mrs. S. R. has gained a total of 8.5 lb. The iron supplement is helping to overcome the lack of dietary iron.*

P: *Dx: none.*

   Rx: Again reviewed the importance of protein and calcium. Told Mrs. S. R. to take only one iron supplement daily. Will recommend community health nurse make a visit to assist client to use food stamps.

   Client Education: Asked Mrs. S. R. to keep another food record for the 2 days prior to her next visit.

   R. Dawson, R.D.

CITED REFERENCES

1. Robinson, C. H. Nutrition education—what comes next? *J. Am. Dietet. A.* 69:126, 1976.
2. Morgan, W. L., and Engel, G. L. *The Clinical Approach to the Patient.* Philadelphia: W. B. Saunders Co., 1969.
3. Enelow, A. J., and Swisher, S. N. *Interviewing and Patient Care.* 2nd Ed. New York: Oxford Univ. Press, 1979.
4. Fletcher, R. H. Auditing problem-oriented records and traditional records. *N. Eng. J. Med.* 290:829, 1974.
5. Rakel, R. E. The problem-oriented medical record (POMR). *Am. Fam. Phys.* 10:3:100, 1974.
6. Normal reference laboratory values. *N. Eng. J. Med.* 302:37, 1980.

7. Thiele, V. F. *Clinical Nutrition*. 2nd Ed. St. Louis: C. V. Mosby Co., 1980.

8. Bennion, M. *Clinical Nutrition*. New York: Harper & Row, Publ., 1979.

9. Christakis, G., Ed. Nutritional assessment in health programs. *Am. J. Publ. Health* 63:Nov. 1973 Suppl:1, 1973.

10. Sauberlich, H. E., Dowdy, R. P., and Skala, J. H. *Laboratory Tests for the Assessment of Nutritional Status*. Cleveland: CRC Press, Inc., 1974.

11. Harvey, A. Mc., Johns, R. J., Owens, A. H., and Ross, R. D., Eds. *The Principles and Practice of Medicine*. 19th Ed. New York: Appleton-Century-Crofts, 1976.

12. Seltzer, C. C., and Mayer, J. A simple criterion of obesity. *Postgrad. Med.* 38:A101, 1965.

13. Thurnhan, D. I. The range and variability of biochemical indices: What is 'normal'? *Nutr.* 29:79, 1975.

14. Ganong, W. F. *Review of Medical Physiology*. 9th Ed., Los Altos, Calif.: Lange Medical Publications, 1979.

15. Zilva, J. F., and Pannall, P. R. *Clinical Chemistry in Diagnosis and Treatment*. 2nd Ed. Chicago: Year Book Medical Publishers, Inc., 1975.

16. Hartshorn, E. A. Food and drug interactions. *J. Am. Dietet. A.* 70:15, 1977.

17. Baumgarten, S., and Collins, M. E. The dietitian in continuing care. *J. Am. Dietet. A.* 67:576, 1975.

18. Weed, L. L. *Medical Records, Medical Education, and Patient Care*. Cleveland: The Press of Case Western Reserve Univ., 1970.

19. Caserta, J. E. A problem-oriented and patient-oriented record system. *In Problem-Oriented Systems of Patient Care*. Publ. No. 21-1522. Department of Home Health Agencies and Community Health Services, National League for Nursing. New York: Nat'l. Leag. Nurs., 1974.

20. Weed, L. The problem-oriented record—its organizing principles and its structure. *In* Visiting Nurse Association, Inc., Burlington, Vt. *The Problem-Oriented System in a Home Health Agency—A Training Manual*. National League for Nursing Publ. No. 21-1554, League Exchange No. 103. New York: Nat'l. Leag. Nurs., 1975.

21. *The Problem-Oriented System—A Multidisciplinary Approach*. Publ. No. 20-1546. Department of Hospital and Related Institutional Nursing Services, National League for Nursing. New York: Nat'l. Leag. Nurs., 1974.

22. Yarnall, S. R., and Atwood, J. Problem-oriented practice for nurses and physicians. General concepts. *In* Atwood, J., and Yarnall, S. R., Eds. Symposium on the problem-oriented record. *Nurs. Clin. N. Am.* 9:215, 1974.

23. Woody, M., and Mallison, M. The problem-oriented system for patient-centered care. *Am. J. Nurs.* 73:1168, 1973.

24. Goldfinger, S. E., and Dineen, J. H. Problem-oriented medical record. *In* Wintrobe, M. H., Thurn, G. W., Adams, R. D., Braunwald, E., Isselbacher, K. S., and Petersdorf, R. D., Eds., *Harrison's Principles of Internal Medicine*. 7th Ed. New York: McGraw-Hill Book Co., 1974.

25. Atwood, J., Mitchell, P. H., and Yarnall, S. R. The POR: A system for communication. *In* Atwood, J., and Yarnall, S. R., Eds. Symposium on the problem-oriented record. *Nurs. Clin. N. Am.* 9:229, 1974.

26. Fowler, D. R., and Longabaugh, R. The problem-oriented record. Problem definition. *Arch. Gen. Psych.* 32:831, 1975.

27. Voytovich, A. E. The dietitian/nutritionist and the problem-oriented medical record. I. A physician's viewpoint. *J. Am. Dietet. A.* 63:639, 1973.

28. Walters, F. M., and DeMarco, M. The dietitian/nutritionist and the problem-oriented medical record. II. The role of the dietitian. *J. Am. Dietet. A.* 63:641, 1973.

SUGGESTED REFERENCES

AMA Department of Drugs Staff. *AMA Drug Evaluations.* 3rd Ed. Chicago: American Medical Association, 1977.

Berni, R., and Readey, H. *Problem-Oriented Medical Record Implementation: Allied Health Peer Review.* 2nd Ed. St. Louis: C. V. Mosby Co., 1978.

Davidsohn, I., and Henry, J. B., Eds. *Todd-Sanford Clinical Diagnosis by Laboratory Methods.* 15th Ed. Philadelphia: W. B. Saunders Co., 1974.

Dorland's Illustrated Medical Dictionary. 25th Ed. Philadelphia: W. B. Saunders Co., 1974.

Faulkner, W. R., King, J. W., and Damm, H. C., Eds. *CRC Handbook of Clinical Laboratory Data.* 2nd Ed. Cleveland: The Chemical Rubber Co., 1968.

Faulkner, W. R., and King, J. W., Eds. *CRC Manual of Clinical Laboratory Procedures.* 2nd Ed. Cleveland: The Chemical Rubber Co., 1970.

Garb, S. *Laboratory Tests in Common Use.* 6th Ed. New York: Springer Publ. Co., 1976.

Goldberg, L., Benoit, C., Docker, C., Hoagberg, E., and Wesselman, J. *The Problem/Need-Oriented Approach to Planning and Evaluating Patient Care.* Minneapolis: Medallion Comm., Inc., 1978.

Goldfinger, S. E. The problem-oriented record. A critique from a believer. *N. Eng. J. Med.* 288:606, 1973.

Goodman, L. S., and Gilman, A., Eds. *The Pharmacological Basis of Therapeutics.* 5th Ed. New York: MacMillan Co., 1975.

Govoni, L. E., and Hayes, J. E. *Drugs and Nursing Implications.* 3rd Ed. New York: Appleton-Century-Crofts, 1978.

Hurst, J. W., and Walker, H. K., Eds. *The Problem-Oriented System.* New York: Medcom Press, 1972.

Joint Committee of the American Hospital Association and the American Dietetic Association. *Recording Nutritional Information in Medical Records.* Chicago: Am. Hosp. Assoc., 1976.

March, D. C. *Handbook: Interactions of Selected Drugs with Nutritional Status in Man*. Chicago: The American Dietetic Association, 1976.

McLeroy, S. L., and Klover, R. V. Implementing Problem-Oriented Medical Records (POMR) in an out-patient clinic. *J. Am. Dietet. A.* 72:522, 1978.

Mitchell, P. H., and Atwood, J. Problem-oriented recording as a teaching-learning tool. *Nurs. Res.* 24:99, 1975.

Moore, A. O., and Powers, D. E. *Food-Medication Interactions*. Tempe, AZ: Powers and Moore, 1978.

Physicians' Desk Reference. 35th Ed. Oradell, N.J.: Medical Economics Co., 1981.

Roe, D. A. *Drug-Induced Nutritional Deficiencies*. Westport, CN.: Avi Publ. Co., 1976.

Steen, E. B. *Medical Abbreviations*. 3rd Ed. Philadelphia: F. A. Davis Co., 1971.

The Medical Letter on Drugs and Therapeutics. New Rochelle, N.Y.: The Medical Letter, Inc. Published bi-weekly.

Thomas, A. E., McKay, D. A., and Cutlip, M. B. A nomograph method for assessing body weight. *Am. J. Clin. Nutr.* 29:302, 1976.

Tilkian, S. M., Conover, M. B., and Tilkion, A. G. *Clinical Implications of Laboratory Tests*. 2nd Ed. St. Louis: The C. V. Mosby Co., 1979.

Wallach, J. *Interpretation of Diagnostic Tests. A Handbook Synopsis of Laboratory Medicine*. 3rd Ed. Boston: Little, Brown and Co., 1978.

Walter, J. B., Pardee, G. P., and Molbo, D. M., Eds. *Dynamics of Problem-Oriented Approaches: Patient Care and Documentation*. Philadelphia: J. B. Lippincott Co., 1976.

White, W. F. *Language of the Health Sciences: A Lexical Guide to Word Parts, Word Roots, and Their Meanings*. New York: John Wiley & Sons, Inc., 1977.

Widmann, F. K. *Goodale's Clinical Interpretation of Laboratory Tests*. 8th Ed. Philadelphia: F. A. Davis Co., 1979.

Young, C. G., and Berger, J. O. *Learning Medical Terminology Step by Step*. St. Louis: C. V. Mosby Co., 1979.

5
The Interview

The professional relationship . . . is recognized as essential to sound medical practice and the optimal well-being of the patient. Mutual trust and respect are basic characteristics of this relationship. The interview is the medium for the development of the professional relationship.

Lewis Bernstein and Rosalyn S. Bernstein,
**Interviewing: A Guide for Health
Professionals,** 3rd Ed. (New York:
Appleton-Century-Crofts, 1980).

The interview is a process by which clinical dietitians collect data that are relevant to assessment and frequently are unobtainable by any other means. It is an experience within which clients and practitioners develop a trusting, nonjudgmental relationship in order to collect data about behavior, past and present. The desired data are so often related to the client's feelings of self-worth that he may be able to share only what he thinks will be acceptable to the clinician.[2] The more data he feels able to reveal, the more reliable will be the decisions about his real needs. The goal of nutritional counseling, the facilitation of behavior change, is seldom achieved unless these assessment data are reliable. Even the more open clients may not communicate well. Thus, it is best to corroborate interview data with data from other sources.

THE PURPOSES OF THE INTERVIEW

The first, and most basic, purpose of the interview is for the clinical dietitian to establish a safe, trusting, and caring environment for the client. This environment should be one in which the client feels able to take risks, to be honest about himself, and to make decisions that affect him.[3] Such an atmosphere encourages the client to feel accepted as he is, and not judged as good or bad, right or wrong. Attitudes developed during the interview in regard to the client-clinician relationship set the tone for success or failure of counseling. Even with clients who view the practitioner as competent, and who are also highly motivated to care for their own health needs, there is still the preference on the part of clients that health professionals demonstrate human warmth and caring as well as competence.[4]

Relationships between client and counselor have been described as fitting one of four models.[5] The Engineering Model describes a relationship in which the counselor treats the client like a subject in a scientific experiment. The counselor makes the decisions about client care based on what he thinks will work, with neither consultation with the client on choices, nor acknowledgement of ethical considerations. In the Priestly Model, the counselor becomes the savior, doing what he deems best, making decisions heavily imbued with moral judgments. The third model, the Collegial Model, exemplifies the counselor and client as colleagues working together to achieve client goals. The clinician using this model tends to overestimate the expertise of the client in planning his own care. A more effective kind of participation in health care is the Contractual Model. This last model does not imply that the counselor and client are equivalent in skill, as does the Collegial Model, but recognizes the counselor as the expert and the client as the decisionmaker. As such, the latter must achieve as much independence as possible in his own health care. The client can select from alternatives, but probably does not have the knowledge to propose feasible solutions. For example, the physician counsels the client that he needs to follow a particular regimen. The client then may choose whether or not he will follow through, and if so, he will select the options most acceptable to him. The Contractual Model, or one similar to it, has been proposed by several theorists[5,6] and supported by practitioners.[7-9]

The importance of client independence is stressed even more emphatically by Dyer and Vriend as they believe that:

The client who leaves counseling and feels that the counselor deserves the credit, who feels the counselor has accomplished the seem-

ing miracle of producing the more effective life-handler that she or he has now become, has met a counselor lacking effectiveness in the most crucial dimension of all: psychological and physical dependency.[4] (p. 21)

The Contractual Model,[5] one of mutual participation,[6] addresses pragmatically the most effective form of health care. Certainly there are times when the client is unable to participate in his own care in a crisis situation, but the nonparticipatory approach tends to permeate all aspects of health care. Hence, noncompliance is often the result.[10] There are, of course, instances of coercive, judgmental environments in which some clients will condescend to adhere to a regimen. More often the result is noncompliance as contact with the supervisory health worker is reduced.[11]

A second purpose of the interview is to ascertain from the client a description of his food intake patterns and the bases for the patterns. Although some counselors believe that it isn't necessary to know why a person behaves as he does in order to change, there are many others who would disagree with that approach.[12] At the very least, some knowledge of the reasons certain behaviors are maintained is helpful, even though analysis of their early development may not be required. The interviewer will seek to discover the client's own *modus operandi* in meeting his socioemotional, intellectual, and physical needs as they relate to his food behaviors.[13]

THE PROCESS OF THE INTERVIEW

Preparing for the Interview

If the client is perceived as an unique individual, functioning in his own environment, the clinician needs to obtain basic information about that person and his environment.[1,14] This implies both current and historical information concerning his family, occupation, economic status, religion, culture, residence, education, physical condition and health status, and social and recreational preferences.

If the interview is to take place in an acute or chronic care facility, it should be arranged in advance for the client's convenience and in harmony with other professional plans.

The first step is to obtain a profile of the client so that preparation for interviewing may be personalized to the client's needs. If the client is in traction, he obviously will be unable to come to a counseling office.

The medical record, if available, is a good source for some of the profile information. Additional data may need to be obtained from the client and can be readily collected on a form designed for such a purpose (a sample is shown in Appendix J). If the client shows hesitancy in responding to a questionnaire, it is necessary to determine if there is a language barrier, illiteracy, or a physical disability problem. If so, alternate means of data gathering may be employed. This information regarding a client's language and physical capabilities (e.g., vision, hearing) should also influence the selection of learning objectives and strategies.

In scheduling the interview, several factors need to be considered. The location should be as conducive as possible to confidentiality, concentration, comfort, and caring (the four "Cs" of an interviewing environment). A client may be very reluctant to be open and honest about his behavior if he feels that others will overhear. Counseling should be confidential both during and following client contact. Distractions are also detrimental to effective interviewing. Television, telephone calls, visitors, note-taking, or visual distractions, such as activity in the halls and outside windows or book titles to peruse, can provide undesirable interference in the interviewing process. Physical comfort also contributes to the success of interviewing.[15] Levels of heat, light, and noise require attention. The softness and height of the chair or angle of the head section of the bed will contribute to the comfort level of the client.

The fourth characteristic of an effective environment is caring. This characteristic is exhibited in the nonverbal messages sent by the location of furniture and other cues. A large desk positioned between the client and counselor may be perceived as a "wall." Clinicians who sit in imposing chairs seem to convey the message to the client, "I'm more important than you." A clock facing the client or one with an alarm may say, "My time is more important than yours." A practitioner standing over an immobilized client may also send the message that the clinician is an authoritarian or in a hurry. Nonverbal behaviors may be easily misinterpreted. The clinician must take responsibility for being aware of these environmental factors, what they are intended to mean, and how they are received by the client.

In an ambulatory unit, HMO, or private practice setting, an appointment can be made by the client just as he makes his other health care appointments, or he may be referred by another professional who makes the appointment. The same four Cs of the interviewing environment are applicable. They need only to be translated.

The acquisition of profile data may be limited to a client questionnaire for a new client unless the setting has access to medical records of other primary care providers and care facilities.*

Interviewing Skills

To achieve the two major purposes of the interview (building a relationship and gathering significant data), there exists a need for a variety of interviewing skills and theoretical knowledge in the behavioral sciences. Although our understanding of human behavior is incomplete, there is a growing body of knowledge in interpersonal communications that can enhance the success of a clinical dietitian.

A number of interviewing skills have been developed and tested by communication and counseling experts.[16-18] To achieve the intended purposes of the interview, the clinical dietitian needs to learn these responses and substitute them for the familiar but relatively ineffective responses so indigenous to human communication.[8,19] Each skill is a way of demonstrating to the client that he has been heard and an earnest attempt is being made to understand his problems.

Verbal skills   The verbal skills include both listening and sharing responses. Listening responses, used to indicate to the client that she has been heard, include exploratory, clarification, and empathy responses. Sharing responses are meant to convey to the client either the counselor's thoughts and feelings, or general knowledge. The sharing responses are information giving, confrontation, and self-disclosure. Table 5.1 illustrates the relationships of the six basic responses and highlights their purpose.

The most commonly used and least helpful of the acceptable interpersonal communication responses are the general responses. The responses that focus on thoughts and behaviors are more useful in achieving effective communication. The most effective responses, however, are the responses that highlight feelings as they focus on the meaning of client experiences.

Listening responses.   Many of the listening responses can be categorized as active listening, meaning that the counselor/clinician demonstrates by his responses that he is actively involved in the dialogue. The *exploratory responses*, however, are passive. Common passive responses are: "I see", "Yes", "Um-huh", or "I understand". They are brief acknowledgments of a pause in the client's narrative, but they

* Written permission of the client may be required.

TABLE 5.1   Verbal Communication Skills of Clinicians

		Type of Response	
		Listening	Sharing
NATURE OF RESPONSE	General	Exploratory	Information Giving
	Thoughts/Behavior	Clarification	Confrontation
	Feelings	Empathy	Self-Disclosure

do not demonstrate any real understanding of content or its meaning. Other responses in this category include: "Please tell me a little more", "I'd like to hear more about that", or "Go on". Open-ended questions such as, "How did you feel when that happened?" or "Would you like to tell me about it" are also effective.[13] Because these passive responses permit the client to go in the direction of his own choosing and to share what he feels comfortable sharing at that point, they are often referred to in the literature as nondirective.

Occasionally, more direct questions and requests are necessary. Danish and co-workers[13] have referred to direct questions as closed-ended responses. These directive responses can be effective in gaining specific information if used judiciously. Early in the counseling sessions, however, before trust is established, they may be viewed as probing and thus serve as a roadblock to counseling. Exploratory responses (passive listening) can be useful, but if they are the only types used, there is frequently a sense of monotony as well as a perceived lack of clinician involvement.

In contrast to the passive exploratory responses, clarification and empathy are active listening responses. They overtly demonstrate the clinician's attempt to receive and understand the client's messages. Both clarification and empathy are also considered nondirective.

The active listening response, *clarification*, is directed to the thoughts and behaviors expressed by the client. To clarify is to restate or reflect the content. The response begins with leads such as, "you are . . . ," "you think . . . ," "you seem to be . . . ," "you have . . . ," and so on. A complete response is "You are planning to leave your job next week." Such a response demonstrates that the clinician has heard what was said as well as encourages the client to continue. It also allows the client to rephrase herself if she has not said what she really meant, as well as to correct the clinician if he didn't interpret the message properly.

Reflection is a mirror image of the client's words: restatement puts the client's thought into new words. The latter is probably more useful to the client and conveys better understanding of the content. Reflection can sound parrotlike, unless used very infrequently and interspersed with a variety of other responses. Clarification is a response that is used throughout the interview.

The two types of clarification, reflection and restatement, are illustrated in the following example of a client-clinician exchange:

Client: There seems to be no reason for me to adhere to this plan.

Dietitian: You don't see any reason to adhere to the plan. (*reflection*)
or
    You can't understand why the plan is important to you. (*restatement*)

Empathy is not an easily acquired active listening skill, but is of tremendous value when it finally becomes a part of the clinician's expertise. Empathic listening involves relating back to the client the feelings the clinician believes he has identified in the client's discussion of his problem. He does so by naming the feeling he perceives and the circumstances in which the feeling is elicited. As an example, in response to a client who says, "I just don't know if I can possibly adhere to this plan," an appropriate response might be, "You seem to be pretty discouraged about your plan." The response, then:

1. Labels the feeling—"discouraged"
2. Describes the situation—"your plan"
3. Keeps the focus on the client—"you"

Although empathy responses seem unnatural at first, such a skill can be learned and used effectively.[3,20-22] Empathic listening achieves the desired goals of client-counselor rapport and client self-examination.

Clarification statements are often confused with empathy responses, but can be distinguished readily by the presence of a labeled feeling in empathy. One reason confusion occurs is that the word "feel" is often used when the speaker really means "think." For example, when saying "You *feel* you are having a difficult time understanding your wife's problem," the words used really should be, "You *think* you are having. . . ." These are both clarification responses. A useful test of whether "feel" really implies feelings or thoughts is to substitute the word "think" for "feel." If they interchange readily, the response is probably clarification.

If the content of a client's statement appears to have a significant emotion attached to it, empathy is the preferred response. The example above incorporates an element of emotion. Therefore, a better response might be the empathic, "You feel terribly confused [feeling word] by your wife's problem." Empathy, also nondirective, is the most powerful response for obtaining significant personal data; clarification is the next most valuable.

There are practitioners who believe that empathy can not be taught. It is true that just repeating the empathy response is not the equivalent of being empathic. There are people skilled in the technique who are not sensitive to others' feelings. Conversely, there are people who are sensitive, but use ineffective means of conveying their sensitivity. Both can benefit from the application of the technique because the feedback given by the client on the accuracy of the counselor's perceptions can help to sharpen those perceptions and facilitate in the clinician increasing ability to empathize.

Sharing responses.   Although most information should be dispensed during the implementation (instruction) phase of counseling, there are times when a client needs specific information or an answer to a question he asks. An example of *information giving* is the structure provided at the initiation of the interview and the closure statements at the end. If the client is asking questions, the clinician must determine when these are legitimate questions requiring answers, and when they are diversionary tactics. The client may also perceive the interview time as instruction rather than assessment. This difference should have been made clear during structuring and may need to be reiterated during the interview if the client appears to be confused. The clinician may say, "I know you have lots of questions and I will try to answer all of them a little later. Right now I need to know as much about your problem as you can tell me. Unless you feel uneasy not knowing the answer right now, I'd like to postpone answering your question." Information giving turns the client into the interviewer, which is not in concert with the original purpose of the relationship at this stage in counseling.

Another form of response that can contribute to the interview, if used with care, is *confrontation*. To confront, the clinician shares with the client some perceptions he has about the client's problem. Then the focus goes immediately back to the client, as lengthy descriptions or analyses are inappropriate in the interview. An example of confrontation follows:

Client: I'm not interested in staying healthy.

Dietitian: I heard you say earlier you cared about being well. I think there is some conflict in what you're telling me.

Confrontation is a useful response when the clinician needs to deal with client resistance, as humans use a number of behaviors to resist self-analysis and change. Silence, changing the subject, talking too much, speaking in the third person, denial of feelings and/or responsibility, or even agreement with suggested changes are typical resistant behaviors. The counselor may wish to say something like, "I have observed that you change the subject when we talk about your father and I think there may be something related to him that is difficult for you to express." A note of caution: delaying the confrontation response to the later part of the interview promotes more effective client participation.

During the interview the clinician is experiencing feelings, thoughts, and behavior while listening to the client. At appropriate points, the clinician may choose to share these with the client. Such a response is labeled *self-disclosure* and is a statement of clinician feelings about the client-counselor relationship.[13] For example, "I'm really upset by what's happening here because I think I hear you blaming me for your problem" is self-disclosure. The clinician must judiciously use this response as it increases the risk of client withdrawal. Self-disclosure, even more than the other responses, is dependent upon the trust base. The client needs to feel that the clinician accepts and understands his behavior without rejecting him as a person before he can handle the clinician's feelings about their relationship.

Self-disclosure can also have a positive perspective, such as the clinician saying to the client, "I'm really pleased with the progress you've been making." Efforts to provide more positive than negative self-disclosures are very effective. Most clients can only tolerate negative feedback when it is well tempered with the positive. Self-disclosure is best deferred beyond the initial interview, however, so that it does not interfere with the client's self-examination.

When the clinician uses self-disclosure, he then returns to the listening mode as the client responds. This turns the focus back to the client. It is very easy, but unproductive, to become drawn into a defense of the self-disclosure statement instead of working on the client's reaction to it.

Roadblocks. In contrast to effective interpersonal responses, Gordon has defined 12 roadblocks to good communication. [19] These roadblocks include responses such as ordering, moralizing, lecturing, judging, and so on. Although many of these responses may be appropriate in other settings, roadblock responses will influence what a client is willing to reveal and are best not used in counseling interviews during the assessment phase. When there are action plans being developed, then suggestions or warnings of negative consequences can be offered with benefit. A few roadblock responses, such as ridiculing, have little redeeming value.

Nonverbal skills. In addition to verbal communication skills, there are nonverbal behaviors that convey to the client that the clinician is listening. One is silence. Silence allows the client to set his thoughts straight, or it serves to tell him that the practitioner is not ready to jump in with a comment every time there is a short pause, thus indicating that periods of silence are acceptable and valuable in the interview. The client will soon learn that he can continue after he has thought out what he wants to say. Clinicians need to be aware of the tendency to avoid the discomfort of periods of silence.

There are other nonverbal behaviors that set a tone of attentiveness and concern. The use of eye contact communicates an attempt to "be in touch." A forward-leaning posture suggests acceptance instead of rejection or disinterest. A gentle touch, sensitively offered, can speak silently of empathy. Such behaviors must be used judiciously, as too much eye contact may make a client feel "exposed," leaning too close may invade personal space, and touch may be interpreted as a sexual advance, manipulation, or parental control. The most important point to remember about all of these responses is that there is no absolute formula for implementation. Their value will increase as the clinician's continued practice enhances his ability to use them appropriately. Clinicians must be aware of the nonverbal messages they send and receive, and the effects they are having on the client.

Initiating the Interview

A few directive statements to provide the client with structure will be needed at the first contact. Structure is the presentation of an overview of the counseling process to the client as it relates to his needs. This includes an introduction of the clinician and his function, the purpose of the interview, the intended outcomes, and the constraints. By orienting the client to the who, why, what, and how long, the clinician helps reduce the client's anxiety and directs his thoughts to his nutritional needs and potential means of addressing them. In this regard, the clinician might say, after introducing himself and stating he is a dietitian: "I would like to discuss with you your concerns about what you've been eating. What you tell me will help me discover what we really need to focus on."

Often, but not necessarily, the introductory statement is followed by a question asking the client how he is feeling today, and listening to his general concerns, even though they may seem unrelated to the client's nutritional problem in the beginning. To ask a client how he is feeling, and then not to respond demonstrates a clear lack of interest in the client. Indeed, he may tell you some very significant information about himself in that exchange. It is unfortunate that the common greeting of "How are you today?" is usually understood to be only a social ritual. In a similar vein, it is inappropriate to begin the interview with small talk. This behavior tends to make the client feel the clinician is reluctant to deal with his concerns.

In order to set the tone for interviewing, the clinician usually begins the actual interview with an open-ended question or statement, which means there is no specific answer or response sought. An example of an open-ended statement is, "I'd like you to tell me something about your concerns about your food;" of a nondirective question, "What can you tell me about your problem?" This approach allows the client to explore those issues and concerns that seem most important to him. The concerns may not be the most important in terms of the nutritional care problem, but they are what the client feels comfortable sharing at this point. As a consequence, the client is not threatened. As he senses that he can trust the dietitian to accept somewhat undesirable behavior without making him feel he is guilty of misbehavior, the client will be more willing to share more significant undesirable behaviors. As with any other risk-involved experience, most people attempt increasingly risky behaviors and, as long as they are successful and can handle the consequences, will take on increasingly risky challenges.

Implementing the Interview

Since the goals of interviewing are to build relationships and to gather as much data as possible, it is imperative to use an interviewing approach that will optimize the chances of achieving those goals. There are several basic approaches to interviewing that range from a very structured question-answer session (directive) to an interaction in which the counselor only listens (nondirective).[23] Most practitioners use a systhesis of the two extremes.

A recently proposed model of interviewing for the medical profession combines these two techniques.[7] This format is viewed by the authors as viable in interviewing for nutritional counseling as well. The proposed model subscribes to an interview begun in the nondirective style, providing the client an opportunity to talk about his perceptions of his problem. The nondirective approach, by its very nature, facilitates the development of rapport and trust between client and clinician, a major reason for using the technique in the beginning of the interview. The crucial development of a working relationship is the result of communication of empathy, concern, withheld judgment, and sincere interest in the client's problems. A well-laid foundation in the beginning supports a productive counseling experience.

The importance of placing the direct questioning at the end of the interview lies in the fact that the nature of directive questions will indicate to the client the content that the clinician values most. Some clients consequently will tend to focus on data emphasized by the clinician rather than what is most important to them. Thus the nondirective approach is strongly recommended for the early part of the counseling session.

Closing the Interview

As the interview nears its conclusion, the practitioner may be more directive by asking the client specific, probing questions, or confronting, if necessary. Doing so, however, involves the risk of terminating interpersonal communication prematurely. The clinician may prefer to delay directive responses to later sessions. At least 5 minutes prior to termination, the practitioner should give an indication of closure by saying, for example, "We have just 5 more minutes today. Is there anything else you would like to tell me before we close?" When the last few exchanges are completed, the arrangements for the next contact should be initiated, and the task or purpose of the next meeting clearly defined. With the purpose established, the client may benefit from having an assignment to prepare for the next contact. This may be the collection of food intake data, or recording of related food behaviors.* Such data become a part of the diet history and are discussed in subsequent interviews.

A SAMPLE INTERVIEW

Let's now examine a brief client-clinical dietitian dialogue in which the described responses are illustrated.

Dietitian: "Why don't you tell me a little bit about the problems you've been having planning meals for your family." (*exploratory response—nondirective*)

---

* Formalized guides to food behavior data collection are available in the literature.[24,25]

Client: "Oh, some days I get so discouraged. I guess I've never really learned to plan meals. I just go to the grocery store, buy what looks good, and then come home. Other times I just fix whatever I have in the house. I just can't seem to stay within the budget that way. It just takes all the fun out of preparing meals."

Dietitian: "It sounds like preparing meals has become a drag for you." (*clarification response—restatement*)

Client: "Oh, it really has. Just the other day the family was asking for pot roast and I had this terrific new recipe for a salad, so I ran to the store to get what I needed and discovered I didn't have enough left in my grocery budget for the roast, let alone the artichokes for the salad. I felt like crying right there in the store. We ended up having hot dogs and applesauce."

Dietitian: Silence. (*nonverbal response*)

Client: "I just don't know. I sit down and make lists and try to plan, but I always end up unable to take advantage of sale items and having to buy the more expensive small sizes because I don't have enough money to buy the larger size. I guess I've gotten to the point where I don't even like to cook anymore. The family just complains all the time because they don't have their favorite dishes."

Dietitian: "You seem almost depressed by the thought of meal planning and cooking." (*empathy response*)

Client: "I think you're right, I think I don't care if I never have to prepare meals again. I would just as soon take them all to a hamburger place. They prefer that anyway."

Dietitian: "You don't even care to prepare meals again." (*clarification response—reflection*)

Client: "You'd better believe it's the easy way! Everybody gets what they want and I don't have to do anything but pay for it. Of course, the budget doesn't stretch very well to do that but at least 4 nights a week they're happy."

Dietitian: "Have you considered any other alternative?" (*exploratory response—directive*)

Client: "Not really, I don't even like to think about it."

Dietitian: "Um-huh." (*exploratory response—nondirective*)

Client: "Well, I can't help it if I never really learned to cook. Most of the time my food budget won't make it because I have to use so many mixes and things."

Dietitian: "You don't feel competent as a cook." (*empathy response*)

Client: "I can't even read a recipe."

Dietitian: "I think this might be the reason you have such a difficult time with meal planning." (*confrontation response*)

Client: "You know, I guess it really is!"

The foregoing is an example of a client interview in which the clinical dietitian has used examples of the listening responses. As a result of this short dialogue, we already know some very important facts that pertain to the client's motivation as related to her nutritional behavior. At the conclusion of this interview, the client may be asked to record the contents of the meals eaten by her family for the week prior to the next counseling session, if she is agreeable and understands the purpose.

For other types of concerns, various forms and techniques can be used to record food intakes and food behaviors, based on the problem identified in the interview. Samples of these forms are included in Chapter 6 or related appendices. The resulting data are incorporated into the analysis of food intake (Chapter 10).

SUMMARY

The interview is the keystone to nutritional counseling. It is the major tool in defining the client's problems. A problem well-defined is a problem at least half-solved. An effective interview process builds a constructive working relationship, and provides significant assessment data. The interview evolves from a very nondirective format to a directive one as it concludes.

In order to achieve the desired outcomes there are skills that, although difficult, can be learned. These skills include verbal and nonverbal responses, based on intellectual and emotional understanding of behavior. All clinical dietitians can enhance their professional practice by acquiring these skills.

CITED REFERENCES

1. Bernstein, L., and Bernstein, R. S. *Interviewing: A Guide for Health Professionals*. 3rd Ed. New York: Appleton-Century-Crofts, 1980.
2. Schafer, R. B. The self-concept as a factor in diet selection and quality. *J. Nutr. Educ.* 11:37, 1979.

3. Benjamin. A. D. *The Helping Interview*. 3rd Ed. Boston: Houghton-Mifflin, 1981.

4. Dyer, W., and Vriend, J. *Counseling Techniques That Work: Applications to Individual and Group Counseling*. Washington: APGA Press, 1975.

5. Veatch, R. Updating the Hippocratic Oath. *Med. Opinion* 8:56, 1972.

6. Szasz, T., and Hollender, M. A contribution to the philosophy of medicine: The basic models of the doctor-patient relationship. *Arch. Int. Med.* 97:585, 1956.

7. Enelow, A. J., and Adler, L. Basic interviewing. *In* Enelow, A. J., and Swisher, S. N., Eds. *Interviewing and Patient Care*. 2nd Ed. New York: Oxford Univ. Press, 1979.

8. Brill, N. I. *Working with People: The Helping Process*. 2nd Ed. Philadelphia: J. B. Lippincott Co., 1978.

9. Brammer, L. M. *The Helping Relationship: Process and Skills*. 2nd Ed. Englewood Cliffs, NJ: Prentice-Hall, Inc., 1979.

10. Evans, R. I., and Hall, Y. Social-psychologic perspective in motivating changes in eating behavior. *J. Am. Dietet. A.* 72:378, 1978.

11. Haynes, R. A critical review of the "determinants" of patient compliance with therapeutic regimens. *In* Sackett, D., and Haynes, R., Eds. *Compliance with Therapeutic Regimens*. Baltimore: The Johns Hopkins University Press, 1976.

12. Zifferblatt, S. M., and Wilbur, C. S. Dietary counseling: Some realistic expectations and guidelines. *J. Am. Dietet. A.* 70:591, 1977.

13. Danish, S. J., Ginsberg, M. R., Terrell, A., Hammond, M. I., and Adams, S. O. The anatomy of a dietetic counseling interview. *J. Am. Dietet. A.* 75:626, 1979.

14. Woolley, F. R., Warnick, M. W., Kane, R. L., and Dyer, E. D. *Problem-Oriented Nursing*. New York: Springer Publ. Co., 1974.

15. Anthony, W., and Carkhuff, R. R. *The Art of Health Care*. Amherst, MA: Human Res. Dev. Press, Inc., 1976.

16. Kagan, N., "Influencing human interaction: Eleven years of IPR." Paper presented at the Annual Meeting of the Am. Educ. Res. Assoc., New Orleans, 1973.

17. Garrett, A. *Interviewing: Its Principles and Methods*. 2nd Ed. New York: Family Serv. Assoc. Am., 1972.

18. Truax, C., and Carkhuff, R. R. *Toward Effective Counseling and Psychotherapy*. Chicago: Aldine, 1967.

19. Gordon, T. *P.E.T. Parent Effectiveness Training: The Tested New Way to Raise Responsible Children*. New York: Peter H. Wyden, Inc., 1970.

20. Payton, O. D., Beale, A. V., Munson, P. J., and Morriss, R. L. Student produced empathic responses: The second step in teaching communication skills to allied health supervisors. *J. All. Health* 7:302, 1978.

21. Gazda, G. M. *Human Relations Development: A Manual for Educators.* 2nd Ed. Boston: Allyn and Bacon, Inc., 1977.
22. Sydnor, G., Akridge, R., and Parkhill, N. *Human Relations Training: A Programed Manual* Minden, LA: Human Rel. Dev. Train. Inst., 1973.
23. Rogers, C. R. *Client-Centered Therapy: Its Current Practice, Implications, and Theory.* Boston: Houghton-Mifflin Co., 1951.
24. Ferguson, J. M. *Learning to Eat: Behavior Modification for Weight Control. Leader Manual.* Palo Alto, CA: Bull Publ. Co., 1975.
25. Stuart, R. B., and Davis, B. *Slim Chance in a Fat World: Behavioral Control of Obesity.* Champaign, IL: Research Press, 1978.

6
The Diet History

The collection of meaningful dietary history information is a challenging and extensive task for the clinical dietitian.

Nancy Hsu and Annette Gormican, **The computer in retrieving dietary history data. II. Retrieving information by summary generation.** (*J. Am. Dietet. A.* 63:402, 1973).

The diet history is *the* unique assessment contribution that clinical dietitians make in client-centered health care. The diet history represents both a *tool* and a *process* used by practitioners.

The diet history is the special *tool* by which data describing a client's past and/or current food intake and food behaviors are collected. The description of food intake should provide an estimation of the typical intake of an individual and should be both qualitative and quantitative in nature. A client's food behaviors are characterized by his usual pattern of food and nutrient consumption, variation of that intake, and the impact of other significant variables (physiologic, psychologic, and environmental).

As a *process,* the diet history represents the procedure for collecting the desired data. The interview is one of the methods by which the collection of meaningful information about the client is obtained.

The assembly and evaluation of the information contained in the diet history permits the clinician to make statements about dietary status. In the case study contained in Chapter 4, R. Dawson, the Registered Dietitian, wrote assessment statements about dietary status.

Dawson's status remarks, contained in the SOAP notes, are in accordance with our earlier definition of dietary status:

> "Dietary status" tells us only what the individual has been eating; it gives no direct indication of nutritional status—only presumptive evidence if his nutritional requirements are average and there are no conditioning factors present.[2] (p. 98)

All of Dawson's comments pertaining to kilocaloric and iron intakes are statements about dietary status, based on assessments of the diet history.

The term "nutritional history" is not interchangeable with the term "diet history." The former usually means the assembly and subsequent evaluation of a great deal more information than that incorporated in the diet history. Properly executed, a nutrition history will contain the elements of the diet history in addition to the results of specific laboratory assessments and evaluations of physical signs and symptoms of inadequate nutrition. Such clinical studies may include examinations of the hair, face, eyes, and so forth. Laboratory assessments may include those discussed in Chapter 4 (e.g., blood-forming nutrients). All of the foregoing activities that support statements about the nutritional history fall under the umbrella term, "nutritional assessment*".

In 1973, a most useful guide to nutritional assessment in health programs was published.[3] This document adds to the definition of nutrition history a fourth dimension, community assessment. Such an assessment gives an overview of the nutritional life of a given community, incorporating those variables affecting the nutritional health of its citizens. Combining all four assessment procedures—diet histories, clinical evaluations, laboratory investigations, and community assessment— allows for statements about the nutritional status of a community. The first three procedures may be applied to single individuals or small groups. Earlier we accepted the definition of nutritional status as:

> . . . the actual nutritional condition of the patient as measured by physical examination, laboratory determinations, pathologic morphology, and therapeutic response under controlled conditions. Nutritional status is influenced not only by dietary intake but also conditioning factors, such as increases in nutrient requirements, excretions, or destruction and interferences with nutrient intake,

---

* This term is often misused in practice as clinical dietitians frequently are not professionally able to perform all those varied activities.

TABLE 6.1 Information Needed For Assessment of Nutritional Status

Sources of Information	Nature of Information Obtained	Nutritional Implications
1. Agricultural data Food balance sheets	Gross estimates of agricultural production Agricultural methods Soil fertility Predominance of cash crops Overproduction of staples Food imports and exports	Approximate availability of food supplies to a population
2. Socioeconomic data Information on marketing, distribution, and storage	Purchasing power Distribution and storage of foodstuffs	Unequal distribution of available foods between the socioeconomic groups in the community and within the family
3. Food consumption patterns Cultural-anthropological data	Lack of knowledge, erroneous beliefs, prejudices, and indifference	
4. Dietary surveys	Food consumption	Low, excessive, or unbalanced nutrient intake

5. Special studies on foods	Biological value of diets Presence of interfering factors (e.g., goitrogens) Effects of food processing	Special problems related to nutrient utilization
6. Vital and health statistics	Morbidity and mortality data	Extent of risk to community Identification of high-risk groups
7. Anthropometric studies	Physical development	Effect of nutrition on physical development
8. Clinical nutritional surveys	Physical signs	Deviation from health due to malnutrition
9. Biochemical studies	Levels of nutrients, metabolites, and other components of body tissues and fluids	Nutrient supplies in the body Impairment of biochemical function
10. Additional medical information	Prevalent disease patterns, including infections and infestations	Interrelationships of state of nutrition and disease

NOTE: Reprinted by permission of the publisher from *WHO Report of Expert Committee on Medical Assessment of Nutritional Status.* (World Health Organization Technical Report Series 258, 1963).

absorption, or utilization which may be operating either currently or in the past.[2] (p.98)

The assessment of the data contained in the nutrition history permits statements about nutritional status. The diet history is but one component of the nutrition history.

Additional refinements and extensions of the assessment components of nutritional status have been described[4] and are shown in Table 6.1. Such an elaborate assessment process is inappropriate in the everyday practice of clinical dietitians, as the client-counselor relationship is of an entirely different nature than community-wide surveys.

The primary purpose of the diet history is to enable the clinician to assemble part of the data base necessary for the execution of the two distinct roles delineated in Chapter 1. Briefly, those roles are:

1. Provision of nutritional counseling

2. Provision of nutrient sources

In our hierarchy of nutritional care priorities (Fig. 1.1), the diet history serves as an assessment tool for those clients who:

1. Are capable of self-determination, but are unable to be totally self-sufficient, or

2. Are capable of self-sufficiency and self-determination.

The diet history is also a basic assessment tool for those clients in practitioner-managed settings. The history, therefore, serves as a vital part of the data base in the assessment component of all health maintenance and health improvement programs.

The diet history has two distinct features. The first is information or data about actual food and nutrient consumption. The history attempts to answer the question *"What* is the client ingesting?" The second feature is information or data about some of those variables that dictate what foods and nutrients are consumed. The second feature is designed to partly answer the question *"Why* does the client choose as he does?" In the following pages, we shall examine both features of the diet history, and then discuss the methods by which the history is evaluated (Chapter 10).

ASSESSING FOOD CONSUMPTION: WHAT IS THE CLIENT INGESTING?

In a now classic document,[5] Becker, Indik, and Beeuwkes point out that there are a number of considerations to be made in the data collection phase of a study of food consumption. Writing about epidemiologic studies, Young and Trulson remarked that food consumption data may be recorded as:

1. *Intake at specific meals recorded concurrently by means of:*
   (a) *weights*
   (b) *household measures, or*
   (c) *estimates of quantity of specific foods.*
2. *Intake at specific meals recorded by recall in terms of:*
   (a) *estimates of quantity of a specific food, or*
   (b) *frequency of occurrence of food item.*
3. *Current usual intake recorded by recall in terms of:*
   (a) *estimates of quantity of specific foods, or*
   (b) *frequency of occurrence of food items.*
4. *Past intake over specific period recorded by recall in terms of estimates of quantity of specific foods.*
5. *Past changes in intake recorded by recall in terms of frequency of occurrence of food items.*[6] *(p. 805)*

The methods cited above, appropriate for large scale surveys, may be adapted for use with individual clients.

A review of the five ways of recording food consumption data shows that the first reflects current activity in relation to food intake. That is, what is the client doing now? The other items ask what the food intake has been in either the recent or distant past.

To elicit responses to the queries, "What *is* the client ingesting?" or "What *has* the client ingested?" a series of questions may be posed, each of which is related to the others[5]:

1. What foods are or were eaten?
2. How much food is or was eaten?
3. When are or were the foods eaten in relation to other foods?
4. When are or were the foods eaten in relation to physical activity?
5. Where are or were the foods eaten?
6. Under what conditions are or were the foods eaten?

We may add a seventh question: "How is (or was) the food prepared?" All of the responses are of considerable value to the clinical dietitian when she is compiling the diet history. The seven questions above should be incorporated into whichever assessment method is being used by the clinician.

To facilitate clinical practice and to objectively derive answers to these questions, Young and Trulson's categories[6] are reorganized for use in this text. Therefore, for individual clients, there are two basic categories of food consumption reviews. They are:

1. Retrospective reviews, recalling *past* intakes. They are retrospective in that the client will be asked to refer back, or to go back in thought, to recall what foods were consumed

2. Inspective reviews, recording of *current* intake. Such reviews are inspective in that the client will be asked to view closely what he is now consuming

We shall examine these methods in ensuing pages. There are, of course, other and more elaborate ways in which methods of collecting food consumption data may be categorized.[5,6] The determination of the right procedure, or method, for assessing the food history data of an individual in a particular care setting is most appropriately made by the clinical dietitian practicing in that site.

Retrospective Reviews

Retrospective reviews of food and nutrient consumption are reviews of *past* food intake. Such reviews may consider what was eaten yesterday, last week, or even last year; in all cases, the data are historical and do not necessarily represent present intake. Like other human behaviors, food consumption behaviors are subject to change. Some of the variables responsible for change will be examined in the next section of this chapter.

The collection of retrospective data may be conducted in a variety of ways. For clarification, the two most common routes for the collection of such data by clinical dietitians are:

1. By *informal* exchanges of information, in client-clinician counseling sessions

2. By *formal* recording of client responses to clinician-prepared questionnaires

Each route has more than one way or method by which data may be collected.

Informal route.   The collection of retrospective data within the counseling process may be thought of as part of that assessment component which we have termed "the interview." An interview is defined as a purposeful conversation between the client, or the client and his significant others, and the clinician. In the last chapter (Chapter 5), we examined the purpose, process, and content of the interview in depth.

In a counseling setting, the clinical dietitian may obtain food history information by asking the client to recall exactly what he has eaten within a specified 24-hour time frame (e.g., from midnight Monday to midnight Tuesday): Such a method is termed the *24-hour recall*. The basic structure of the 24-hour recall technique is as follows:

Clinician: I would like you to recall for me everything that you ate or drank all day yesterday, from the time you woke in the morning until the time you went to sleep at night. Include everything you ate away from home, at school, or at work, or any other place you visited. Tell me about any special food supplements you might be consuming, and anything else you actually swallowed.

To begin, tell me about your day. What time did you get up? Is that your normal time? When did you first eat or drink, and what was it that you had? Did you eat this food at home or away? How much of this food did you consume?

And so on, through the day. The skilled clinician will conduct the interview in such a manner that the client is not faced with a barrage of closed-ended questions, but rather is guided to respond freely, leading the dietitian through his day. The resulting information may be recorded, as shown in Figure 6.1, in a manner designed to organize the data.

Time	Eating Location	Name Of Food or Supplement	How Prepared?	Amount

FIGURE 6.1   24-hour diet intake record.

The 24-hour recall method is a fairly simple technique that is in great use in a variety of clinical sites. The data generated from the use of this technique are primarily qualitative; that is, the recall method yields casual information only about the kinds of foods and supplements consumed within a specified time frame. Quantification of the data is difficult, if not impossible, in most circumstances, as clients frequently are unaware of the amounts of food they have eaten.

One helpful technique in the attempt to quantify food consumption information is the use of food models.[7,8]* Lifelike models of food are helpful to clients in establishing portion sizes and methods of preparation. Along with food models, simple tools such as drinking glasses of various sizes, measuring cups and spoons, plates of differing dimensions, and rulers may be employed with the recall technique.

The recall method is highly dependent on the ability of the client to remember what has happened and his willingness to reveal the information. Recollection can be a difficult task for many, especially those who are older.[9,10] Beal underscored this point by noting that "A 24-hr. recall without advanced warning to the subject is a simple test of memory. . . . Most people have little reason to remember what they have eaten"[11] (p. 427). In contrast, one might argue that, with advance notice, clients may give information that is not truly reflective of their food behaviors. Such information, then, may be biased in that it is reflective of what the client wants the clinician to know.[12] (Even without prior warning, some clients may "code" their responses.) Of the utmost importance is the fact that such a recall method supplies data for only 1 day, and that particular day may not be representative of "usual" food practices. Meals on weekend days can be different from those eaten on weekdays. One solution to this problem is to repeat randomly the 24-hour recall history over time, thus high-lighting those great variations in intake not apparent in one interview.[13] In any event, in some clinical sites, and with certain clients, the 24-hour recall method may be the most highly satisfactory method of assessing food and food supplement consumption.

A variation of the 24-hour recall method is to ask the client to give a summary of his "normal" or "usual" food intake. This is a retrospective means by which general information is solicited about food and food supplement intake. To recall *"usual" food intake,* the clinician asks the client to state what his usual day is like, what he usually consumes first in the day, and so on. The format of the usual food intake recall may be like that of the 24-hour recall, but both questions

* One source of food models is Nasco, Fort Atkinson, Wisc. 53538.

and answers are stated in terms of *usual* practices. Once again, the problems of quantities of foods may arise (e.g., "half a glass of milk" instead of 6 ounces). In many instances, the two recall methods may be used together to aid in the assessment process. This is one of the ways that great variations in intake from day to day may be ascertained and evaluated.

A second retrospective method used for the collection of food ingestion data is that of *food frequency*. In this method, the frequency of use of foods and food supplements is recorded for assessment purposes. Both frequency of use and frequency of purchase may be estimated; for the latter, the clinician must account for food brought into the client's home from his own farm, garden, or other source. Such foods are not usually considered to be among regular food budget items. Most avid vegetable gardeners never consider the purchase of seeds, plants, fertilizer, or even garden tools as part of their grocery budget; the results of their efforts are thought to be means by which food expenditures are controlled.

Formats for collecting food frequency data are usually formally constructed. Foods are organized into groups that have similar nutrients in common. Armstrong[14] reports the use of nine such groups:

1. Milk, milk products
2. Meat, poultry, fish, eggs, related products
3. Dried beans and peas, nuts, related products
4. Vegetables, vegetable products
5. Fruits
6. Breads
7. Grain products (excluding breads)
8. Fats, oils
9. Sugars, sweets

Other workers have devised a great many variations of food groupings; in fact, the variations seem to be endless. Many are regional, accounting for the food customs of the geographic area. The major deviations from Armstrong's groups are primarily subdivisions of one of the nine. Milk and milk products, for example, may be further divided into milk, ice cream, cheese, yogurt, and other dairy products. An example of a food frequency tool is shown in Appendix E.

The frequency of use of the food groupings is ascertained by asking, "Do you drink milk? If so, how much milk do you drink every day?" or "How much milk do you buy each week?" In that manner, a day's or a week's use frequency is established. Generally, quantities expressed for a week are often more reliable than a single day's food intake. For assessment purposes, the evaluation results of the week's food usage may be divided to show one-seventh of the total. The food frequency tool differs from the 24-hour recall method in that it does not ask about the specific foods consumed in a limited time period; it asks more generally about the frequency of usage of food groups. Ascertaining food frequency usage is a retrospective review technique that may be used either formally or informally.

The 24-hour recall or the "usual" food intake method may be used with the frequency tool to validate the information obtained in the assessment phase.[15-17] Using the food frequency data to verify the recall method information is termed the "cross-check." By carefully examining each food group listed in the frequency tool in relation to the food quantities given as "usual," or "yesterday's" intake in the recall method, the usefulness of the history is greatly enhanced. The final result of all this activity can be a reasonable description of the client's intake for the specified period of time.

Formal route.   A client may provide retrospective food consumption data by recording his responses in a structured manner. Currently, there are at least two methods by which the client may do this. One method is the *questionnaire*. Usually this tool is a paper-and-pencil device, self-administered by the client. The questionnaire has a distinct advantage in that it serves as a means of determining literacy of clients. Since clients are usually reluctant to disclose overtly that they are unable to read and/or write, the printed questionnaire, which requires a written response, allows the clinician to note illiteracy with a minimum of negative overtones. The experienced clinical dietitian will then move to assessment procedures that do not require a command of the written language.

Questionnaires may be designed to ask about food consumption in a variety of ways. Schedules (questionnaires) constructed to elicit yes-or-no answers are appropriate only for large-scale surveys; schedules constructed for use by clients in nutritional counseling environments should be designed to ask open-ended questions. In that manner, clients have the greatest freedom in responding, thus affording opportunities for self-expression. The formats of most questionnaires are primarily adaptations of the recall method: recalls of recent food intake, food frequency, "usual" food intake, and so on. Added to some schedules are questions designed to gather data about food preferences.

In addition to ingestion data, questionnaires may also be designed to elicit information about food practices and food behaviors.[18-20] That is, questions regarding attitudes about food, food purchasing practices, and so on, may be placed in the schedule. An example of a food practices schedule is shown in Appendix F.

A recent event in clinical dietetics is the use of *computers* for eliciting food history and practices data.[1,21,22] In the limited number of clinical sites where such programs are currently available, clients actually become involved in responding to queries presented to them on a computer terminal screen. Such automated reviews have the distinct advantage of being well-conceived (as they must be!) and requiring an active participation on the part of the client. The major disadvantage is that the client must be literate. Some practitioners would argue that automated reviews are deterrents to client-counselor relationships. The apparent solution is a compromise—an integration of the informal exchange and the automated review components of this phase of assessment.

Hunt and co-workers[23] have reported using a computerized food frequency questionnaire and the 24-hour recall method with 50 adult subjects. The recall method was repeated in five successive weekly interviews; the questionnaire technique was administered on the first visit of the subject to the study site. Except for vitamin A, the data for the five 24-hour recalls were similar. There was a striking difference *between* methods, however; except for caloric and carbohydrate intake, mean intake data for other nutrients varied from 6 to 68 percent greater for the computerized method. Hunt et al. conclude that " . . . it does not appear that the computerized food frequency questionnaire accurately estimates dietary intake as compared with the determinations resulting from the average of five 24-hr. recalls"[23] (p. 659). This study points out the great need for further research in clinical methodology.

Inspective Reviews

The second basic category of collecting food consumption data is the keeping of current food diaries or records. Such inspective records are usually kept for a period of 3 or 7 days; the time span over which the records are maintained is varied according to the interests of both the client and the clinician. There are a number of studies that support either a week's record[24-28] or the abbreviated period of 3 days.[29-31] In general, the length of the recording period depends primarily on the purpose of the record, the nutrients or foods being assessed, and the interest and abilities of the clients.[32-38]

Current food and supplement consumption may be recorded in one of three ways: by weights, measurements, or estimation. The weighing of food is usually done on a household gram scale. Such scales are readily available to clients in drug, department, or cut-rate stores. Foods may be weighed either before or after cooking; the latter weight is usually recorded, except for foods normally eaten raw (e.g., salad greens, fresh fruit).

Foods are measured with such household tools as measuring spoons and measuring cups. Measurement is most appropriate for liquids of all types, fats, grain products, and so on.

Estimation of food portions is the least fruitful method of the three ways to record food intakes, but is often the only appropriate one. Estimates of food consumed are recorded by clients eating meals in restaurants, in college cafeterias, and other meal sites away from home. For this method, it is best for the clinician first to show the client models of food before the recording phase actually begins so that the client has some idea of what a 3 ounce (90 gram) portion of cooked ground beef or a 1 ounce (30 gram) portion of cheddar cheese looks like.

The format of a consumption record is fairly simple; the most important part is the directions given to the recorder. An example of a record format follows in Figure 6.2. In the figure, the directions given in statement no. 5 of the instructions must necessarily be modified to accommodate the manner in which the food quantities will be recorded.

Another variation of the food intake record is designed to measure that which is procured and consumed in a specified time frame, usually a week. In this variation, records are not kept of day-to-day or meal-to-meal consumption. Instead, what results is information about total food and food supplement consumption in a week's time. Often this type of record keeping activity is useful for studies of a whole household's intake.[3] The format of the weekly food summary record is shown in Figure 6.3.

There are, of course, objections to the inspective method of collecting food consumption data. Such objections include the inability or unwillingness of a client to participate because of the amount of time and energy needed to record. Although the food record presumably produces data more meaningful than the recall method in terms of actual quantitative consumption, there exists the possibility that clients change their food behaviors simply because they *are* keeping records.[39] Clients may modify their intake because of a growing awareness of their food

Instructions

1. Use the attached pages to record your food and food supplement intake for _____ days. Use a new page for each day.
2. Record everything you eat, drink, or swallow in each 24-hour period (column 1).
3. Remember to record when you ate or drank (column 2), and where this occurred (column 3).
4. Describe each food and indicate (column 1) whether it is cooked or raw. If cooked, tell how it was prepared (for example, boiled, baked, fried). Tell also how it was served (for example, with french dressing, with cream sauce).
5. Record the amount of everything you ate, drank, or swallowed (column 4). Weigh on the gram scale, or measure with measuring cups or spoons, each of these foods. If you eat away from home, estimate to the best of your ability the portion sizes of everything you consume.

Record

Name:

Day And Date:

1 Food	2 Time	3 Place	4 Amount

FIGURE 6.2 Daily food consumption record.

Instructions

1. Use the attached pages to write down the amounts of food on hand (in the house) that you may use during the week.
2. When food is brought into the home, either from the store or from the garden or elsewhere, record the food and amount on the record.
3. Record the amount of food (column 1), kind of food (column 2), and the source of food (column 3) on the Food Record.
4. At the end of the week, write down the amounts of food left from those you put on the record (bottom of the record, columns 1 and 2).
5. Fill in daily the form asking for a record of meals eaten at home and meals eaten away from home (Meals Record).

Food Record

Name: Date:

1 Amount	2 Kind Of Food	3 Source

End of the week: List those leftover from the record above:

Amount   Kind Of Food

FIGURE 6.3   Weekly food consumption record.

Meals Record

Person	Number meals eaten at home or made at home (brown-bag lunches)	Number meals eaten away from home and not made at home

FIGURE 6.3   (Continued)

practices or because they wish to present only certain kinds of information to the counselor. In contrast, Adelson[40] has published the results of a study with adult men in which she found little or no difference in the results obtained by using either the 24-hour recall or the 7-day food record. Furthermore, in a sample of 65 older subjects at five separate congregate meal sites, Gersovitz and co-workers found that the 24-hour recall and the 7-day food record methods " . . . provide about equally accurate estimates of the mean intake"[41] (p. 54). In this study, however, the 24-hour recall method tended to inflate low or inadequate intakes and deflate high or excessive intakes

In the final analysis, the choice of the method is a highly individualized one in which all of the variables of client interest and awareness, and the reasons for the assessment are considered.

ASSESSING FOOD BEHAVIORS: WHY DOES THE CLIENT CHOOSE AS HE DOES?

So far in this text, the authors have purposely avoided the use of the phrase "food habits" to describe those behaviors associated with the food acquisition and ingestion activities of people. We shall continue to do so, as we believe that an alternate phrase, "food behaviors," provides a more flexible and comprehensive framework in which to develop and test ideas about clients and their food selections.

In an excellent and unique text in the field of nutrition, food habits are described as:

> ... *the characteristic and repetitive acts that he [an individual]*
> *performs under the impetus of the need to provide himself with*
> *nourishment and simultaneously to meet an assortment of social*
> *and emotional goals. By the choices he makes which become habit*
> *on repetition, he strives to achieve such satisfactions as security,*
> *comfort, status, pleasure, and enhancement of his ego. Once formed,*
> *food habits tend to control behavior.*[42] (*p. 29*)

It is probably reasonable to assume that repetitive choices do become habits over time, but such a view tends to overlook the possibility of emergence of new behaviors. Nutritional counseling, the primary responsibility of clinical dietitians, is a process by which new behaviors can and do develop from the combined activities of the client and the clinician. Therefore, in keeping with the principal theme of this text, we shall address ourselves to "food behaviors" rather than to "food habits." The former provides us with the latitude to develop and test ideas about the nutritional counseling process; the latter tends to restrict us to the view that food choices are relatively fixed beyond the childhood years.

Assessing food behaviors is not an easy task! The academic study of food behaviors has, within recent years, become a fruitful activity of many behavioral scientists.[43,44] There are any number of anthropologists, psychologists, and sociologists studying various facets of this particular human behavior. We shall not, therefore, attempt to deal with the many theories of food behaviors, but rather we shall examine some of the variables that are universally accepted as affecting the food choices of individuals.

One of the most readily available sources of information that the clinical dietitian may use to collect assessment data is the medical record. In Chapter 4, we explored the contents of both the SOR and POR. The face sheet or front sheet of the record contains a wealth of SES (socioeconomic status) information important to the clinician, as it usually lists:

Name

Address (indicating neighborhood or town)

Age and sex

Birthplace

Insurance carrier or Medicaid number (economic indicators)

Marital status

Religion

Occupation and place of work (economic indicators)

These data may be used for a beginning profile of the client. For example:

> Mr. McC. is 74 years old, a widower who lives on the south side
> of the city. He was born in Toronto, is a member of a Protestant
> church, and has retired from his job as a factory foreman. His
> health care bills are paid by an insurance carrier, one of his re-
> tirement benefits.

From this beginning profile, the clinician knows that the client is an older gentleman, perhaps preparing his own meals, English-speaking, most likely literate, and probably financially independent. In addition, his food choices are unlikely to be governed by religious tenets.

A second major source of information about food selection variables is the client himself, or his significant others. Clients are often eager to talk with clinical dietitians about such matters as who carries the responsibility for food preparation in the household, who does the shopping, and so on. Such data may be collected during the course of interviews about food and food supplement intake, or may be solicited in questionnaires (Appendices F and J).

There are, of course, many different kinds of information the clinician needs to know about the client in order to advance the assessment process. For the sake of clarity and discussion, Table 6.2 lists seven broad categories of food selection variables. Each category contains a few basic statements about behaviors, achievements, or constraints that directly or indirectly influence food choices.

It seems an impossible task to incoporate the enormous number of variables presented in Table 6.2 into the ·diet history, but it is both essential and feasible to do so! If we extend the beginning profile of the client, Mr. McC., to include a consideration of those food selection variables that have been enumerated, the profile might expand as follows:

> Mr. McC. is 74 years old, a widower who lives on the south side
> of the city. He was born in Toronto, is a member of a Protestant
> church, and has retired from his job as a factory foreman. His
> health care bills are paid by an insurance carrier, one of his re-
> tirement benefits.
>
> Mr. McC. has come regularly to the Old Town Health Center for
> the purpose of general, preventive health care for the past 8 years.
> In that time, he has gained approximately 8 kg (17.6 lb), so that he
> now weighs 79 kg (173.8 lb). He is 172 cm tall (5 ft 9 in); his ideal
> body weight is about 70 kg (154 lbs). The results of all routine
> laboratory tests have fallen into the ranges for normal.

TABLE 6.2 Categories of Food Selection Variables

Categories	Food Selection Variable	Descriptors
General health practices	Oral hygiene	Mouth care, dental visits
	Physical handicaps	Mobilization and/or feeding aids
		Environmental barriers
	Use of nonprescription drugs	Laxatives, sleeping aids; frequency of use
	Use of tobacco, alcohol	Frequency of use
	Appetite	Changes in weight and appetite
Health attitudes, beliefs, and information	Attitudes about health care	Access to and use of health care delivery systems
	Nutrition beliefs	Use of "fad" diets
		Use of "health" foods
		Excessive vitamin and mineral supplement use
	Nutrition information	Knowledge of nutritional quality of foods
		Application of that knowledge in food choices
	Past experiences	In nutritional counseling
		Health care delivery in general
Physical activities	On-the-job exercise	Type of activity
		Frequency of activity
		Caloric expenditure
	Household activities	Type of activity
		Frequency of activity
		Caloric expenditure

Category	Subcategory	Details
	Recreational activities	Type of activity Frequency of activity Caloric expenditure
Educational achievements and language skills	Formal education	Grade or degree achieved
	Other education	Evening school, high school equivalency
	Language	English: first or second language, or not at all Other languages: first or second language, or not at all Literacy: English or other, or not at all
Economic considerations	Employment	Occupation: percentage of full-time work If unemployed: retired or public assistance
	Food programs	Eligibility for assistance Use of such programs
	Other financial resources	Availability and use
Environmental considerations	Household members	Age and responsibilities Contributions to overall health and welfare of basic living unit Delegated responsibilities for food procurement, preparation, service Skills in food activities

TABLE 6.2 (Continued)

Categories	Food-Selection Variable	Descriptors
	Household facilities	Adequate storage, refrigeration, preparation facilities
	Neighborhood facilities	Barriers for physically handicapped persons Shopping and banking areas Public transportation
Social considerations[a]	Attitudes and beliefs	Religious, ethnic, or other similar influences on food selection Attitudes toward client, the process of nutritional counseling, and health care in general
	Household members	Attitudes, knowledges, and beliefs about food, nutritional counseling, and health care in general
	Social groups, peers	
	Mass media	Exposure to, and belief in, information presented in newspapers, magazines, and on radio and television

[a] For a thorough and enlightening discussion of this topic, see Chapters 1–3 of *Nutrition, Behavior, and Change.*[39]

The client lives with his daughter (Mrs. D.) and her family (hus-
band and three sons, aged 22, 19, and 14 years). Their home is
large, about 20 years old, and is well equipped. Mrs. D. does all
the food budgeting, buying, and preparation. Mr. McC. occasionally
goes to the market with Mrs. D.; he does not like to prepare meals,
but always helps to clean the kitchen after breakfast and dinner.
He makes a monthly financial contribution towards the upkeep of
the house and to pay for his food. Mrs. D. says it is not necessary
for him to do so, but Mr. McC. insists on "paying his own way,"
so they have agreed for him to continue his contribution as long as
he is able.

The one recreational activity that Mr. McC. enjoys most is bowl-
ing; before he retired, he bowled in three leagues, each meeting once
a week. Now he bowls only infrequently because it has become "too
hard to follow through on my swing." As a consequence, Mr. McC.
is considerably less active physically. On his job, Mr. McC. walked
a great deal; in retirement, he walks daily to the park with his dog,
Pepper, but this walk is probably only half the exercise that he once
had.

From this extended profile, the clinician has available a great deal of
information that is useful in the assessment process. From the profile
of Mr. McC., the practitioner has learned that the client is financially
independent, relatively healthy except for an insidious weight gain,
and leads a life that includes limited physical activity. He lives with
a family who seem to view him as an important part of the family unit.
There are, for this client, relatively few economic, socioemotional, intellectual, or physical constraints on his activities.

In alliance with the food consumption data, the food behavior variables compose the diet history. Both of these distinctive features of
the history interact with one another. The adequacy of storage space,
for example, directly affects whether or not a client can take advantage
of food market sales of important food sources of nutrients such as
ascorbic acid. The willingness of significant others to be supportive of
clients in food behavior changes can be a major determinant of the
success of nutritional counseling. In any event, the interface between
the two features is of great significance in the client's food choices.

SUMMARY

The diet history is *the* unique contribution that clinical dietitians make
in client-centered care. The history is both a tool and a process. As a

tool, the diet history is composed of two parts: reviews of food intake, and summaries of food selection variables that guide or dictate food intake. As a process, the diet history may be conducted in a variety of ways: by collecting retrospective or past intake data, or by summarizing inspective or current intake data. Once food intake data are gathered, they are subjected to evaluation. The evaluation, to be discussed in Chapter 10, consists of two parts: the determination of the nutrient content of the food intake, and a subsequent scrutiny of the appropriateness of the nutrient intake for the client. The former requires a knowledge of the sources of food composition data and skills in using such information; the latter requires intelligent and thoughtful decisions. The properly executed diet history is a vital component of the assessment process in client-centered nutritional counseling, as well as in provision of nutrient sources to clients.

CITED REFERENCES

1. Hsu, N., and Gormican, A. The computer in retrieving dietary history data. II. Retrieving information by summary generation. *J. Am. Dietet. A.* 63:402, 1973.

2. Young, C. M. The therapeutic dietitian—a challenge for cooperation. *J. Am. Dietet. A.* 47:96, 1965.

3. Christakis, G., Ed. Nutritional assessment in health programs. *Am. J. Publ. Health* 63: Nov. 1973 Suppl.:1, 1973.

4. *WHO Report of Expert Committee on Medical Assessment of Nutritional Status.* World Health Organ. Tech. Rep't. Series No. 258, 1963.

5. Becker, R. C., Indik, B. P., and Beeuwkes, A. M. *Dietary Intake Methodologies—A Review.* Tech. Rep't. 03188-2T. Ann Arbor: Univ. Mich. School Publ. Health, 1960.

6. Young, C. M., and Trulson, M. F. Methodology for dietary studies in epidemiological surveys. 2. Strengths and weaknesses of existing methods. *Am. J. Publ. Health* 50:803, 1960.

7. Youland, D. M., and Engle, A. Practices and problems in HANES. Dietary data methodology. *J. Am. Dietet. A.* 68:22, 1976.

8. Moore, M. C., Judlin, B.C., and Kennemar, P. McA. Using graduated food models in taking dietary histories. *J. Am. Dietet. A.* 51:447, 1967.

9. Campbell, V. A., and Dodds, M. L. Collecting dietary information from groups of older people. Limitations of the 24-hr. recall. *J. Am. Dietet. A.* 51:29, 1967.

10. Madden, J. P., Goodman, S. J., and Guthrie, H.A. Validity of the 24-hr. recall. Analysis of data obtained from elderly subjects. *J. Am. Dietet. A.* 68:143, 1976.

11. Beal, V.A. The nutritional history in longitudinal research. *J. Am. Dietet. A.* 51:426, 1967.

12. Snowman, M. K. Nutrition component in a comprehensive child development program. II. Nutrient intakes of low-income, pregnant women and the outcome of pregnancy. *J. Am. Dietet. A.* 74:124, 1979.

13. Balogh, M., Kahn, H. H., and Medalie, J. H. Random repeat 24-hour dietary recalls. *Am. J. Clin. Nutr.* 24:304, 1971.

14. Armstrong, H. Nutritional status of black preschool children in Mississippi. Assessment by food frequency scale. *J. Am. Dietet. A.* 66:488, 1975.

15. Burke, B.S. The dietary history as a tool in research. *J. Am. Dietet. A.* 23:1041, 1947.

16. Blecha, E. E. Dietary study methods. IV. The dietary history for use in diet therapy. *J. Am. Dietet. A.* 27:968, 1951.

17. Mann, G. V., Pearson, G. Gordon, T., and Dawber, T. R. Diet and cardiovascular disease in the Framingham study. I. Measurement of dietary intake. *Am. J. Clin. Nutr.* 11:200, 1962.

18. Maternal and Child Health Unit, California Department of Health. *Nutrition During Pregnancy and Lactation.* Rev. Ed. Sacramento: Calif. Dept. Health, 1975.

19. Browe, J. H., Gofstein, R. M., Morlley, D. M., and McCarthy, M. C. Diet and heart disease study in the Cardiovascular Health Center. 1. A questionnaire and its application in assessing dietary intake. *J. Am. Dietet. A.* 48:95, 1966.

20. Kaufman, M. A food preference questionnaire for counseling patients with Diabetes. *J. Am. Dietet. A.* 49:31, 1966.

21. Evans, S. N., and Gormican, A. The computer in retrieving dietary history data. I. Designing and evaluating a computerized diabetic dietary history. *J. Am. Dietet. A.* 63:397, 1973.

22. Witschi, J., Porter, D., Vogel, S., Buxbaum, R., Stare, F. J., and Slack, W. A computer-based dietary counseling system. *J. Am. Dietet. A.* 69:385, 1976.

23. Hunt, I. F., Luke, L. S., Murphy, N. J., Clark, V. A., and Coulson, A. H. Nutrient estimates from computerized questionnaires vs. 24-hr. recall interviews. *J. Am. Dietet. A.* 74:656, 1979.

24. Eppright, E. S., Patton, M.B., Marlatt, A. L., and Hathaway, M. L. Some problems in collecting dietary information about groups of children. *J. Am. Dietet. A.* 28:43, 1952.

25. Flores, M. Dietary studies for assessment of the nutritional status of populations in nonmodernized societies. *Am. J. Clin. Nutr.* 11:344, 1962.

26. Consumer and Food Econ. Res. Div., Agric. Res. Serv. *Food Consumption of Households in the United States, Spring, 1965. Household Food Consumption Survey, 1965-66,* Rep't No. 1. Washington: U.S. Dept. Agric., 1968.

27. Hankin, J. H., and Huenemann, R. L. A short dietary method for epidemiologic studies. I. Developing standard methods for interpreting seven-day measured food records. *J. Am. Dietet. A.* 50:487, 1967.

28. Hankin, J. H., Rhoads, G. G., and Glober, G. A. A dietary method for an epidemiologic study of gastrointestinal cancer. *Am. J. Clin. Nutr.* 28:1055, 1975.

29. Grotkowski, M. L., and Sims, L. S. Nutritional knowledge, attitudes, and dietary practices of the elderly. *J. Am. Dietet. A.* 72:499, 1978.

30. Kerry, E., Crispin, S., Fox, H. M., and Kies, C. Nutritional status of preschool children. Dietary and biochemical findings. *Am. J. Clin. Nutr.* 21:1274, 1968.

31. Owen, G. M., and Kram, K. Nutritional status of preschool children in Mississippi. Food sources of nutrients in the diets. *J. Am. Dietet. A.* 54:490, 1969.

32. Chalmers, F. W., Clayton, M. M., Gates, L. O., Tucker, R. E., Wertz, A. W., Young, C. M., and Foster, W. D. The dietary record—how many and which days? *J. Am. Dietet. A.* 28:711, 1952.

33. Kelsay, J. L. A compendium of nutritional status studies and dietary evaluation studies conducted in the United States, 1957–1967. *J. Nutr.* 99: Supp. I, Part II: 123, 1969.

34. Trulson, M. F. Assessment of dietary study methods. I. Comparison of methods for obtaining data for clinical work. *J. Am. Dietet. A.* 30:991, 1954.

35. Trulson, M. F. Assessment of dietary study methods. II. Variability of eating practices and determination of sample size and duration of dietary surveys. *J. Am. Dietet. A.* 31:797, 1955.

36. Young, C. M., Chalmers, F. W., Church, H. N., Clayton, M. M., Tucker, R. E., Wertz, A. W., and Foster, W. D. A comparison of dietary study methods. 1. Dietary history vs. seven-day-record. *J. Am. Dietet. A.* 28:124, 1952.

37. Young, C. M., Hagan, G. C., Tucker, R. E., and Foster, W. D. A comparison of dietary study methods. 2. Dietary history vs. seven-day-record vs. 24-hr. recall. *J. Am. Dietet. A.* 28:218, 1952.

38. Young, C. M., Franklin, R. E., Foster, W. D., and Steele, B. F. Weekly variation in nutrient intake of young adults. *J. Am. Dietet. A.* 29:459, 1953.

39. Marr, J. W. Dietary survey methods: Individual and group aspects. *Proc. Roy. Soc. Med.* 66:639, 1973.

40. Adelson, S. F. Some problems in collecting dietary data from individuals. *J. Am. Dietet. A.* 36:453, 1960.

41. Gersovitz, M., Madden, J. P., and Smiciklas-Wright, H. Validity of the 24-hr. dietary recall and seven-day-record for group comparisons. *J. Am. Dietet. A.* 73:48, 1978.

42. Gifft, H. H., Washbon, M. B., and Harrison, G. G. *Nutrition, Behavior, and Change*. Englewood Cliffs, NJ: Prentice-Hall, Inc., 1972.

43. Foley, C., Hertzler, A. A., and Anderson, H. L. Attitudes and food habits—a review. *J. Am. Dietet. A.* 75:13, 1979.

44. Wilson, C. S., Ed. Food—Custom and Nurture. An annotated bibliography on sociocultural and biocultural aspects of Nutrition. *J. Nutr. Ed.* 11: Supp. 1:211, 1979.

SUGGESTED REFERENCES

Baird, P. C., and Schutz, H. G. Life style correlates of dietary and biochemical measures of nutrition. *J. Am. Dietet. A.* 76:228, 1980.

Beaton, G. H., Milner, J., Corey, P., McGuire, V., Cousins, M., Stewart, E., de Ramos, M., Hewitt, D., Grambsch, P. V., Kassim, M., and Little, J. A. Sources of variance in 24-hour dietary recall data: Implications for nutrition study design and interpretation. *Am. J. Clin. Nutr.* 32:2546, 1979.

Bowering, J. Morrison, M. A., Lowenberg, R. L., and Tirado, N. Evaluating 24-hr. dietary recalls. *J. Nutr. Ed.* 9:20, 1977.

Bryan, A. H., and Anderson, E. L. Retrospective dietary interviewing. A technique. *J. Am. Dietet. A.* 37:558, 1960.

Christakis, G. How to make a nutritional diagnosis without really trying. A. Adult nutritional diagnosis. *J. Fla. Med. A.* 66:349, 1979.

Epstein, L. M., Reshef, A., Abramson, J. H., and Bialik, O. Validity of a short dietary questionnaire. *Israel J. Med. Sci.* 6:589, 1970.

Huenemann, R. L. Interpretation of nutritional status. *J. Am. Dietet. A.* 63:123, 1973.

Kafatos, A. G. How to make a nutritional diagnosis without really trying. B. Pediatric nutritional diagnosis. *J. Fla. Med. A.* 66:356, 1979.

Lowenberg, M. E., Todhunter, E. N., Wilson, E. D., Savage, J. R., and Lubawski, J. L. *Food and People*. 3rd. Ed. New York: John Wiley and Sons, Inc., 1979.

Räsänen, L. Nutrition survey of Finnish rural children. VI. Methodological study comparing the 24-hour recall and the dietary history interview. *Am. J. Clin. Nutr.* 32:2560, 1979.

Reaburn, J. A., Krondl, M., and Lau, D. Social determinants in food selection. *J. Am. Dietet. A.* 74:637, 1979.

Report of the Committee on Food Habits. *The Problem of Changing Food Habits*. Nat'l. Res. Coun. Bull. 108. Washington: Nat'l. Aca. Sci., 1943.

Report of the Committee on Food Habits. *Manual for the Study of Food Habits*. Nat'l. Res. Coun. Bull. 111. Washington: Nat'l. Aca. Sci., 1945.

Rhee, K. S., and Stubbs, A. C. Health food users in two Texas cities. Nutritional and socioeconomic implications. *J. Am. Dietet. A.* 68:542, 1976.

Schafer, R. B. Factors affecting food behavior and the quality of husbands' and wives' diets. *J. Am. Dietet. A.* 72:138, 1978.

Slack, W., Porter, D. Witschi, J., Sullivan, M., Buxbaum, R., and Stare, F. J. Dietary interviewing by computer. An experimental approach to counseling. *J. Am. Dietet. A.* 69:514, 1976.

The validity of 24-hour dietary recalls. *Nutr. Rev.* 34:310, 1976.

7
The Scientific Literature

We like to think of exploring in science as a lonely, medi-
tative business, and so it is in the first stages, but always,
sooner or later, before the enterprise reaches completion,
as we explore, we call to each other, communicate, publish,
send letters to the editor, present papers, cry out on finding.

Lewis Thomas, **The Lives of a Cell: Notes**
of a Biology Watcher (New York: The
Viking Press, 1974).

The daily practice of clinical dietitians is enhanced by a working knowledge of recent advances in the discipline of nutrition, in other sciences,
and in the applied fields of dietetics, education, health care, and so on.
Keeping abreast of the literature is virtually a full-time occupation,
but is nonetheless a primary responsibility of all clinicians.

There are two major activities associated with literature use, which
will be examined in this chapter. The first of these is the *discovery* or
unearthing of the sources of literature appropriate for clinical practice—where does the clinical dietitian look for written communications
on the subjects of interest? The second activity follows the first, and
is the *understanding* of what is read—how does the clinical dietitian
interpret, evaluate, and apply what is read? We shall attempt to examine these activities from the perspective of client-centered care. The
objective of the planning component of clinical practice is to plan—
either *with* the client (as in preventive or maintenance care) or *for* the
client (as in a health crisis)—those strategies and resources that permit

the achievement of mutually derived goals. The clinician maintains or increases his expertise in the planning phase through effective and continual use of the literature.[2]

SEARCHING THE LITERATURE*

There are few published guides to actually performing a search of the literature,[3–5] but seemingly endless sources of abstracts, reviews, research reports, commentaries, theses, and bibliographies housed in every quality library. The most successful approach to a literature search is first to establish the limits of the topic of interest, and then proceed to the many available guides to current literature.

One helpful guide to establishing topic limits, or finding key words for use in mechanized retrieval systems is *A Guide to Nutrition Terminology for Indexing and Retrieval*. Although the publication was ". . . prepared as a resource for those who are responsible for indexing, storage and retrieval of information in the broad field of nutrition"[6] (p. 1), it is useful for the systematic development of finite topic areas. The guide is designed to be compatible with the listing of topics appearing in *Index Medicus*.[7]

Once the topic is well defined, the clinician's next step is to search the guides to the periodical literature. There are a variety of useful resources, the first of which is abstracting services. Abstracts themselves are concise statements of the salient features of a journal paper, usually indicating the importance of the reported work. The abstract serves the purpose of assisting the clinician to select papers of interest, which then should be read in the original publications. A listing of pertinent abstracting services may be found in Appendix G.

A second general source of information leading eventually to the original literature is the index service. Unlike the abstract, the index is designed as a compilation of article listings focusing on particular topics or key words. Included in this category is the important publication of the National Library of Medicine, *Index Medicus*.[7] *Index Medicus* is a compilation of over 2600 journal titles[8] and, more recently, selected monographs,[9] a feat accomplished by technical innovations in data storage and retrieval systems. The major section of the index is the subject heading listing; under each such heading are found the authors and titles of papers pertaining to that subject. The names of

* This section was reviewed and written, in part, by M. Cherie Haitz, M.S., of the New England Regional Medical Library Service (Region I), Francis A. Countway Library of Medicine, Boston.

the journals listed in *Index Medicus* are cited in the publication, *List of Journals Indexed in Index Medicus*.[9] The alphabetical listing of topics used in the *Index Medicus* is published in the index itself, and also as a separate document by the National Library of Medicine and is called *Medical Subject Headings (MeSH)*.[10] It can be used when attempting to explore the topic headings that are available prior to an *Index Medicus* search. *Index Medicus* is used extensively in the health disciplines as a reliable guide to the orderly searching of biomedical literature. An annual compilation of the information found in *Index Medicus* is published under the title of *Cumulated Index Medicus*.

Two other important indexes are the publications, *Hospital Literature Index* and *Science Citation Index*. The former is a publication of the American Hospital Association and includes many journal titles not found in *Index Medicus*. Since 1978, *HLI* has been produced in cooperation with the National Library of Medicine. Its subject headings, therefore, conform to *MeSH*, which has been expanded to accommodate this literature. *Science Citation Index* is a unique service, in that it is keyed according to references rather than topical words. A primary reference is followed in each instance by the list of papers that have cited that particular article. The object of this arrangement is to lead the reader from a key article to other articles that have referred to it, on the assumption that they will be relevant.[8]

Current Contents is yet another publication designed to lead readers to the original literature. Although it is used primarily by researchers, it is of great help to clinicians in keeping abreast of new papers. This publication, shaped like a pocket-sized popular magazine, actually reproduces the tables of contents of hundreds of journals. As such, it is not an index, but is considered to be a "Current Awareness" source.[11] There are six separate editions of *Current Contents*, each having its own title and distinct areas of interest. Appendix H lists the indexing and *Current Contents* services relevant to the daily practice of clinical dietetics.

Clinicians will frequently make use of the literature for the primary purpose of surveying a number of journals just to see what is being published. As the reader well knows, there are virtually dozens of journals that publish papers of interest to clinical dietitians. The most important publication in the field is *The Journal of The American Dietetic Association*, which is issued monthly by the parent organization, The American Dietetic Association. The journal contains not only original communications, but commentaries on practice, association news and announcements, and periodical, film, and book reviews. Many other journals, published by a variety of professional societies and publishing companies, contain papers that are applicable to clinical dietetics. For a more comprehensive listing of journals, the clinician should consult *Ulrich's International Periodicals Directory*.[12] This reference is arranged according to disciplines; Nutrition and Dietetics is one of the many categories listed. Each category is cross-indexed with related disciplines.

There are, of course, many other sources of information that are useful to the clinician. These include reference books, theses, research reports, bibliographies, reviews, dictionaries, directories, reports of congresses, and so on. The reader is directed to use the services of the reference librarian, a most valuable human resource for finding the appropriate literature.

Readers' services librarians can also be most helpful when a mechanized search of the literature is warranted. Such retrieval systems are invaluable aids to literature surveys, as they save countless hours of time and effort. The librarian's role in such searches is to assist the reader in specifically defining the topic and then suggesting the appropriate means of search.

One of the most widely used on-line network of data bases in the United States today is MEDLARS* (Medical Literature Analysis and Retrieval System), the automated searching and printing program of the National Library of Medicine[13]. It contains over 4,500,000 references to journal articles and books in the field of biomedicine published after 1965. MEDLARS now encompasses 16 data bases or files; the largest and most frequently used is MEDLINE (*MED*lars on-*LINE*). This file is a compilation of bibliographic materials found in *Index Medicus, Index to Dental Literature*, and *International Nursing Index*.

Access to computerized literature searching has grown from MEDLARS availability only at large academic medical centers in 1970 to the present diversified network of over 1000 on-line centers in community hospitals, industry, and specialized information centers. If this service is not available locally, clinicians may contact any of the 11 Regional Medical Libraries who handle search requests (see Appendix I for a listing of Regional Medical Libraries).

In addition, a number of other mechanized retrieval systems are available in libraries throughout the country. Such systems include data bases from MEDLARS, Biological Abstracts, Psychological Abstracts, ERIC (Educational Resources Information Center), and the National Agricultural Library (NAL). Still other mechanized systems use data bases from Chemical Abstracts, Institute for Scientific Infor-

---

* A registered acronym.

mation, Excerpta Medica System, and Smithsonian Science Information Exchange.[4] In all cases, the relevance of what is issued by the
retrieval system is determined by the careful selection of the key words
to be searched.

Once the literature search is begun in earnest, a major activity of
organization begins. There is nothing so frustrating or wasteful of time
as going back through journal after journal trying to find that one
particular statement that was of interest 2 months ago. Thus, the
clinician must develop those bibliographical habits that will keep his
literature efforts relatively well organized. This is as true of the ongoing perusal activity as for the in-depth literature search.

There are a number of ways in which literature information may be
stored. Taylor demonstrated a technique that is useful when the focus
of attention is on a particular indexing or abstracting service.[5] In that
method, the years of publication of the service (going back to any
desired date) are listed across a 5 × 8 card, with the key subject
headings listed vertically. Then, once a particular year is reviewed for
those key headings, a check is made on the card indicating that all
titles of interest have been duly noted on a "to-be-read" list. This
method is extremely useful for an organized search with very well-
defined limits.

When the clinician finds a paper of interest, the next step is to make
a citation card for it. The best plan is always to prepare the card
immediately, as if it were to be given to a typist for the preparation
of a citation list of a paper or thesis or even a book! A very useful
scientific style of citation listings is given in the section "Guidelines
for Authors," found in the first issue of each volume of *The Journal
of The American Dietetic Association.* There, examples of citation styles
for periodical articles, books, citations from compilations or books of
readings, bulletins or books in a numbered series, and theses are demonstrated. A more comprehensive guide for form and style both of
citation listings and papers themselves is that published by the Council
of Biology Editors, the *CBE Style Manual.*[14]

The citation may be recorded on a 3 × 5 card; notes about the paper
may be made on a 4 × 6 or larger card. An alternate method is to
record both the citation and desired information on the same card. The
advantage to the former system is that the cards may be quickly filed,
given to a typist, or shuffled about easily while preparing a listing.
The disadvantage is that both the small and large cards must be carefully coded so that inadvertent mixing of titles and comments does not
occur.

In the event that a paper does not contain useful information, the reader should prepare a citation card for it anyway. Then, on the bottom of the card, the notation "not useful" should be made, along with a statement of the reason for rejection. This will also save the clinician time when he forgets that he has already examined a paper and spends more time finding and reading it again.

As the number of citation cards grows, the clinician must face the next organizational problem, filing. The most appropriate method of filing is to sort the cards according to subject matter; the *Medical Subject Headings (MeSH)* publication is a useful tool in designing a filing system. Some clinicians may wish to devise their own system or use that suggested by Todhunter.[6] Each of these systems requires frequent duplication of cards for cross-filing purposes, since papers often focus on more than one topic.

A filing system for reprints may be devised along similar lines; papers may be filed according to subject headings. The problem of multiple topics is not easily solved, however. A good method, designed to avoid the problem of "losing" papers in filing systems, is to number them consecutively as they are received. The number is then simply marked on the citation card(s) and the paper filed in numerical order.

Searching the literature is sometimes tedious and sometimes frustrating, but is *always* useful to the clinical dietitian in his practice. Understanding what is read and then making the appropriate application are the more difficult tasks of the practitioner.

UNDERSTANDING THE LITERATURE

Innumerable kinds of communications are published in the journals that appeal to the clinical dietitian. Commentaries on a wide variety of clinical practice subjects are frequently seen. They are not "true" reports of research activities, but may be accounts of new ways to deal with old problems, insights gained through observations made in clinical practice, or even editorial remarks about the state of the art. The commentary paper is written primarily to give notice to practitioners that the author has something to say about a specific topic.

A research report, in contrast, is an article written at the conclusion of an experiment that was designed, hopefully, to answer a very specific question. There are nearly as many ways of conducting an experiment as there are scientific disciplines. Research in the field of psychology, for example, often requires very different techniques than those applied in food science. Basic to all disciplines, however, is the assumption that the investigator begins the experiment with no preconceived ideas about the outcome; his biases are put aside so that he may proceed with the work in a fair and nonprejudicial manner.

In the first of a series of excellent papers, Ethridge and McSweeney deal with varying types of research in one health discipline.[15] They describe three distinct kinds, analytic, descriptive, and experimental, which are shown in Table 7.1. In this chapter, the attention of the reader will be directed to the type of research labeled by Ethridge and McSweeney as "experimental," since basic nutrition experimentation tends to follow along those classic lines.

Perhaps the most simplistic approach to evaluating and interpreting the scientific literature is to examine the basic components of a research paper. The major sections of such papers usually include:

Introduction
    A statement of purpose
    The statement of the problem
    The hypothesis
    Review of literature
Methodology
    Methods
    Materials
Results
    Presentation of data
    Analysis of data
Discussion
    Meaning of the results
    Inadequacies, if any, of the study
    Conclusions
Summary
    A brief overview of the study problem,
        methods and results
Conclusions (if not in discussion section)

Not every paper will contain each section listed above; some will merge the results and the discussion sections, while others will begin with an abstract that replaces the summary. In general, the clinician should approach each new paper to be read with the expectation that there will be a degree of order that enables him to understand what is being reported.[16]

TABLE 7.1   Types of Research in Relation to Types of Conclusions Reached

Types of Research	Purpose	Types of Conclusions Reached
Analytic	To arrive at relationships through deduction	Points out assumptions and possible consequences of proposed changes; useful in establishing criteria
Descriptive	To describe existing conditions	Presents an objective analysis of the conditions studied, showing correlation or significant relationships
Experimental	To test causal relationships	Shows the effect of systematically varying conditions of experimental and control groups

NOTE: Reprinted by permission of the publisher from "Research in occupational therapy. I. Introduction," by D. A. Ethridge and M. McSweeney (*Am. J. Occup. Ther.* 24:490, 1970).

Components of a Research Paper

Introduction.   The first section of a research paper, the introduction, tells what the study is about and why it was done (the statement of purpose). The introduction should contain a very well defined statement of the problem investigated, which indicates to the reader immediately what he is about to learn. The statement of the problem may also contain the hypothesis, which is the expectation of the research outcomes.[17]

The hypothesis statement may take one of two forms. A *null* hypothesis states that there is no difference between groups X and Y when X and Y are treated differently. In classic experimental research, the null hypothesis supposes that, given two groups of subjects,* applying a special treatment to one will cause no difference in the outcome measure between the two.[18] Assume for a moment that the researcher wanted to study the effects of a specific drug on the levels of glucose in the blood. The two groups, X (control) and Y (experimental), are selected (by a very carefully designated process, we might add); they are known to be alike in all characteristics that have any bearing

* Subjects may be humans, experimental animals, plants, or any other objects of interest.

on blood glucose levels. One group (Y) is given the drug, while the other (X) is not. Blood samples are drawn from each subject at specified times and the glucose levels measured and compared statistically. In this example, the null hypothesis states that there is no difference between the blood glucose levels of groups X and Y, even though Y is given a particular drug. If this statement turns out to be statistically true, then the researcher accepts the null hypothesis, rejects the drug as a way of manipulating blood glucose levels, and goes back to the drawing boards. If, however, there is a difference in the levels, the researcher rejects the null hypothesis and accepts the *alternate* hypothesis, which states that there is a difference between groups X and Y when the drug of interest is administered to Y. The hypothesis is simply a restatement of the research problem in terms which indicate the anticipated terminal behaviors of the subjects.[19]

The introductory section will also contain the review of the literature pertinent to the research problem. This review will summarize those findings reported previously by the author or other workers in the field. The importance of a literature examination is underscored by Ziman:

> *Scientific papers are derivative, and very largely unoriginal, because they lean heavily on previous research. The evidence for this is plain to see, in the long list of citations that must always be published with every new contribution. These citations not only vouch for the authority and relevance of the statements that they are called upon to support; they embed the whole work in a context of previous achievements and current aspirations. It is very rare to find a reputable paper that contains no references to other research. Indeed, one relies on the citations to show its place in the whole scientific structure, just as one relies on a man's kinship affiliations to show his place in the tribe. All this becomes perfectly natural and proper once one has accepted that normal science is a highly cooperative activity, the corporate product of a vast social institution, rather than a series of individual forays into the unknown.[20]*
> *(p. 318)*

The literature review, an integral component of the introduction, helps to set the stage for the present research problem and provides the rationale for the execution of the study.

Methodology. The second section of a research paper usually contains the statements pertaining to the research design, the plan of execution of the study. Included in such discussions are some details of both the methods and the materials employed for the collection and analysis of the data.

Many kinds of study designs may be used for experimental research, and for the other two types, analytic and descriptive, as well. The design of an individual study must be very specific, as it represents the means by which the hypothesis is to be tested. Guides to planning research designs are available for both the biologic and social sciences, especially the latter.[21-24] Two of the most important characteristics for any research design, regardless of the nature of the problem being explored, are those of reliability and validity.

The term reliability describes the likelihood that the research results are capable of being reproduced (often by another investigator) if the same measuring procedures are applied under similar experimental conditions.[25] When we say that the results are reliable, we mean that those descriptive statements made about the "sample" (the subjects under study) are also applicable to the "target population" (the special group that the sample represents). A major consideration in evaluating the methodology of a study is whether the size of the sample (the number of subjects) is really large enough to merit generalizations and conclusions about the target population of interest.[17]

How the sample was selected is also of concern: the "random" selection of subjects advances the value of the outcome measurements in terms of the probability that the same results would be obtained if another sample was selected from the target population.[26] One of the major problems encountered in working with human subjects, however, is the availability of qualified persons willing and able to participate in the experiment.[27] Investigators reporting results obtained from studies using subjects not randomly selected must carefully define the limitations of their conclusions. The reader, therefore, should examine closely the number of subjects[28] and how they were recruited. *This is a crucial point in the translation of theory into practice.*

The second characteristic of interest, "validity," depicts the likelihood that the outcome measures truly reflect the status of the phenomenon being observed.[25] That is, the term validity is used to describe the actual relationship between what we *believe* is being observed (measured) and what is *actually* being observed. Factors influencing the validity of a study include the measurement methods (e.g., specific laboratory procedures, biologic or social), the time period of the experiment, sample or data storage, and so on. How valid an experiment is depends on the manner in which the methods of assessment actually depict the reality of the problem under study. Ethridge and McSweeney make the point that "Validity is associated with the question, 'Does this instrument measure the trait of interest in its entirety and to the exclusion of other traits,' while reliability deals with the question of 'How consistently is the trait measured by the instrument?'"[29] (p. 93). In our discussions, the term instrument means measuring procedure, while trait is the same as phenomenon or research result.

In the methods section, then, the reader should expect to find an adequate description of the ways the subjects were selected; how the data were collected and assembled; the tools of data evaluation (hypothesis testing); and, in some cases, the hardware (computer systems) employed for the statistical evaluation.

Results.   The next phase of the research paper should contain the sections devoted to the presentation and evaluation of the data. If those paragraphs also contain interpretations of the meanings of the results, the section should be labeled "results and discussion." In our view, it is easier to prepare and to read such a section where interpretation is an integral part of the data presentation.

The results may be presented in a variety of ways. Measurements representing raw data (untreated empiric results) or measures of central tendency (mean, mode, median) can be expressed in tables, figures, charts, graphs, or by other visual means. Such presentations may be handicapped when the sample is large or the number of measurements great, simply because of the problem of economy of space and the limitations imposed on interpretation of the real meaning of the data. In most cases, with the advantages afforded to researchers by technologic advances in data evaluation, appropriate statistics will be employed to expedite the process of hypothesis testing.

At this juncture the authors feel compelled to point out that these pages do not represent a treatise on statistics, or even an attempt to convey some of the basic principles. There are a number of publications on the subject, ranging from the elementary[18] to the advanced,[30] which better serve the needs of clinicians wishing (or needing!) to understand this branch of mathematics. Nonetheless, a discussion of the terms "significant" and "highly significant" is in order.

When an investigator is in the planning stages of a research project, he usually chooses the statistic(s) to be employed in the evaluation of the data at that time. (Hopefully, he seeks out the services of a statistician to help him). In doing so, he also chooses the *level of significance* at which he will reject the null hypothesis.[31] That is, the investigator selects, ahead of time, the probability level (a real number) at which a true null hypothesis will be rejected. The most common probability level selected by nutrition researchers is p (for probability) ≤ 0.05.

Thus, if $p \leq 0.05$ *and* if the statistic indicates the null hypothesis is not true, the alternate hypothesis is accepted and the results are said to be "significant." Furthermore, if $p \leq 0.01$ and the alternate hypothesis is accepted, it is customary to say that the results are "highly significant." As the reader can see, by setting the probability level low, the chance of rejecting a null hypothesis that is true is considerably reduced.* This is a definite advantage in many situations, but places restrictions on what may be said about the data.

In the language of statistics, rejecting a true null hypothesis is called a "Type I" error; accepting a false null hypothesis is a "Type II" error.[18] By setting the probability level quite low, the investigator reduces his chances of making a Type I error while *at the same time* he increases his chances of making a Type II error. These concepts are demonstrated in Table 7.2. Recall, for a moment, the investigator working with a drug that he suspects may have an effect on blood glucose levels. The hypotheses are written as follows:

Null hypothesis (H_0): There is *no* difference in the blood glucose levels of two groups of subjects when one group is given a particular drug.

Alternate hypothesis (H_A): There *is* a difference in the blood glucose levels of two groups of subjects when one group is given a particular drug.

TABLE 7.2   Type I and Type II Errors

		Decision	
		Reject	Accept
Null	True	Type I error	Correct
Hypothesis	False	Correct	Type II error

SOURCE: John L. Phillips, Jr., *Statistical Thinking: A Structural Approach* (San Francisco: W. H. Freeman & Co., 1973).

Assume that these subjects all have a disease that affects their blood glucose levels. The results of making a Type I error are more serious in this case than those of a Type II error *if* all patients with the disease are given the drug, and *at the same time*, all other forms of treatment are omitted. Why? Because the drug is ineffective (remember, the H_0

* In this case, $p \leq 0.01$ is lower than $p \leq 0.05$, making it even less likely that the null hypothesis will be rejected.

was true, yet rejected) and the patients being treated with the drug are, in effect, receiving no treatment!

In this example, the results of making a Type II error are considerably less serious. Suppose the investigator's primary purpose in conducting the experiment was to find a drug that would be taken orally once a week, and would absolutely replace all other forms of therapy, some of which may involve daily administration of a hormone. The clinician will undoubtedly see that convenience is one of the primary features of this drug. If a Type II error is made, however, the subjects will not receive the convenient drug, but *will* continue their other forms of treatment, which are known to be effective in controlling blood sugar levels! The problems created by no treatment are, therefore, avoided, while what is lost is an item of convenience. What happens next is that eventually the investigator or someone else will repeat the study and, hopefully, come up with the right conclusions (depicted in the upper right or lower left corners of Table 7.2).

In any event, the levels of significance attached to the reporting of the results are helpful guides in understanding and interpreting the experiment. The clinician's responsibility in reading the results section of a research paper is to look for the *meaning* of data in their proper context.

Discussion.   This section of the research paper, if separate from the results section, should serve the purpose of comparing the results with those obtained by other workers. The review of literature is again featured in the paper as the similarities or diagreements between two or more experiments are compared.

The primary role of the discussion section is to allow the investigator to ". . . report, analyze, interpret, and draw conclusions from his findings"[17] (p. 175). In order for him to do so, the results section must be lucid and explicit. The writer, furthermore, has the opportunity in this section to point out the failings of the study, if such occurred (and they often do). The limitations of the experiment must be made perfectly clear! The reader has a right to know how he may use the information generated by the research. The clinician must recognize that while the investigator's *recommendations* are his suggestions about the applicability of the findings, the *conclusions* he reaches are his own judgments about the outcome of his work.[32]

Summary.   The summary section should contain no information not presented elsewhere in the research paper. It should be a clear and concise statement of the problem, the basic methodology, and the results. Successful writers realize that this section is read more than the other parts of the paper, so they go to great extremes to express their ideas clearly and explicitly here. In many journals today, the summary is replaced by an abstract which may appear at the beginning of the paper, just underneath the title, or in a separate abstract section of the journal.

Evaluation of a Research Paper

In 1978, Jacox and Prescott[33] published a paper for the nursing profession that details some of the major dimensions of a research report, underscoring areas where practitioners not educated in the actual conduct of research can and should judge clinical relevance. In that paper, the authors present some basic rules in the form of questions to which critical readers should respond:

> *Questions to Ask Yourself . . .*
>   *About the statement of the problem:*
>   *Is there a complete statement of the problem early in the report?*
>   *Is the problem placed within the context of a conceptual framework?*
>   *Are the concepts used in the study clearly defined?*
>   *Are the research questions and/or hypotheses clearly stated, directly related to the conceptual framework used, and testable?*
>   *Does the researcher relate the study to other relevant research?*
>   *About the research design:*
>   *Is the research-design approach clearly identified and appropriate for the problem being studied?*
>   *Are the population and sample clearly described, with the sampling plan identified?*
>   *Are the methods of data collection clearly described, including information about the data-collection instruments?*
>   *About the analysis of data and discussion of the study findings:*
>   *Is the data-analysis approach appropriate for the research question or hypothesis?*
>   *Are the findings or results of the study clearly presented?*
>   *Are the conclusions drawn supported by the study's findings?*[33]
>   *(p. 1884)*

Application of these questions to papers read by clinical dietitians can serve as a useful activity in literature evaluation.

SUMMARY

Reviewing the literature is an ongoing responsibility of the clinical dietitian. When the appropriate tools are available and utilized, it becomes an opportunity as well as a responsibility.

The efforts of the clinical dietitian to discover and understand the literature are rewarded when practice is enhanced by the introduction of new ideas and techniques in client-centered care. What is served are the best interests of the client, which is, after all, what we're about.

CITED REFERENCES

1. Thomas, L. *The Lives of a Cell: Notes of a Biology Watcher.* New York: The Viking Press, 1974.

2. Owen, A. L., and Owen, G. M. Training public health nutritionists: Competencies for complacency or future concerns. *Am. J. Pub. Health* 69:1096, 1979.

3. Baker, D. B. Communication or chaos? *Sci.* 169:739, 1970.

4. Beatty, W. K. Searching the literature and computerized services in medicine. Guides and methods for the clinician. *Ann. Int. Med.* 91:326, 1979.

5. Taylor, S. D. How to search the literature. *Am J. Nurs.* 74:1457, 1974.

6. Todhunter, E. N. *A Guide to Nutrition Terminology for Indexing and Retrieval.* Washington: Dept. Health, Educ. and Welfare, 1970.

7. *Index Medicus.* DHEW Publ No. (NIH) 80-252. Washington: National Library of Medicine, 1980.

8. Sutherland, F. M. Indexes, abstracts, bibliographies and reviews. *In* Morton, L. T., Ed. *Use of Medical Literature.* 2nd Ed. London: Butterworth and Co. (Publishers) Ltd., 1977.

9. *List of Journals Indexed in Index Medicus.* DHEW Publ. No. (NIH) 80-267. Washington: National Library of Medicine, 1980.

10. *Medical Subject Headings, 1980.* DHEW Publ. No. (NIH) 80-265. Washington: National Library of Medicine, 1980.

11. Dannatt, R. J. Primary sources of information. *In* Morton, L. T., Ed. *Use of Medical Literature.* 2nd Ed. London: Butterworth & Co. (Publishers) Ltd., 1977.

12. *Ulrich's International Periodicals Directory.* 18th Ed. New York: R. R. Bowker Co., 1979.

13. *MEDLARS: The Computerized Literature Retrieval Services of the National Library of Medicine.* DHEW Publ. No. (NIH) 80-1286. Washington: National Library of Medicine, 1980.

14. CBE Style Manual Committee. *Council of Biology Editors Style Manual: A Guide for Authors, Editors, and Publishers in the Biological Sciences.* 4th Ed. Arlington, VA: Council of Biology Editors, 1978.

15. Ethridge, D. A., and McSweeney, M. Research in occupational therapy. I. Introduction. *Am. J. Occ. Ther.* 24:490, 1970.

16. Ethridge, D. A., and McSweeney, M. Research in occupational therapy. VI. Research writing. *Am. J. Occ. Ther.* 25:210, 1971.

17. Fleming, J. W., and Hayter, J. Reading research reports critically. *Nurs. Out.* 22:172, 1974.

18. Phillips, J. L. *Statistical Thinking: A Structural Approach.* San Francisco: W. H. Freeman & Co., 1973.

19. Ethridge, D. A., and McSweeney, M. Research in occupational therapy. II. The hypothesis. *Am J. Occ. Ther.* 24:551, 1970.

20. Ziman, J. M. Information, communication, knowledge. *Nature* 224:318, 1969.

21. Ethridge, D. A., and McSweeney, M. Research in occupational therapy. III. Research design. *Am. J. Occ. Ther.* 25:24, 1971.

22. Campbell, D. T., and Stanley, J. C. *Experimental and Quasi-Experimental Designs for Research.* Chicago: Rand-McNally & Co., 1966.

23. Miller, D. C. *Handbook of Research Design and Social Measurement.* 3rd Ed. New York: David McKay Co., Inc., 1977.

24. Webb, E. J., Campbell, D. T. Schwartz, R. D., and Sechrest, L. *Unobtrusive Measures: Nonreactive Research in the Social Sciences.* Chicago: Rand-McNally & Co., 1966.

25. Enelow, A. J., and Swisher, S. N. *Interviewing and Patient Care.* 2nd Ed. New York: Oxford Univ. Press, 1979.

26. Weinstein, M. C. Allocation of subjects in medical experiments. *N. Eng. J. Med.* 291:1278, 1974.

27. Fruin, M. F. and Davison, M. L. Some considerations in the measurement of change. *J. Am. Dietet. A.* 73:15, 1978.

28. Garn, S. M., Shaw, H. A., Wainright, R. L. and McCabe, K. D. The effect of sample size on normative values. *Eco. Food Nutr.* 6:153, 1977.

29. Ethridge, D. A., and McSweeney, M. Research in occupational therapy. IV. Data collection and analysis. *Am. J. Occ. Ther.* 25:90, 1971.

30. Snedecor, G. W., and Cochran, W. G. *Statistical Methods.* 7th Ed. Ames, IA: The Iowa State Univ. Press, 1980.

31. Ethridge, D. A., and McSweeney, M. Research in occupational therapy. V. Data interpretation, results and conclusions. *Am. J. Occ. Ther.* 25:149, 1971.

32. Ward, M. J. and Fetler, M. E. Research Q & A. What guidelines should be followed in critically evaluating research reports? *Nurs. Res.* 28:120, 1979.

33. Jacox, A. and Prescott, P. Determining a study's relevance for clinical practice. *Am J. Nurs.* 78:1882, 1978.

SUGGESTED REFERENCES

Barber, B. The ethics of experimentation with human subjects. *Sci. Am.* 234:2:25, 1976.

Chernin, E. A worm's-eye view of biomedical journals. *Fed. Proc.* 34:124, 1975.

Davidoff, F. Medical therapies for Diabetes: Do they work? *J. Am. Dietet. A.* 71:495, 1977.

Day, R. A. *How to Write and Publish a Scientific Paper.* Philadelphia: ISI Press, 1979.

Fox, T. *Crisis in Communication: The Functions and Future of Medical Journals.* London: The Athlone Press, University of London, 1965.

Ingelfinger, F. J. Using the library without pain. *N. Eng. J. Med.* 290:460, 1974.

O'Connor, M., and Woodford, F. P. *Writing Scientific Papers in English.* New York: American Elsevier, 1975.

Sackett, D. L., and Gent, M. Controversy in counting and attributing events in clinical trials. *N. Eng. J. Med.* 301:1410, 1979.

Woodford, F. P. Sounder thinking through clearer writing. *Sci.* 156:743, 1967.

8

Instructional Resources

New procedures for instructional development place emphasis upon the need to consider alternative means of providing instruction and choosing from these alternatives on the basis of criteria which will maximize learning.

W. H. Levie and K. E. Dickie, *in* **Second Handbook of Research on Teaching** (Chicago: Rand-McNally & Co., 1973).

There is an axiom among educators that is well-founded, but not always followed: The more involved the learner can become in the learning process, the more effective the learning will be. Involvement increases with each sensory dimension experienced, as alluded to in the old adage, "I hear, I forget; I see, I remember; I do, I understand." Thus, the closer to reality an experience can be, the better it will be remembered. A real or concrete example will be recalled more readily than a representation such as a picture. In turn, representations will be remembered better than word descriptions.

Real experiences, requiring active participation on the part of the client, will be recalled better than those she only observed. There are a wide variety of representations, from movies that seem almost real, to still photos, to line drawings that may be difficult to interpret. There is a difference, however, in the power of those representations to be engraved on the memory. This difference depends on the proximity of the representation to a real experience.

Instructional technology is a relatively new discipline in the educational world. The history of its development has recorded many successes and failures, the latter stemming from the tendency to see a promising new development as a panacea. Failure has occurred, in part, from the expectation that technological advances could replace the human element in teaching. If all teachers do is give information, then books and technology can replace them. If, however, teachers are facilitators, motivators, and planners, then technology has its limitations. Thus, it is important to remember that instructional technology supplements rather than supplants the work of anyone involved in the instructional process.

The major resources of the technological field are hardware and software. Hardware includes the many varied pieces of equipment designed to deliver instruction or information such as projectors, computers, and recorders. Software is the specific instructional materials that are placed in or on the hardware. Software includes tapes, films, discs, or other materials containing instructional content. In addition, there is printed matter that does not require the use of hardware, the major resource of pretechnologic instruction.

HARDWARE AND RELATED SOFTWARE

There are many types of hardware and related software available for clinicians to consider in the planning and development of learning experiences. Such hardware and software may be readily accessible in a media center of the practice site, or available on loan from a local library or media center. If not, the purchase of such equipment and materials should be considered in terms of their cost/effectiveness in client care. The use of audiovisual equipment for basic information giving, repetitive learning, and even learner evaluation can free a clinician for more important aspects of human interaction, as well as increase the number of clients instructed.[2] Machines cannot respond to feelings, solve problems, or make decisions without human intervention. In these areas, a clinician's skills can best serve.

Projectors

A well known piece of hardware is the film projector designed to show 16mm films. Projectors have been around for a number of years, particularly in school systems. Newer models are automatically loaded and relatively easy to handle and operate. Although they may be used to show a film to one person, projectors are most frequently used to screen a movie for a large group. If used for individual viewing, films can be projected on a small screen (e.g., 18″ × 18″) in an individual learning booth called a carrel.

The software includes black and white, or color films. Films may be purchased, rented, or borrowed from a variety of sources.* The advantage of movies is that, along with television and video tapes, they are the closest to reality without being real. The disadvantage is their cost. Software (i.e., films) obtained from government sources, however, is frequently less expensive than materials produced by the private sector. To assist in identifying films and other software that are of high quality, the *Journal of Nutrition Education* publishes monthly critiques as a service to readers.

Another form of hardware is the filmstrip projector. Filmstrip projectors may vary from a simple, hand-operated unit to a totally automatic one that coordinates a cassette tape for sound with the filmstrip. These projectors are more effective for individuals and small groups, but may be used as the movie projector. Some models are especially designed for use in individual study carrels.

Film strips are less realistic than 16mm films or video tapes, but they are more versatile in use. A filmstrip can be used with the narrative presented *ad lib* by an instructor, or a prepared narrative can be recorded on a cassette tape or record for coordinated accompaniment to the filmstrip. Advantages include lower costs and the increased ability of the client to learn to handle the equipment, thus freeing the clinician from serving as an audiovisual technician. Another advantage of filmstrip technology is that strips may be made with fairly basic cameras and processed locally so that clinicians can develop their own filmstrips when commercial ones are not available to meet needs. Finally, filmstrip units can be assembled in a way that permits them to be started and stopped on command so that a learner can see a portion of the strip and then pause to do some paperwork or manipulation of materials before proceeding.

A very similar type of equipment is the slide projector, which uses 2 × 2 slides. These slides are the common household variety, allowing ready development by clinicians. Anyone with the ability to use a 35mm camera can prepare an instructional slide tape unit on his own,[3] but knowledge of some basic principles of artistic design and photographic know-how is helpful in developing quality slides.[4] An audiotape player unit can be attached to one or more slide projectors to

---

* The resource catalogues and professional journals listed at the end of the chapter provide an extensive review of sources and materials.

permit coordination of slides and tape for a sound-slide presentation. Such a mutlimedia unit is an excellent resource for individual study carrels and transportable learning units as well as for group projection. There are units available that, rather than projecting on a screen, include a built-in television-like screen for individual viewing. This type of unit is often fitted with earphones so that the user does not disturb others with the sound track.

A fourth type of projector is called the overhead projector. This tool is designed to be used either with transparencies or a special writing instrument permitting recording on a roller of transparent film. The major use of this sophisticated blackboard is to display illustrations of an oral presentation either prepared in advance, or drawn as the speaker presents. Overhead projectors are of limited value in individual instruction as the information source is required to be present. Thus, this type of hardware does not free the clinician from being the basic information giver.

Overhead projectors can be used where blackboards are not available; however, a screen of some sort is required. The advantage of this projector is that the speaker may write while facing the audience. The disadvantage is that it will usually hold less information than a blackboard.

Transparencies, the related software of overhead projectors, are sheets of clear film that are available in several colors. When run through a special copy machine with a master print, the machine will make a copy of the print on the film. The resultant sheets may then be encased in cardboard frames. Like other learning aids, transparencies should be pilot tested for ease of reading. A large audience will not be able to read standard typing or print. In addition, certain colors project better than others.

A less frequently used machine is the opaque projector. Its major use is to project images from an opaque object or surface, such as a book page. It may also be used to project relatively flat objects, such as coins or stamps. Generally, these machines are bulky and, with the prevalence of copy machines, the need for projection of a written page is not great. If available, however, an opaque projector could be a useful tool for certain instructional strategies such as projection of nutrition labels.

A sixth type of projector is designed to handle film loops. The loops are enclosed in cassettes, thus protecting the film from damage and making them more appropriate for learner handling. The projector is also simple to load. The film loops are usually very short, single concept films. They are continuous run, which means that, if the viewer stops in the middle of the film, the next viewer will begin at that point. There is no rewind or fast forward capacity; however, since film loops are usually short, this may be only a minor drawback.

Recorders

For audio instruction only, the tape recorder is a very common type of hardware. Audio recorders are available in many styles and sizes, such as reel-to-reel recorders and single unit cassette machines. There are also machines especially designed to make multiple tapes simultaneously and others that "mark" tapes with inaudible pulses that direct the recorder to operate slides or filmstrips automatically.

Audio recorders are excellent tools for use in interviewing or other interactive settings. When used in such encounters, clients must know that the recorder is "on." Furthermore, they must agree to the taping process and to the use of the material.* In addition, instructional tapes may be purchased or prepared by the clinician to meet his own special needs.

Another form of audiovisual hardware that is becoming more popular is the video-tape recorder. This type of equipment incorporates advantages of many other types of hardware. Video-tape images are animated, realistic, and frequently in color. The tapes may be made locally, "developed" immediately, and then projected at will. As desired, the recorders can be stopped and restarted, as well as rerun. The equipment can project on a large movie screen or be displayed on a television monitor. Individual viewers can also use earphones to eliminate sounds distracting to others.

Calculators and Computers

Calculators are another type of hardware that are helpful in instructional strategies. The small, portable calculator, now a common household item, is useful in teaching clients to calculate meal costs, unit pricing, recipe revision, caloric intake, and other calculations common to food and nutrition practices. Some calculators also perform metric conversions. Another type can be programmed to do nutrient analyses.[5]

The most sophisticated and expensive educational hardware available on a large scale is the computer.[6] Early computers were enormous complexes that often took up complete floors of office buildings. Over

---

* Written permission of the client will usually be required if the tapes are heard by persons other than the original interviewer/clinician.

time and with advancing technology, computers have become reduced in size, but are still permanent, expensive operations. Users may be located floors, blocks, or states away. To utilize the computer, the terminal, located at the user's site, hooks into the computer center via the telephone system. (The terminal is the instrument used to send and receive information to and from the computer.) As a phone call activates the system, the user must pay both for phone service and computer time, calculated by the minute. These computers can store vast quantities of data, however, and serve a large number of users.

Since large computers are unwieldy, very expensive, and have the capacity to provide for extensive use, they are not practicable for small business ownership and operation. In time, the minicomputer was developed, streamlined eventually to be the size of a large console television set. With its reduced price, size, and capacity, it became feasible for a small business, school, or other institution to purchase and operate its own minicomputer.[7] Such computers are small enough to be located on the premises, thus eliminating phone bills and computer time charges. All of the equipment, including a keyboard and processing unit, and a printer and/or display screen are housed on site. Minicomputer owners may need to employ a computer programmer either full time or as a contracted service if "canned" programs are unsuitable.

The newest member of the computer family is the microcomputer. With its appearance, computers have become practicable for personal and instructional use, appropriate for clinic, small office, or home. The microcomputer is composed of a typewriter-like keyboard and a television-like screen called a cathode ray tube (CRT) for information display. A tape recorder can be added to these basic units to permit the owner to design his own programs and "load" them. A printer can also be attached to permit paper recording of displayed information; other equipment can be added to make them even more versatile. Microcomputers are no larger than a 12" television screen and an electric typewriter, so they are quite portable and manageable. As a result, however, they have even less storage capacity than a minicomputer.

Computers can be used for a variety of purposes.[7] They have been demonstrated to be very effective instructional tools as they can play games, do calculations, give tests, convey information, and give immediate feedback. The learner sits at the terminal or keyboard and "talks" to the computer. The computer responds by "asking questions," giving information, accepting responses, and reacting to asnwers, with feedback on correctness.

The computer must be given directions on how to process input data. This is done in one of several ways, depending on the type of computer. Information and instructions that are typed on the keyboard may be stored on tape, punch cards, or discs. Prepared programs may be purchased ready to use (i.e., "canned"), or skilled programmers may be hired to design needed programs. With some instruction, laypersons can learn to program, particularly in some of the less complex computer languages such as BASIC, which is well adapted for the microcomputers and for educational purposes. With specially designed programs, known as nutrient data bases, the computer can analyze food intakes and menus.* They can also analyze, for example, a sample of written work for its reading level. In fact, there seems to be no end to what computers can perform, from artwork and calculus to diagnosing disease and problem solving.

The computer is able to perform all of these seemingly miraculous feats because some human wrote instructions for the machine, specifying exactly what she wants done. The instructions are called programs and the writers are programmers. Instructional programs can be very sophisticated, but require someone with programming skill to write them. The practitioner can benefit from knowing what computers can do and how to tell the programmer what he wants. If a computer and/or terminal is available to clinical dietitians at the practice site, the possibility of using that computer for instructional purposes should be investigated. With the advent of computer technology and its projected impact on society, every dietitian should be conversant with computer specialists.[8]

OTHER TYPES OF SOFTWARE

Not every effective instructional strategy requires hardware, expensive or not. Books, workbooks, and pamphlets have been around for a very long time and are often effective sources of information. Printed materials are not, however, the only or always the best means of providing information. Lack of understanding or fear of technology tends to cause overutilization of printed materials, frequently to the exclusion of other very effective instructional resources.

A recent modification of the workbook is a programmed instruction manual.[9,10] A workbook provides blanks to be completed, and occa-

---

* The major available data bases at present are designed for larger computer systems and thus contain too much information for the microcomputer. Undoubtedly, there will be a time in the near future when a base is prepared for the microcomputer.

sionally provides answers in the back. A programmed manual is designed to give immediate feedback (correction) as each response is recorded. In linear programming, the responses are progressive with planned repetition and cues. In a branched program, the answer a learner records determines the next question she is to answer or task she is to do. If she is correct, she may be directed to go to the next page. If not, she may be requested to read something or go back a page. Branched programs are designed to communicate specific information until the learner can demonstrate that she can provide suitable answers, at which point she is permitted to proceed. Branched programs are also adaptable to computerization. Programmed instruction can be effective in small doses, but it is not the panacea of learning that was proposed when it first made its appearance. (This is true of all instructional strategies.) As human beings thrive on variety and also have preferred learning styles, any one strategy will not be effective with all learners.

Charts and posters presenting nutrition information are useful and inexpensive (and sometimes free) resources. For example, a specialized set of nutrient content cards has been developed by the National Dairy Council. A more sophisticated form of cards utilizes the concept of nutrient density.[11]* These software tools are very useful in helping clients visualize and make decisions about food selection.

Both children and adults alike enjoy games, and there are numerous ones on the market related to nutrition.[12] Common games, as well, can be adapted to utilize nutritional content. One desirable element of learning games is the socialization they provide. Thus, learning is fun and acquired with less effort, as the required repetition is not boring with competition.

Puppetry is an excellent teaching medium for children. Puppet shows can be presented to children, clinicians can use the puppets to communicate directly with the child on a spontaneous, one-to-one basis, or the children themselves can develop their own show based on their learning about nutrition. This latter approach is based on the axiom that "teaching something is the best way to learn it."

Another effective instructional resource falls under the heading of models and realia. Remembering the value of learning with resources that approximate the real world, real materials or lifelike models are valuable tools to incorporate into instruction. Food models are available that approximate standard serving sizes. A small scale model grocery in a classroom or health care facility can be instructive, with

* To be discussed in Chapter 10.

real cans, boxes, and bottles displayed. Using the real world of a cafeteria or school lunchroom is also very useful.

Models are usually thought of as three dimensional visual replicas, but there are other models that are designed to enhance the learning of activities or skills. Such models may be drawn, as flowcharts or diagrams,[13] experienced as in role-playing (simulation) or in simulation games designed to replicate reality.[14] These models are the next best thing to experiencing reality and sometimes safer during the learning phase (i.e., the simulator for training jet pilots). Since the provision of reality experiences is frequently not within the province of the clinician, simulations can be structured in a teaching environment to ensure a fair degree of success in teaching clients.

SUMMARY

We do not presume to be all inclusive in this discussion of instructional resources. Our purpose is to convey some sense of the scope of instructional resources with the hope that clinicians will be curious about and desirous of using the most effective means of instruction for their clients.

CITED REFERENCES

1. Levie, W. H., and Dickie, K. E. The analysis and application of media. *In* Travers, R. M. W., Ed. *Second Handbook of Research on Teaching.* Chicago: Rand-McNally & Co., 1973.

2. Hutton, C. W., and Davidson, S. H. Self-instructional learning packages as a teaching/learning tool in dietetic education. *J. Am. Dietet. A.* 75:617, 1979.

3. Herrick, K. L., Scott, L. W., Weaver, F. J., Foreyt, J. P., and Gotto, A. M. Developing and evaluating audiovisual media for dietetic education. *J. Am. Dietet. A.* 73:660, 1978.

4. Am. Assoc. Agric. College Eds. *Communications Handbook.* 3rd Ed. Danville, IL: Interstate Printers & Publ., 1976.

5. Kee, B. L., and Kilby, M. E. Use of a programmable calculator for nutrient analysis. *J. Am. Dietet. A.* 72:571, 1978.

6. Wade, C. W., and Thiele, V. F. Computer-assisted instruction in a college nutrition course. *J. Nutr. Ed.* 5:246, 1973.

7. Willis, J. *Peanut Butter and Jelly Guide to Computers.* Portland, OR: dilithium Press, 1978.

8. Billings, K., and Moursand, D. *Are You Computer Literate?* Portland OR: dilithium Press, 1979.

9. Epsich, J. E., and Williams, B. *Developing Programmed Instructional Materials: A Handbook for Program Writers.* Palo Alto, CA: Fearon Publ., 1967.

10. Marino, M. A. Developing and testing a programmed instruction unit on PKU. *J. Am. Dietet. A.* 76:29, 1980.

11. Hansen, R. G., and Wyse, B. W. Expression of nutrient allowances per 1000 kilocalories. *J. Am. Dietet. A.* 76:223, 1980.

12. Zifferblatt, S. M., Wilbur, C. S., and Pinsky, J. L. Changing cafeteria eating habits. *J. Am. Dietet. A.* 76:15, 1980.

13. Monteith, M., and Nakagawa, A. A flow chart approach to nutritional screening and assessment in long term care facilities. *J. Am. Dietet. A.* 75:685, 1979.

14. Gillespie, P. H. *Learning Through Simulation Games.* New York: Paulist Press, 1973.

SUGGESTED REFERENCES

A Reference List of Audiovisual Materials Produced by the United States Government
    General Services Administration
    National Archives and Record Service
    National Audiovisual Center
    Washington, DC 20409

Audiovisual Resources in Food and Nutrition
    The Oryx Press
    2214 N. Central at Encanto
    Phoenix, AZ 85004

Catalog of Food and Nutrition Information and Educational Materials Center
    Food and Nutrition Information Center
    National Agricultural Library
    United States Department of Agriculture
    Room 304
    Beltsville, MD 20705

Index of Nutrition Education Materials
    Office of Education and Public Affairs
    The Nutrition Foundation, Inc.
    888 Seventeenth Street NW
    Washington, DC 20006

The print, film, and sound reviews of the *Journal of Nutrition Education* and the *Journal of The American Dietetic Association.*

PART
III
Process for Nutritional Counseling

9
A Systems Approach to Nutritional Care

*Counseling is not simply conveying set plans to clients
. . . counseling involves knowing clients' needs and developing strategies which enable them to meet those needs.*

Steven J. Danish, Mark R. Ginsberg, Ann
Terrell, Marian I. Hammond, and Simone O.
Adams, **The anatomy of a dietetic
counseling interview** (*J. Am. Dietet. A.*
75:626, 1979).

A systems approach is one of the most effective ways of achieving a goal. In clinical dietetic practice, the goal is quality nutritional care that has identifiable objectives leading toward the realization of that goal. Nutritional counseling, the process through which we work toward the goal, is expressed in these pages as a model utilizing a systems approach.

A systems approach is defined by several distinct attributes. First, a clearly identified change is described in a stated objective. In the system presented here, the subject is a human being who changes behavior as a result of entering the nutritional counseling system. Secondly, the system itself is developed by a task analysis, which carefully delineates the component parts and identifies the manner in which they are related to one another. Each step in the process is clearly stated, with information on how to progress to the following step. Thirdly, the system is designed to be responsive to feedback at a number of points, so that when evidence illustrates that the outcomes are not being achieved, it is relatively simple to identify and alter individual components without scrapping the whole system.[2]

AN OVERVIEW OF THE SYSTEM

A systems approach is based on a pattern of progression of related components that are implemented sequentially.[3] The components of the system employed here are:

1. *Assessment,* a gathering and analysis of the data related to the status of the subject prior to entering the system
2. *Planning,* a statement of the specific outcomes, a description of the strategies for achieving the stated outcomes, and a clear means of evaluating the outcomes and success of individual components
3. *Implementation,* the process of putting the plans into action
4. *Evaluation,* an examination of the results of implementation and the contribution of the system components to those results

To clarify these technical statements, a look at the implications for nutritional counseling is in order. The general system has been designed and is presented in Fig. 9.1. For each individual client and circumstance, a specific, personalized system is developed according

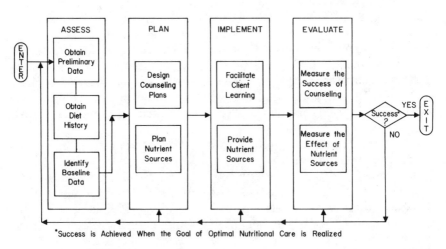

*Success is Achieved When the Goal of Optimal Nutritional Care is Realized

FIGURE 9.1   A model for the provision of nutritional care.

to the components of the general system. Activation of the system occurs when a client decides to "enter the system" (elect counseling). During the *assessment* phase, the practitioner must gather all relevant data about the client's present problem, including the behaviors that contribute to that problem. In the *planning* phase, a determination of the need for intervention is made. When this is accomplished, the counselor continues by writing a specific goal or outcome for client behavior. Then a selection of learning experiences that would best facilitate the behavior change must be identified. (Remember that learning is defined as a rather permanent change in behavior.) At the same time, arrangements must be made for evaluating learner achievement.

With the completion of tailoring the general system to a given client (planning), the step of *implementation* is begun by consulting with the client on the appropriateness of the plan. If the client was intimately involved in the interview process during the assessment phase, he should find only minor adjustments needed in the plan. The presentation of alternative plans allows the client the opportunity to feel that he has an increased level of participation and usually promotes better client adherence to selected plans.[4] Once client acceptance is achieved, the learning experiences are provided. These learning experiences frequently are most effective when they provide the client the opportunity to evaluate his own progress.

At the completion of the learning experiences, an *evaluation* of the client's behavior is conducted. It is important for the client to know that he has succeeded so he feels confident in going out on his own. The evaluation step is followed by the steps of revision (replanning), reimplementation, and reevaluation when the outcomes indicate that success, the achievement of optimal nutritional care, is not realized. Revision is alteration of the plans to increase successful outcomes; reimplementation is putting the revised plans into action; and reevaluation is checking out the success of the revision.

At this juncture in the presentation of the model (and in the development of the principal theme of this text), it is important to reiterate the philosophy expressed in Chapter 1. The primary professional role of clinical dietitians is the process of nutritional counseling. This role does not negate the other important role in nutritional care, the provision of nutrient sources to clients. Indeed, Figure 9.1 demonstrates the systematic steps in such provision: that of identifying client needs, planning and providing nutrient sources to meet those needs, and evaluating the effectiveness of the care plan. The ideas presented in Chapter 1 are embodied in the steps above and carefully delineate how the components of clinical practice structure the rational provision of nutrient sources. Another example of a systematic model, but with delineation of its component parts for educational purposes,[5] confirms the viability of our model.

In the remaining pages of this chapter, and in all chapters to follow, the focus of attention will be on nutritional counseling and not on provision of nutrient sources. Therefore, the philosophy, major themes, and examples will be directed to the counseling role of clinical dietitians. In all instances, both dietetic learners and practitioners will find that the basic ideas are applicable to the provision of nutrient sources, but every reader will have to make the transition for herself. The literature dealing with specific principles of the provision of nutrient sources is abundant; the reader is directed to find that which is most suitable for her own needs.

ENTERING THE SYSTEM

Entry into the nutritional counseling component of the system occurs when the clinical dietitian makes the initial contact with the client through a process defined as client referral. Referrals may originate in several ways. The most obvious and perhaps frequent referrals come from physicians and other primary care providers. In addition, other members of the health care team may suggest that a client needs to be contacted if they become aware of significant data relevant to the clinical dietitian's responsibility. Referrals may also come from such significant others as parents, spouse, or friends, who bring to the dietitian's attention a possible need for counseling. More important and yet rather rare to date is client self-referral. A client who has chosen counseling himself has a degree of motivation based on a feeling of self-determination, enhancing the possibility of goal achievement.

At this point, if there is not a nutritional care prescription and adequate evidence is available to suggest that one is indicated, the clinical dietitian should determine the prescription, following the policies of the institution. In the event that there *is* a prescription, the dietitian has the responsibility to determine if it is correct.[6] An inappropriate prescription should be challenged, giving the rationale for the challenge as well as the rationale for the substitute prescription.[7]

Once the prescription for the nutritional care plan is established, the clinical dietitian may proceed to contact that client for whom nutritional counseling is indicated. That is, clients capable of at least self-determination, if not self-sufficiency, should be offered the opportunity to work towards independence in healthful nutritional behaviors (Figure 1.1). For those clients who refer themselves, an appointment to begin the counseling process is made and the nutritional care prescription established.

The client who is referred by someone other than himself must be given the choice whether or not he wishes to be counseled. If the introductory explanation was adequate, he is able to make a reasonably sound judgment as to whether he wants or needs counseling. *Even if he needs counseling, but does not want it, the client has the right to make that decision.* If it is feasible to work with the client's significant others, such persons may become secondary clients who serve as additional resources to working with the primary client. In a situation where a child is the client, both parent(s) and child are the primary clients (conjoint counseling).[8]

In the event that the client appears to have firm convictions that he does not wish counseling, then communication to the primary care provider or other referral source is in order. A summary of the procedures followed from referral to closure is recorded in the health record. Since no follow-up is needed under these circumstances, the client leaves the system, hopefully to return at a later time when the relevancy of the counseling process has become apparent to him.

THE SYSTEM COMPONENTS

For those clients who choose to enter the counseling process, the next step is to obtain a data base (discussed in Chapter 4 through 8). Early in this *assessment* phase, the clinical dietitian gathers some general background information called "preliminary data." Preliminary data can most profitably be collected from the medical record or from the client himself. The medical record, if available, gives a rather brief but useful profile of socioeconomic status, primarily on the patient identification form. The body of the record describes the medical history of the client. Together these give the clinical dietitian a beginning profile of the client upon which to build counseling. Preliminary data may also be collected during an interview with the client, or even prior to the interview, using a form specifically designed for the purpose (a sample is shown in Appendix J).

Following in the assessment process is an interview with the client to establish the counseling relationship and to obtain an overview of the client's nutritional problems, particularly the behavioral aspects. At the conclusion of the interview the client should provide specific diet history information, perhaps best obtained on a tool designed for that purpose.

Upon completion of the data base, the final step of the assessment process is to identify the baseline data (Chapter 10). *The analysis of data and identification of baseline data step is a crucial one in the successful completion of the counseling process.*

As experienced clinicians know, there is always the possibility that what was initially perceived as a problem turns out not to be one. The clinical dietitian may decide that nutritional counseling is not needed. If so, this is an appropriate time to give the client a vote of confidence that supports what he is doing.

For the client whose needs are real, the clinical dietitian prepares a nutritional care plan in collaboration with the client. The *plan* is designed to reflect the most recent advances in the disciplines of food and nutrition, and in the related behavior and biologic sciences (Chapter 11). It includes competence (cognitive and psychomotor) objectives, and motivational (affective) objectives. Each objective will require learning experiences to be planned, which help the client meet the objectives. If possible, several alternatives within the plan itself are desirable to provide the client with choices. The evaluation instruments and strategies must be developed at this stage in order to evaluate the behavior change.

Since most health care delivery systems have teams of workers or other health personnel involved with any given client's care, it is important to coordinate the nutritional care plan with other plans, including the nursing care plan, physical therapy care plan, and so on.

If the care plan is compatible with the care plans established by others, then the client should be given the opportunity to peruse it carefully, including examining the objectives and the learning experiences. He then makes his decision to accept all, part, or none of the plan (Chapter 12). As client adherence is influenced extensively by feelings of self-determination, the extra time spent consulting with the client during the *implementation* phase is time well invested. If the client selects what seems to the counselor to be the less important objectives, then the others can be filed to be pulled out later when the client has tasted success and is ready to take on bigger tasks.

Whatever instruction has been arranged should be implemented either by or for the client. The emphasis should be on "by the client," as one motivation goal is to give him the confidence to be a self-directed learner. This instruction should include periodic opportunities for self-evaluation as learning progresses. By a predetermined time or when the client decides he's ready, he will be *evaluated* for his level of success in meeting the objectives (Chapter 13). The clinical dietitian will also evaluate the counseling process to decide where improvements can be made for that client. If the client demonstrates that he has acquired the know how, then arrangements are made for further contact to discover how successful he is in applying these skills in his life style. The client is also given feedback to reinforce his skill success. In the event that the plan fails, the processes of revision, reimplementation, and reevaluation should occur.

As *all* clinical dietitians are working with more than one client at a time in the counseling process, the effective management of resources is basic to successful practice. The practitioner who directs a unit will have even greater need for management skills. The systems model represents the core activities of the manager. To facilitate the successful achievement of the goals of the system, the clinician needs the skills required to manage resources such as personnel, time, money, materials. The more complex the system and extensive the demands, the more important the management skills become. A more comprehensive survey of management is presented in Chapter 14.

DATA CATEGORIES

In the model of nutritional care presented in this chapter, four components are identified (assessment, planning, implementation, and evaluation). In each of the segments of the counseling process, four major data categories are emphasized. The categories are biologic, food intake, environmental, and behavioral, as depicted in Figure 9.2.

The sequence of data collection and analysis presented in the next chapter provides the most effective means of processing the data. First, a knowledge of the client's *biologic* or physical status provides a focus for the assessment of *food intake*. When the food intake patterns are known, the *environmental* factors that impinge on client decisions need to be understood. Ultimately, then, the *behaviors* that contribute to the biologic and food intake concerns, and that are not controlled by environmental factors, can be assessed. A more complete description of the analyses of these data categories, hopefully, will illustrate the value of the preferred order of analysis.

Biologic Data

The biologic data that are evaluated in the assessment process are found in the medical record. Such data include objective measures of

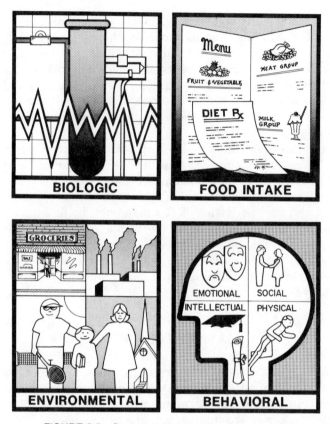

FIGURE 9.2   Content categories of nutritional data.

present height and weight, and often a historical recounting of these parameters; laboratory test results that serve as indexes of general health and well-being (e.g., hemoglobin, blood glucose levels); specific laboratory determinations of nutrient levels (e.g., folic acid, ascorbic acid values); diagnosis or reason for seeking health care. Additional biologic data of use include skinfold thickness measures; records of body temperature and fluid intake and output; and medication records.* Precisely which data are the most meaningful to the dietitian is primarily determined by the original need for the nutritional counseling process, whether the prevention of future problems or the modification of present problems.

* See especially the SOR and Case Study sections of Chapter 4 and Appendices B, C, and D.

Food Intake Data

During the preliminary data collection period, the medical record may be a source of information related to the client's food intake. In some cases a nutritional care prescription may have been written. Other health care providers may have recorded either food intake data or information that alludes to the client's food intake. Identification of the data available from this source will assist the dietitian in clarifying the need for information from the client when planning the next major step of the assessment, the diet history. Surveying the medical record at this time may reveal that there is no reference to food intake at all.

The acquisition of food intake data is of utmost importance in the diet history interview or in conjunction with it. Information about a client's food intake may be collected by observing his choices from menus, observations of his tray after meals, or by using more formal inspective or retrospective review techniques. A combination of all of these approaches is most effective. These techniques were discussed in detail in Chapter 6.

Environmental Data

Following the collection of biologic and food intake data, the clinician needs to be alert to the availability of environmental data. Appendix J, "Preliminary Data Schedule," includes such information as place of residence, marital status, family, occupation, education, sociocultural background, and religious preference. The medical record will often have these kinds of data recorded as well. In preparation for the diet history assessment phase, the practitioner needs to be alerted to those environmental factors that may be alterable and those that are relatively inflexible in the client's life style.

During the diet history phase, the clinician may wish to ask specific questions about such items as availability of cooking facilities, food preparation responsibilities, financial resources, and job constraints. This is also the time to follow up on hunches made during the preliminary data phase.

Behavioral Data

The availability of behavioral data early in the assessment process may be limited, but nonetheless should be sought. The Preliminary Data Schedule (Appendix J) may again serve as a resource. In that questionnaire, the client is requested to record food related concerns or needs, hobbies, recreation, and preference for kinds of activities, size of groups, frequency of participation, and nature of the activity (e..g., sports, educational). In addition, commercially prepared inventories and clinician prepared questionnaires that have been designed to assess attitudes and values can be used to plan and predict compliance.[9,10] Such information provides leads for planning strategies that the client will consider acceptable, both in the counseling itself and when he goes into his world to comply with the mutually agreed-upon regimen.

In the diet history interview, the clinician will begin to gain a sense of the client's food behaviors and attitudes, as well as an understanding of the accuracy of his nutrition knowledge. Extensive acquisition of food behavior information at this point, however, is premature. The crucial decision to make here is whether or not the client knows and understands how to eat for his own health. If it is determined that he does not know how to select food appropriately, there is no need to deal with motivational concerns unless he expresses dissatisfaction with his prescribed plan. If he does know how to consume an appropriate diet but doesn't do it, and there are no extenuating circumstances, then additional information must be obtained as to *why* he is not eating appropriately.

SUMMARY

The systems approach to nutritional care is *the* most viable means of ensuring comprehensive client care. The value of the systems approach demonstrated in the decision-making model is that it not only permits but actually demands continual alteration of the system toward the realization of the client's goals. The four major components of the process of nutritional care are identified as assessment, planning, implementation, and evaluation. The importance of management skills to successful application of the systems approach to clinical practice is also underscored. Biologic, food intake, environmental, and behavioral content are the four major data categories emphasized in the total counseling process. A synthesis of these processes and data categories provides clinicians with the foundation for effective nutritional care.

CITED REFERENCES

1. Danish, S. J., Ginsberg, M. R., Terrell, A., Hammond, M. I., and Adams, S. O. The anatomy of a dietetic counseling interview. *J. Am. Dietet. A.* 75:626, 1979.

2. Kaufman, R. A. *Educational System Planning*. Englewood Cliffs, NJ: Prentice-Hall, Inc., 1972.

3. Banathy, B. S. *Instructional Systems*. Palo Alto, CA: Fearon Publ., 1968.

4. Johnson, D. W., and Matross, R. P. Attitude modification methods. *In* Kanfer, F. H., and Goldstein, A. P., Eds. *Helping People Change: A Textbook of Methods*. New York: Pergamon Press, Inc., 1975.

5. Burg, F. D., Brownlee, R. C., Wright, F. H., Levine, H., Daeschner, C. W., Vaughan, V. C., and Anderson, J. A. A method for defining competency in pediatrics. *J. Med. Educ.* 51:824, 1976.

6. Hasson, W. E. Legal issues facing dietetic practice. *J. Am. Dietet. A.* 70:355, 1977.

7. Monteith, M., and Nakagawa, A. A flow chart approach to nutritional screening and assessment in long-term care facilities. *J. Am. Dietet. A.* 75:684, 1979.

8. Satir, V. *Conjoint Family Therapy. A Guide to Theory and Technique*. Rev. Ed. Palo Alto, CA: Science and Behavior Books, Inc., 1967.

9. Schutz, H. G., Moore, S. M., and Rucker, M. H. Predicting food purchase and use by multivariate attitudinal analysis. *Food Tech.* 31:8:85, 1977.

10. Hewitt, M. I., O'Dell, D. S., Schellhas, K. P., and Kotnour, K. D. Predictability of patient compliance with a weight reduction program. *Obesity & Baria. Med.* 6:218, 1977.

10

Assessment

> . . . *assessment involves the systematic collection of sub-jective and objective data from and about the client, his or her environment, and his or her support systems. This is done with a view of gaining knowledge about two sides of an equation. . . . The two sides of the equation would seem to be What are the coping challenges to be met? What are the abilities and resources for effectively coping with these challenges?*
>
> Doris Carnevali, *in* **Dynamics of Problem-Oriented Approaches: Patient Care and Documentation** (Philadelphia: J. B. Lippincott Co., 1976).

In the model of nutritional care proposed in Chapter 9, assessment is presented as the first component and is defined as the process of data gathering and analysis. An important principle of assessment is that data gathering and analysis never really end. Applying that principle throughout the provision of nutritional care is critical to success.

The goal of collecting and recording assessment data is to arrive at an adequate base of information about the client that provides the foundation for the next step, planning. Planning and implementation should never be delayed in anticipation of acquiring all of the data; a professional decision must be made as to the point in the assessment process when there is adequate wisdom to proceed. The clinician must be flexible enough to modify plans in the course of counseling when the present plans show evidence of being inappropriate or ineffective. One of the major reasons for applying a systems approach to a task is the emphasis on obtaining feedback that, in turn, may prompt a response to alter the system until the desired outcomes are achieved.

PROCESS OF ASSESSMENT

The acquisition of assessment data involves not only tools and techniques but process. The major tools and techniques have been presented in Part II; this chapter focuses on the process that utilizes these tools.

Assessment in nutritional counseling includes three basic steps (Figure 10.1). The first step is to obtain preliminary data, the client profile. The second step is to obtain the diet history. When the assessment data have been collected and analyzed, the third step involves identification of the baseline data, those that determine the need for intervention.* From the baseline data, needs are identified and goals and objectives are specified (planning). Baseline data are then used as the factors or criteria against which the evaluation data are compared (evaluation) in order to ascertain the value of intervention strategies (implementation).

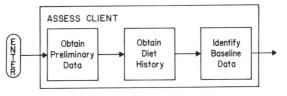

FIGURE 10.1   The process of assessment

The four specific data categories that are evaluated throughout the assessment process were illustrated in Figure 9.2.

OBTAINING PRELIMINARY DATA

A collection and subsequent analysis of information about the client is helpful in providing the clinical dietitian with a cursory understand-

---

* We choose to avoid the term "problem" since an intervention may be designed to reinforce and thus increase desirable behavior.

ing of the client and his environment prior to the first encounter.[2] This prior information has been labeled "preliminary data" by the authors.

The steps involved in the preliminary data phase are illustrated in Figure 10.2. In summary, the data are *collected* from a variety of sources. They are subsequently *recorded* on a form such as the preliminary data schedule (Appendix J). The next step is to *analyze* the pertinent factors. The factors are then *synthesized* or combined into a profile of the client's nutrition-related health status. The diamond box (*decision* step) asks whether or not there are adequate data with which to proceed. If the answer is yes, *plans* and preparation* for the diet history are effected. If the answer is no, then the clinician returns to the first step.

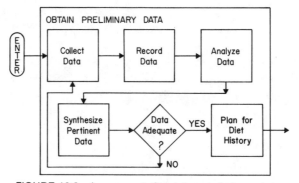

FIGURE 10.2 Assessment: Obtaining preliminary data

Collect, Record, and Analyze Data

One of the primary sources of preliminary data is the medical record. The medical record and the other data sources discussed at length in Chapter 4 contain a great variety of information about the client. An immediate source of data is the face sheet contained in both the SOR and the POR.

If the client comes for counseling to an ambulatory site where no health record is on file, he may be given a preliminary data schedule to complete before seeing the dietitian. The completed schedule allows the nutrition counselor to rapidly develop a profile of the client before the first encounter.

---

* Preparation involves such things as scheduling the first encounter and acquiring related materials.

In an acute or chronic care facility, the clinical dietitian may wish to use the schedule as a guide to recording important information extracted from the medical record and/or cardexes for the preliminary data base. With an analysis of these data, the clinician can then meet her client with some sensitivity to problems she might encounter.

Data may also be collected from human sources such as the client himself, his significant others, and/or health team members. The practitioner must remember that, in acute care facilities, clients may be too ill to be responsive to written inquiries.

When the preliminary data have been obtained, they may be recorded in several ways. These ways are best determined by the setting, the policies and procedure of the care facility, and the clinician's mode of operation. An example of a recording form that addresses the significant preliminary data highlighted in this text is shown in Appendix J. Dietetic practitioners should take the initiative to prepare forms that achieve their purposes when existing forms do not.

When examining the collected data, each factor is considered for its potential impact on nutritional health. For example, if a client is 5 feet 10 inches tall and weighs 245 pounds, a notation can be made that the client is more than 25 percent above ideal body weight. The client complains of constipation; the immediate suspicion of a diet low in fiber and/or fluids may be noted. In addition, muscle cramps are reported. The possibility of inadequate intake of calcium is considered. Other data noted are that the client is 25 years old and a football player. The occupation of professional athlete suggests frequent travel and eating out, as well as a high pressure schedule and life style. In this example, there are at least four preliminary data factors to be considered.

In the analysis of data, it is important to remember that there may be a need to consult the scientific literature. When the implications of the data are unclear or unknown, the clinician has the professional responsibility to examine the available literature for the purpose of resolving the uncertainty. In addition, it is critical that the practitioner continue to monitor new literature because of the frequent revisions and discoveries in the fields of nutritional, behavioral, and other sciences.

Synthesize Pertinent Data: Are They Adequate?

To synthesize means to combine parts or elements to form a whole. At this step in the process, the practitioner must examine the analyzed data and determine their relationships. In reviewing the analysis of data for the client in our example, it is likely that he is not overweight, but has extensive musculature because he is a football player. This can be verified with skinfold calipers if personal observation of the client indicates otherwise. With the extensive musculature and high level of physical activity, his calcium requirement may be higher than the average person's, particularly as indicated by the leg cramps. The need for dining away from home, along with the gastrointestinal problem and inadequate calcium intake, may suggest either lack of knowledge about an adequate diet or problems with selection at restaurants. Synthesizing the data now establishes the concept of the "whole" person, avoiding a singular focus on weight or calcium intake.

When the data are compiled, early hypotheses about pertinent data may need to be modified. Both the early hypotheses and the modifications, however, remain tentative at this stage of counseling. The decision step asks the practitioner to review the established, though tentative, profile and to determine whether to proceed to planning for the diet history, or to return to the data collection step.

Plan for Diet History

Using the preliminary data synthesis as both an entrée to working with the client and as an indicator of potential concerns that will require attention, a plan is made to obtain the diet history. This plan will include *who* will be involved, *where* and *when* it will take place, *how* it will be done, and *what* will be needed.

The people (*who*) involved may include just the clinician and the client. If there is a possible language problem, a bilingual interpreter may be sought. There may be a "red flag" on the medical record that would indicate a need to consult with the health team before approaching the client. It also may be important to discover how much the client knows about his illness at this point in time. For a variety of reasons, some primary care providers do not choose to tell the client everything about his illness. It would be inappropriate for the clinical dietitian to do so without first consulting with the professional charged with the overall responsibility for the client's care.

The location (*where*) of the diet history interview is important. Can a room where interruptions are controlled be found? Is the environment conducive to relaxed conversation? Multiple-use rooms and patient care units are frequently places of much activity, including television, visitors, and rounds. Distractions interfere with the elicitation of a complete diet history. If there is a designated counseling room, the need for scheduling may exist.

The time (*when*) set for obtaining the diet history should interface with the care of other providers, with the wishes of the client, and with the availability of resources and facilities. Asking a client what he eats when he is in a restaurant while he is being bathed will seldom promote good communication. In addition, when clients are new to the health care facility, they frequently experience enough distress to make them resistant to or very resentful of much interaction; they may want to be left alone. In such an event, the clinician must consider the available options and choose the one that seems best to meet the needs of the client.

The way (*how*) in which the diet history will be conducted needs to be predetermined. The client may complete forms on his own, or he could respond to questions presented to him on a computer video display terminal, or the clinician may conduct an interview. Additional information can be obtained by examining the client's menu choices, either in the facility or at home. The client may also be asked to keep a food diary over a period of time. There is no one right way; usually each way has its own advantages and drawbacks, such that a combination of methods frequently provides the best results.

The last step is to determine which resources (*what*) will be needed to obtain the diet history. There may be forms, computer equipment, food models, or a tape recorder needed. If the client is a young child, a food game or pictures may be used, or puppets to stimulate interaction with a frightened or shy child.[3] These materials need to be gathered before obtaining the diet history. A comprehensive discussion of such resources was presented in Chapter 8.

Preliminary Data Summary

In general, the core of the data is collected and recorded before any analysis is done. As the clinical dietitian examines the recorded data, item by item, an analysis of each datum item is made as to its potential impact. When all data have been analyzed and then integrated or synthesized to produce a profile of the client with a statement of potential concerns, a decision is made as to the need for additional data. If there is such a need, the clinician repeats the process depicted in Figure 10.2. When the data appear to be adequate, potential concerns are noted and the plan is then made to obtain the diet history, based on these concerns.

When the clinician has made all necessary plans for the diet history, the next step is to obtain it as planned. One cautionary note is important at this juncture: Even though good planning is crucial to effective performance, a clinician must be able, sometimes at a moment's notice, to alter plans in order to accommodate the unexpected. If an activity is very important to accomplish and there are risks of interference, a contingency plan made at the same time as the primary one may be advisable. When there are time constraints, an opportunity thwarted may be an opportunity lost. Effective client care cannot occur in "catch as catch can" environments.

OBTAINING THE DIET HISTORY

When the clinical dietitian has collected enough preliminary data to compile a profile of the client that includes potential concerns, the next step is the collection of the diet history data. The history contains all four types of data categories (Figure 9.2) and generally is obtained in a counseling interview setting.

Weed[4] emphasized the importance of acquiring a data base that is standardized (consistent from client to client). It is possible to develop forms that will provide guidelines for collecting the data base. One such form may serve for the collection of food intake data whereas others may be used for recording behavior patterns, feelings, and environmental variables. Examples of these have been developed by Ferguson[5] in his structured program for diet modification.

Using these sources and tools, the process of collecting diet history data continues from the previous flow diagram (Figure 10.2). When the decision has been made that there are adequate preliminary data, and the diet history collection has been planned and necessary preparations made, the next step is to initiate the diet history (Figure 10.3).

The process works in the same manner as the preliminary data collection process, with a cyclic sequence that is pursued until the answer to the "decision step" (diamond) is, "Yes, there are adequate assessment data with which to proceed to identifying baseline data."

The collection of diet history data has been traditionally viewed as an acquisition of facts about physical symptoms, food intake, and occasionally the client's knowledge of nutrition. Although practitioners undoubtedly made subconscious hypotheses about environmental obstacles, and behavioral and attitudinal problems, these data seldom were considered formal components of the diet history. With our increased understanding of the influence of attitudes, values, and ecologic factors on ultimate behavioral expression, such factors need to be included in the analysis of nutritional needs, and in the decision to facilitate or not to facilitate change.

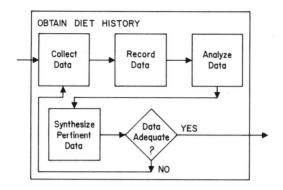

FIGURE 10.3   Assessment: Obtaining diet history

Collect, Record, and Analzye Data

Within an interview structure, diet history data may be collected in one or more sessions with the client. At the conclusion of the first session, a decision is made as to the adequacy of available data. If more data are needed, additional contacts may be planned. The client may also be asked to collect data for himself.

All of the data should be summarily recorded on an assessment worksheet designed for that purpose. Bringing all of this information together enhances the possibility of incorporating all relevant variables. The recorded data should be organized into the four data categories.

The sequence for analyzing the data has been selected with purpose, and is demonstrated in depth in three of the next four sections of this chapter. When organizing the data into four categories, it should become evident that decisions based on each category of data directs the analysis of the next category. It is appropriate at this point to reiterate the importance of consulting the scientific literature to optimize the accuracy of the analyses.

Analysis of biologic data.   An understanding of the client's state of physical health is critical to the effective implementation of nutritional care. To attempt to cover the analysis of biologic data is not appropriate in this text, however. As suggested in Chapters 4 and 7, there are many excellent sources available to clinical dietitians to support this step of the process.

To illustrate the value of specification of biologic data, first consider the analysis of the data for a female client. The fact that she is pregnant will have significant impact on her need for energy and for nutrients.

Exactly what intervention strategy is required, however, will be based on the results of the analyses of food intake data and the other two data categories.

Analysis of food intake data.   Evaluating the adequacy of the food intake history is the next step in assessment. Two questions are associated with this particular analysis: "What nutrients are being consumed?" and "Are the quantities appropriate?"

What nutrients are being consumed?   There are a number of ways the first question may be answered, ranging from the simple (and least meaningful) to the complex. A very common tool, used frequently for evaluative purposes, is the Daily Food Guide,[6] shown in Table 10.1, or its Canadian counterpart, Canada's Food Guide[7].

The Daily Food Guide was originally designed to assist individuals and groups in the selection of foods; its primary purpose was not diet

TABLE 10.1   A Daily Food Guide

Vegetable and Fruit Group:
FOUR BASIC SERVINGS DAILY
Include one good vitamin C source each day. Also frequently include deep-yellow or dark-green vegetables (for vitamin A) and unpeeled fruits and vegetables and those with edible seeds, such as berries (for fiber).

What's a Serving? -
Includes all fruits and vegetables.
Count $\frac{1}{2}$ cup as a serving, or typical portion—one orange, half a medium grapefruit or cantaloupe, juice of one lemon, a wedge of lettuce, a bowl of salad, and one medium potato.

Bread and Cereal Group:
FOUR BASIC SERVINGS DAILY
Select only whole-grain and enriched or fortified products. (But include *some* whole-grain bread or cereals for sure!)
Check labels.

What's a Serving?
Includes all products made with whole grains or enriched flour or meal; bread, biscuits, muffins, waffles, pancakes, cooked or ready-to-eat cereals, cornmeal, flour, grits, macaroni and spaghetti, noodles, rice, rolled oats, barley, and bulgur.
Count as a serving 1 slice of bread; $\frac{1}{2}$ cup to $\frac{3}{4}$ cup cooked cereal, cornmeal, grits, macaroni, noodles, rice, or spaghetti; or 1 oz. ready-to-eat cereal.

TABLE 10.1 (Continued)

Milk and Cheese Group:
BASIC SERVINGS DAILY (Based on servings of fluid milk; for milk product equivalents see below.)

Children under 9   2 to 3 servings
Children 9 to 12   3 servings
Teens   4 servings
Adults   2 servings
Pregnant Women   3 servings
Nursing Mothers   4 servings

What's a Serving?

Includes milk in any form: whole, skim, lowfat, evaporated, buttermilk, and nonfat dry milk; also yogurt, ice cream, ice milk, and cheese, including cottage cheese.

Count one 8-ounce cup of milk as a serving.

Common portions of some dairy products and their milk equivalents in calcium are:

1 cup plain yogurt	$= 1$ cup milk
1 ounce Cheddar or Swiss cheese (natural or process)	$= \frac{3}{4}$ cup milk
1-inch cube Cheddar or Swiss cheese (natural or process)	$= \frac{1}{2}$ cup milk
1 ounce process cheese food	$= \frac{1}{3}$ cup milk
1 tablespoon or $\frac{1}{2}$ ounce process cheese spread; or 1 tablespoon Parmesan cheese	$= \frac{1}{4}$ cup milk
$\frac{1}{2}$ cup cottage cheese	$= \frac{1}{4}$ cup milk

Note: You'll get about the same amount of calcium in each of these portions, but varying amounts of calories.

Milk used in cooked foods—such as in creamed soups, sauces, puddings—can count toward filling your daily quota in this group.

Meat and Poultry and Fish and Beans Group:
TWO BASIC SERVINGS DAILY

What's a Serving?

Includes beef, veal, lamb, pork, poultry, fish, shellfish (shrimp, oysters, crabs, etc.), organ meats (liver, kidneys, etc.), dry beans or peas, soybeans, lentils, eggs, seeds, nuts, peanuts, and peanut butter.

Count 2 to 3 ounces of lean, cooked meat, poultry, or fish without bone *as a serving.* One egg, $\frac{1}{2}$ to $\frac{3}{4}$ cup cooked dry beans, dry peas, soybeans or lentils, 2 tablespoons peanut butter, and $\frac{1}{4}$ to $\frac{1}{2}$ cup nuts, sesame seeds, or sunflower seeds count as 1 ounce of meat, poultry, or fish.

TABLE 10.1   (Continued)

Fats, Sweets and Alcohol Group:
In general, the amount of these foods to use depends on the number of calories you require. It's a good idea to concentrate first on the calorie-plus-nutrients foods provided in the other groups as the basis of your daily diet.

What's a Serving?

Includes foods like butter, margarine, mayonnaise and other salad dressings, and other fats and oils; candy, sugar, jams, jellies, syrups, sweet toppings, and other sweets; soft drinks and other highly sugared beverages; and alcoholic beverages such as wine, beer, and liquor. Also included are refined but unenriched breads, pastries, and flour products. Some of these foods are used as ingredients in prepared foods or are added to other foods at the table. Others are just "extras."

No serving sizes are defined because a basic number of servings is not suggested for this group.

Source: *Food: A Publication on Food and Nutrition* (U.S. Dept. Agriculture, Science and Education Administration, Home and Garden Bulletin No. 228, 1979).

---

history evaluation. Nevertheless, the guide, or adaptations of the guide, are used frequently in a variety of settings as a simple and expedient assessment tool.

There are inherent shortcomings in the guide, which should be recognized when it is used as an evaluative device. For some time now, it has been known that the kilocalories provided by the listed foods in the previous edition[8] were probably inadequate for apparently healthy clients who lead moderately active lives. In addition, the quantity of iron provided in the listed foods may be inadequate for many individuals, particularly females between the ages of 11 and 51 years, unless food sources of iron are carefully chosen.

According to King and colleagues[9], the failings of the Daily Food Guide ("Basic Four Food Guide") to serve in the selection of foods providing those nutrients listed in the 1974 Recommended Dietary Allowances table are probably greater than previously suspected. King et al. report that, in a nutrient analysis of 20 different full-day menus for adults published as examples of well-balanced diets in 10 well-known, authorative references, only 8 of the 17 evaluated nutrients met or exceeded the 1974 RDAs. Five nutrients were provided in quantities less than 60 percent of their respective allowances (vitamins E and B_6, magnesium, zinc, and iron). In response to their findings, King et al. propose a modification of the Daily Food Guide:

> *Modified Basic Four*
> *2 svg. Milk and milk products*
> *4 svg. Protein foods:*
>   *2 svg. animal protein*
>   *2 svg. legumes and/or nuts*
> *4 svg. Fruits and vegetables:*
>   *1 svg. vitamin C-rich*
>   *1 svg. dark green*
>   *2 svg. other*
> *4 svg. Whole grain cereal products*
> *1 svg. Fat and/or oil*[9] *(p. 29)*

These workers suggest that people using the modified guide may find it more restrictive in the variety of food choices, but note that it is more important to have a guide that is "nutritionally sound" than one that caters to food preferences.

When using the guide, the question, "What nutrients are being consumed?" becomes, "What food groups are being consumed?" The answer is forthcoming from those diet histories that are primarily qualitative rather than quantitative. That is, food consumption reviews that yield general, descriptive, nonempiric data may be evaluated by comparing food group intakes to the food groups contained in the Daily Food Guide. The guide, however, is the least useful assessment tool and, therefore, should be used only when other evaluative procedures are inappropriate.

The second way diet histories are evaluated is to determine the nutrient content of each food consumed, in the quantity ingested by the client. Determinations of nutrient consumption may be most effectively done by chemical analyses of small portions (aliquots) of each food consumed.[10] Since this method is not feasible in most practice sites, the next best method of evaluation is the use of food composition tables.

There are a number of widely used food composition tables available to every clinical dietitian. Such composition tables range from broad-scope handbooks[11-21] to the very limited and specific.[22-25] The general handbooks show the known food energy and nutrient composition for most foods found in the "typical" North American diet, while the specific, limited tables show only values for one or a very few nutrients.

To be most effective and efficient, the clinical dietitian should develop worksheets for tabulating the nutrient composition of foods according to the manner in which the nutrients are listed in the selected food composition table. For example, if the table of choice is Table 1 in USDA Handbook 456,[11] the format of the worksheet should be designed along the lines of Figure 10.4. If the clinician wishes information about only certain nutrients, then just those desired may be included on the worksheet. (A note of caution: Read the tables across carefully so that the correct values are recorded in the appropriate column.) The worksheet can serve as a guide for either manual or computer assisted calculation of nutrient content.

Each of the large, comprehensive handbooks of food composition contain certain unique features. A most widely used document, the original USDA Handbook 8,[14] lists the nutrient composition of foods in 100 gram edible portions, and in the edible portion of 1 pound of food as purchased. USDA Handbook 456 gives the nutritive values for household measures and market units of foods, and the gram weight of those measures and units. Thus, the two differ in the units of food measurement. Both handbooks are organized alphabetically so that, for example, honey is followed by honeydew melon.

In the food composition handbook known widely as "Bowes and Church",[12] foods are listed in commonly used portions; the gram weight is given for each portion listed. This handbook is organized into categories of food groups so that, for example, all beverages are listed together.

The smallest publication in this group, USDA Bulletin 72,[13] lists the nutritive values of 615 commonly used foods in both household measures and gram weights.

The foods in both Handbooks 8 and 456 are numbered consecutively in the alphabetical listings. In Handbook 456, there are subsets (letters) of the numbers, which are used to designate various forms of the initial, numbered food. This numbering system, common to both documents, increases the ease with which tabular data can be incorporated into computerized data banks.

In 1976, the first in the series of the long-awaited revised USDA Handbooks was published. At the time of this writing seven handbooks of the series are available.* Each is devoted to a distinct food group. Currently included are the following: dairy and egg products (1976), spices and herbs (1977), baby foods (1978), fats and oils (1979), poultry products (1979), soups, sauces, and gravies (1980), and sausages and luncheon meats (1980). Each is also published in loose-leaf form so

---

* We are informed that there will be at least 20 handbooks in the series.

Name______ Code Number (If Applicable)______ Meal______ Day______ Date______

Food	Approx. Measure Or Unit	Wt. (gm)	Food energy (kilocalories)	Protein (gm)	Fat (gm)	CHO (gm)	Ca (mg)	P (mg)	Fe (mg)	Na (mg)	K (mg)	Vitamin A (IU)	Thiamin (mg)	Riboflavin (mg)	Niacin (mg)	Ascorbic acid (mg)
Totals:																

FIGURE 10.4 Food composition work sheet

that continuous and rapid updating of the tables may be achieved when new data are available.[15-21]

The revised handbooks depart radically from the older USDA Handbook 8 in the organization of the material. First, each page in the table contains data about only one food. The nutrient composition of that single food is listed in 100 gram portions, two common household measurements (which vary from table to table), and the edible portion of one pound as purchased. In addition, for some nutrients, the number of samples tested is also recorded along with the mean and standard error of the resultant values. For example, the recorded water content of 100 grams of butter is 15.87 grams, with a standard error of 0.06 grams, based on analyses of 522 samples.[18]

The initial pages of each of the series contain significant information that the clinician should utilize. Recorded there are limited descriptions of the sources of the data, the format of the table, and some explanation of the laboratory methods employed and the units of expression used. The guide to the table lists each food alphabetically in its appropriate group, its page number, and, whenever possible, the original Handbook 8 page number for that food. In addition, Handbooks 8-3 through 8-7 also record the nutrient data bank number for each of the foods.

Food composition tables, like the Daily Food Guide, have some unavoidable limitations that must be considered by the clinician.[26-28] One constraint is that the calculated amount of a nutrient in a given food is routinely assumed to be absorbed by the organism.[26] In addition, the tabular values are representative of the results of laboratory determinations performed in a variety of settings. The methods used for such determinations are fairly uniform, but not always identical; hence, some variation in results is unavoidable. The published values are *average* values, representing experimental data obtained from analyses of food grown in different regions of the continent and in varying seasons of the year, and food processed and stored in different ways.[27] Thus, the values in food composition tables frequently represent the very best laboratory estimates of nutrient content of foods grown in all areas of North America in all seasons of the year. The actual nutrient content of the food consumed by an individual client may vary.

How food is prepared also contributes to the difference between what nutrients are actually ingested and the tabular nutrient value of that food. Fruits and vegetables, for example, vary widely in their nutrient content according to how they are stored and prepared at home. Mixed dishes, such as casseroles, sauces, stews, soups, and so on, will vary in their content according to the set of directions (the recipe) used for the preparation.[27] Not infrequently, the ingredients of a mixed dish will vary according to what is available for use (as in casseroles or stews) or even whether measuring cups or spoons are used. Thus, the nutrient composition of a food can be easily altered in the preparation.

In addition to food composition handbooks, there are other sources of information available to the dietitian about the nutrient content of foods. It is possible, for example, to find in the literature literally hundreds of research papers which report the content of a particular nutrient in a great many foods, or report all of the known nutrients in a single food. Another source of food composition data is that published by food manufacturing or processing companies. Many such companies in the food industry make available to nutrition professionals the results of their own nutrient analyses of the foods they market. Such information is becoming even more important to clinical dietitians as their clients begin to use, or increase their use of, prepared or partially prepared foods.

In recent years, there has been a great surge of interest in the development of nutrient data banks.[28] Such banks are repositories of nutrient content information and are usually housed in computer centers. Data are stored in various manners (e.g., cards, magnetic tapes), and then are used for a multitude of purposes when commanded by the proper "program" (the set of directions given to the computer). The development of a national nutrient data bank is a current activity of the USDA.[29] Computer data tapes, for example, are available for USDA Handbooks Nos. 8, 456, and 8-1 through 8-7. Such a national (and international) repository will be a significant step toward centralization and standardization of information.

Nutrient data banks can be used in many ways. The primary use of interest to clinical dietitians in nutritional counseling is that of evaluating the adequacy of a client's food intake. Such programs are now available on a limited basis.[30-34]

Are the quantities appropriate? Once the clinical dietitian has a knowledge of what nutrients are being consumed by the client, some decision needs to be made on the appropriateness of the intake. This step is complicated by the fact that differences in the nutrient requirements of individuals are ordinarily unknown and, thus, there are no absolute standards by which the nutritional adequacy of food consumption may be judged for an individual client. It is one thing to have knowledge of a quantitative approximation of nutrients consumed by a client, and an entirely different matter to judge that approximate consumption in terms of meeting individual nutrient needs.

This point was well made by Harper when he discussed nutrient requirements and nutrient allowances:

> The logical starting point for estimating allowances for nutrients other than those that are consumed solely for their energy content is to assemble information about estimated requirements. However, requirements differ with age and body size; among individuals of the same size owing to differences in genetic make-up; with the physiologic state of the individual—growth rate, pregnancy, lactation; and with sex. They also may be influenced by a person's activity and by environmental conditions.
>
> Even when knowledge of human requirements is available, agreement about the criterion for judging when the requirement has been met may still be a problem.[35] (p. 153)

The criteria by which clinical dietitians judge the nutrient quality of the diet consumed by the clients they counsel are, therefore, essentially based on *recommended allowances* of nutrients as opposed to *requirements* for nutrients. In the United States, the guidelines for nutrient allowances are named the Recommended Dietary Allowances; in Canada they are known as the Dietary Standard for Canada. The specific statement of definition accompanying the last revised edition of the U.S. allowances is as follows:

> Recommended Dietary Allowances (RDA) are the levels of intake of essential nutrients considered, in the judgment of the Committee on Dietary Allowances of the Food and Nutrition Board on the basis of available scientific knowledge, to be adequate to meet the known nutritional needs of practically all healthy persons.[36] (p. 1)

The definition of the Canadian standard is essentially the same:

> A dietary standard is a statement of the daily amounts of energy and essential nutrients considered adequate, on the basis of scientific data, to meet the physiological needs of practically all healthy persons in a population. It is not, as many seem to believe, a summary of nutrient requirements for the human. Because recommended nutrient intakes meet the needs of practically all persons, they exceed the minimum requirements of most individuals. However, recommended nutrient intakes are not formulated to cover therapeutic needs, although they are generally considered adequate to maintain reserves of those nutrients stored in the body. The only exception to this approach concerns the recommendations for energy, which are estimates of the requirements of average persons within an age-sex group.[37] (p. 5)

In the 1980 revision of the Recommended Dietary Allowances (RDAs), the Food and Nutrition Board carefully noted what it believes to be the appropriate uses of the RDAs. In doing so, the Board again made the point that the RDAs are recommended intakes of nutrients and not requirements. Among the appropriate uses cited by the Board are[36]:

1. Planning and procuring food supplies for population groups
2. Interpretation of food consumption records in relation to assessment of nutritional status (for groups)
3. As guidelines in establishing policy for health and welfare programs
4. Nutrition education programs
5. Product development, nutritional labeling, and regulation of nutritional quality of foods

For the sake of clarity, the authors have added the phrase "for groups" to the statement about interpretation of food consumption records. We have done so because interpretation of the results of group surveys is an entirely different matter than the interpretation of the record of an individual client. The Food and Nutrition Board speaks very clearly to this point:

RDA should be applied to population groups rather than to individuals. RDA were devised as standards or guides to serve as a goal for good nutrition on the basis that, in population groups consuming a varied diet providing the RDA for all nutrients, there would be few individuals suffering from nutritional inadequacy. RDA are estimates of acceptable daily nutrient intakes in the sense that the needs of most healthy individuals will be no greater than the RDA. The basis for estimation of RDA is such that, even if a specific individual habitually consumes less than the recommended amounts of some nutrients, his diet is not necessarily inadequate for those nutrients.[36] (p. 10)

Sabry, writing about the Canadian Dietary Standard, notes essentially the same point as the Food and Nutrition Board.

The use of the standard should, therefore, be considered with caution. The authors of the standard considered its possible use in planning diets and food supplies for healthy groups or individuals but not in appraising the nutritional status of individuals. They repeatedly stressed the fact that the recommended intakes in the standard were not only above minimum but also above adequate levels.[38] *(p. 195)*

Both sets of guidelines were essentially designed for general uses in evaluating the dietary status of population groups; they were not designed for rigid use in evaluating the dietary status of individuals.

There has been, of course, a great deal of discussion in the literature about the dilemma clinical dietitians face in their everyday practice. One of the major issues discussed is: Is it appropriate to evaluate individual intakes using the RDAs or the Canadian standard? If not, what other criteria are available? In a paper by Hegsted, a similar question is raised:

> *There has always been considerable ambiguity about how the Recommended Dietary Allowances should be used. . . . No instructions are given as to how one evaluates food consumption data of groups of people or the significance of intakes that fall below the allowances. It is stated that one must not assume that an intake below the Recommended Dietary Allowances defines a person as nutritionally deficient.*
>
> *The most recent publication devotes considerably more space to a discussion of the uses and limitations of the allowances. Although these are useful and instructive, it seems to me that they fail to come to grips with the problems the nutritional practitioner faces who must use the dietary standards.*[39] *(p. 14)*

Hegsted's primary hypothesis is that a single set of dietary standards (such as the RDAs) cannot adequately fulfill the two prime purposes for which they are used—that of evaluation of food consumption records, and the planning of diets and food supplies. The authors believe that Hegsted's hypothesis is correct.

In testimony before a U.S. House of Representatives committee in 1978, Robinson spoke for the professional society of dietitians and declared that practitioners use the RDAs in the following ways:

(a) In administration of food services. . . .
(b) As a reference point for the construction of therapeutic diets.
(c) In evaluating diets for individuals and groups.
(d) In evaluating food products.
(e) In the preparation of educational materials.
(f) In the education of consumers and professional persons.[40] *(p. 435)*

In doing so, however, Robinson clearly noted that dietetic practitioners do not make a diagnosis of malnutrition if a person's intake falls below any given allowance. Robinson emphasized the point that the Food and Nutrition Board states clearly: As the intake of any one nutrient decreases over time, the *probability* of the risk of deficiency increases.

In an effort to find ways to evaluate food consumption records of individuals and groups, several investigators have developed methods that are based, for the most part, on the RDAs. In a large food consumption study conducted by the USDA in 1965–1966, approximately 14,500 individual food intake reports were collected from about 6200 households.[41] This sample was drawn to be representative of all housekeeping households in the United States. The basis for evaluation of the food intake records was the revision of the RDAs in effect at the time.[42] The evaluative method and its rationale are described as follows:

> *The Food and Nutrition Board states that the allowances are intended to serve "as guides for the interpretation of food consumption records of groups of people." In the study reported here, they have been considered as reasonable benchmarks to make comparisons among population groups and to indicate trends in dietary quality. Their use has been limited to evaluating diets of groups of persons—those in households, those in income classes, and those in regional and urbanization groups.*
>
> *In this study, a diet was rated good if the nutritive value of the total food brought into the kitchen for use by the household during the week equaled or exceeded the total allowance for each of seven nutrients for all persons eating from the household food supply. A diet was rated poor if it supplied less than two-thirds of the allowances for one or more nutrients. Two-thirds of the allowance has been considered in this and other household surveys of the Department as a level below which diets could be nutritionally inadequate for individuals over an extended period of time.*
>
> *Between the households with good and poor diets were those with diets that provided at least two-thirds of the allowances for all seven nutrients and less than the allowance for at least one nutrient. Such diets were labeled "fair."[42] (p. 3)*

The categories of "good," "fair," and "poor" have been used often in studies of groups selected from the population at large. In 1975, Inano, Pringle, and Little reported the results of a dietary survey of 668 families in Iowa and North Carolina.[43] They used the retrospective method of 24-hour recall to collect family food consumption data. These data were subsequently evaluated by adaptions of either the RDAs or by criteria established for the Ten State Nutrition Survey.[44]

Inano and co-workers describe their evaluative method as follows:

> *Content of the individual nutrients in a family's meals and in the diet as a whole was characterized as "good," "fair," or "poor." When the diet contained 100 per cent or more of the allowance for a nutrient, it was considered "good"; between 67 and 100 per cent of the allowance was termed "fair"; and below 67 per cent, the intake was labeled "poor." In evaluating the total family diet, a diet was "good" if it provided 100 per cent or more of all seven nutrients; "fair" if one or more nutrients was present in an amount between 67 and 100 per cent; and "poor" if one or more nutrients fell below 67 per cent of the standard.[43] (p. 357)*

A similar method was used by Kohrs et al.,[45] although their rating categories were less stringent. "Excellent" was the term assigned to an intake including 67 per cent or better of the nutrients studied, as compared to the RDAs. An intake was labeled "good" if the assessed nutrients met between 50 and 67 per cent of the allowances; "poor" described an intake in which one or more of the nutrients were ingested at a level less than 50 per cent.

Other practitioners have used similar evaluative methods for individual clients. For example, Burke rated diet intakes of pregnant women as excellent to very poor on a scale developed from a very early edition of the RDAs.[46] For a study of older persons, Clarke and Wakefield developed a nutrient intake rating scale, which is described as follows:

> *An individual's nutritional score—ranging from 1 to 8—indicated the number of nutrients consumed in amounts of two-thirds or more of the 1968 Recommended Daily Allowances. . . . Eight, the highest score, indicated that the subject had eaten foods furnishing at least 67 per cent of the allowance for all eight nutrients.[47] (p. 601)*

Note that, in this last rating method, a consumption of at least 67 per cent of the RDAs for all eight nutrients earned the top score. In the other two studies previously cited,[42,43] the label "good" was assigned to intakes of 100 per cent or more of all nutrient allowances evaluated.

In a more recent paper, Shapiro pointed out that ". . . the frequently used 65 to 75 per cent of the RDAs as a dietary norm does not alter (the) principle . . . that intake of one or more nutrients that fails to meet the allowance is not in itself diagnostic of malnutrition"[48] (p. 232). Furthermore, manipulation of the allowances in an effort to define a level of acceptability still does not negate the tenet that the allowances are applicable to groups and *not* to individuals.

To reiterate an earlier passage, making decisions about the appropriateness of nutrient intake is one of the most difficult tasks of the clinical dietitian. Hegsted makes this point very clearly:

It seems entirely logical to most people that if one measures the food eaten and knows the nutrient content of the food, one ought to be able to make a reasonable judgment as to the adequacy of that diet for the individual. If one is to do this, it would appear obvious that the standard used for the evaluation must be somehow related to actual needs. The difficulty, of course, is that even if we knew exactly what the individual consumed, the "minimum no risk standards" are set in excess of the real need of practically everyone in the population being considered. Thus, we arrive at the seemingly inconsistent conclusion that nearly everyone in the population can consume less than the standard yet be adequately nourished. Nor as the RDA Committee has pointed out, is it legitimate to select a lower value, say two-thirds of the RDA, as a cut-off point and conclude that those above this level are adequately nourished. This would presumably be too low for some and too high for others.[49] *(p. 53)*

It seems to the authors that the best answer to the query, "Are the quantities appropriate?" is one that takes into consideration:

1. Human individuality
2. The purposes of the Recommended Dietary Allowances or the Canadian Dietary Standard
3. The number of repetitive food intake assessments for any one individual client
4. The validity and reliability of the methods used to collect and assess intake data.*

The most recent RDA revision does state:

However, since the requirements of each individual are not known, it is clear that the more habitually intake falls below the RDA and the longer the low intake continues, the greater is the risk of deficiency.[36] *(p. 10)*

Thus, a clinical dietitian may wish to circumscribe the evaluation of intake by indicating the method of assessment used to determine in-

---

* See Chapter 7 for a discussion of the terms "validity" and "reliability."

take and the deviation from the RDAs. Until a system is devised to more nearly approximate individual nutrient requirements, the RDAs will, by default, serve as the standard for evaluation. One should use caution in arbitrarily assigning a quality judgment (good, fair, or poor) to intakes that do not meet the RDAs.

Nutrient density* is an approach that can assist clinical dietitians in judging the nutritional quality of a diet and as a basis for developing nutritional care plan strategies.[50,51] Rose [52] was one of the first to apply the concept of nutrient density to human dietaries. Hansen[53] developed a quantitative and qualitative measure of nutrient-to-calorie density, termed an Index of Nutritional Quality (INQ), which may be calculated for each nutrient in a diet as follows:

Equation 1:

$$INQ = \frac{\text{Amount of a nutrient in a diet/kilocalorie}}{\text{Human allowance for nutrient/kilocalorie}}$$

or

Equation 2:

$$INQ = \frac{\text{Percentage of nutrient allowance supplied by a diet}}{\text{Percentage of energy allowance supplied by a diet}}$$

Foods must be consumed within narrow quantitative limits if body weight is to be maintained. Either energy or kilocalories therefore seems an appropriate common denominator for relating human nutrient allowances to the capacity of a diet to provide those nutrients. When energy allowances are met, all other nutrients must be present in recommended amounts for a diet to be balanced. Expressing the nutrient composition of a diet *and* the human dietary allowance for individual nutrients on the same basis, for example, calories, allows a direct comparison between the two parameters, and quality judgments may be derived.

For example, if a diet for a 35-year-old woman provided 2500 kilocalories and 800 mg of calcium, a comparison with the RDA alone would indicate calcium supplied in amounts equal to the RDA. However, if the 2500 kilocalories diet provided calories in excessive amounts and if the client *proportionately* decreases all of her food intake to 2000 kilocalories, calcium would not be provided in amounts

* This section was written by Bonita W. Wyse, Ph.D., R.D., Associate Professor of Nutrition, Department of Nutrition and Food Sciences, Utah State University, Logan.

equal to the RDA. This can be seen from the nutrient density or INQ ratio:

Equation 1:

$$INQ = \frac{640 \text{ mg calcium in 2000 kcal of diet}}{800 \text{ mg calcium in 2000 kcal of diet}} = 0.8$$

Equation 2:

$$INQ = \frac{800 \text{ mg calcium in diet/800 mg calcium RDA for 2000 kcal diet}}{2500 \text{ kcal in diet/2000 kcal for RDA}}$$

$$= \frac{1}{1.25} = 0.8$$

An INQ of "1" for a given nutrient in a diet indicates that the amount of a diet necessary to provide energy in quantities equal to the RDA will also provide the appropriate allowance for that nutrient. Conversely, values less than "1" identify nutrients in a diet where an excess of calories must be eaten to fulfill the standards. The approach will accommodate any number of nutrients for which there are adequate food compositional data, such as vitamin B_6, folacin, and zinc.

Computer programs available for comparing dietary intake with nutritional standards can be easily modified to yield nutrient density ratios as well. Nutrient density profiles for the individual foods in USDA Handbook No. 72 are available[54]. With this reference, using a clear plastic overlay and a water-soluble marker, a clinical dietitian can "add" the calorie and nutrient contents of foods consumed during the day. The energy line is shown first, so the nutrient density relative to calories can be visualized.

Recapitulation. As the reader now knows, the assessment of food intake is usually a time consuming task that requires considerable skill and attention to detail. There are two questions associated with this phase of the data assessment process: "What nutrients are being consumed?" and "Are the quantities appropriate?"

The first question may be answered by comparing the client's food intake to the Daily Food Guide (resulting in a restatement of the question), by calculating the nutrient content of the intake using any one of a number of food composition tables, or by submitting the intake data to computer analysis.

The second question, "Are the quantities appropriate?" is much more difficult to answer. The evaluation standard most commonly used in the United States was never designed to serve as a reference norm for individuals, yet the Recommended Dietary Allowances are commonly used for this purpose. A newer technique, the Index of Nutritional Quality (INQ), has recently been developed in response to the need for an evaluative tool for judging the adequacy of nutrient intakes. At present, this serious problem in food intake assessment has not been entirely resolved to the satisfaction of clinical dietetic practitioners.

Analysis of environmental data. Environmental factors are those elements presently in the environment that are interacting with the client's internal world. Environmental factors in the past may have influenced the client's behavior, but once their effects have been internalized, they become behavioral elements, that is, thoughts, attitudes, values, beliefs, and actions. For example, the fact that a client attends Jewish synagogue renders the synagogue an environmental factor in his life. His Jewish beliefs, however, are part of his behavioral repertoire.

The paragraphs that follow describe some of the hypotheses that could be made about the influence of the environment on a client's food behavior. The examples demonstrate the analysis of a few of the factors earlier identified as food selection variables (Table 6.2).*

Family status. Families may be defined as married couples with or without children (nuclear families) or as extended families (relatives in addition to the nuclear group). Families may also be a group of two or more significant others who may not be relatives, who have elected to establish a mutual home. Members of all kinds of families often play important roles in the food selection process.[55]

A number of factors in the family system affect the client.[56] For example, the number of dependents influences the cost of maintaining the family. Ages of dependents affect the time demands on the parents, and attention given to children. If the client is a child, his behavior may be intensively controlled by a parent.

Marital status of adults in the family influences the children as well as the adults involved. A divorced parent may be breadwinner *and* homemaker, thus creating problems with time allocation. In addition, separated parents can give children contradictory guidance, as can united couples.

Occupation(s). The work a person does for monetary reward provides a number of constraints as well as stimuli for his food behavior.

---

* We again refer the reader to *Nutrition, Behavior, and Change*, by Gifft, Washbon, and Harrison (Englewood Cliffs, NJ: Prentice-Hall, 1972), Chapters 1–3.

The responsibility inherent in the client's job may predict the frequency of dining out and the kind of restaurant he selects. The same level of income will also affect the purchase of foods, and the quality and quantity of material resources required for food handling and preparation. Included in such resources are availability of transportation to stores, a freezer for storage, a range for preparation, and china for service. These factors are influenced by other variables, such as recreational, social, and educational choices, which can use varying proportions of income.

A person's occupation can indicate potential physical and psychologic stress, as demonstrated by a relatively high rate of cardiovascular disease among executives and the high energy expenditure required in certain manual labor jobs. (The type of occupation, ranging from sedentary to highly active, is a major influence on energy needs.)

Other influences associated with occupation are considered. Time commitment can vary from one client's part-time job to another who is a professional, working 60 or more hours a week. The working woman or single head of household often carries the home responsibility in addition to work, which will affect the nature of the meals prepared.

Unemployment may have even greater influence unless the client has a source of income unrelated to employment. Older clients, for example, often have very limited incomes, which put great stress on food intake.

Education. If the client is enrolled in an educational institution, there are obvious and some not so obvious influences on his behavior. The client may have little or no choice in his food selection or he may have a reasonably wide selection. He may or may not have easy access to vending machines, fast food restaurants, and alcohol, all of which may impact on desirable food behaviors. Length of lunch hours, study demands, and quality of food are other factors that influence decision making. A newer example, surfacing in the study of school lunch programs, is the plate waste occurring because children have such short meal hours that they bolt a little food and discard the rest in order to allow time for play. Some schools have reduced plate waste by lengthening the lunch hour, staggering the times classes are sent to lunch so the children don't spend time in long lines, and letting them play first[57].

Ethnic Orientation. The place of birth, citizenship, ethnic name, and racial heritage can suggest particular food preferences and preparation techniques. Methods of preparation may affect the caloric content and nutrient value. Preferences influence the quality of foods selected, as well as the ability to purchase foods, because the desired foods may be unavailable or prohibitively expensive.

The clinician's acquaintance with customs and mores of the significant cultural groups in the community can increase her effectiveness in working with persons of cultures other than her own.[58] In adjusting nutritional care plans to clients' personal life styles, the clinician is not only pragmatic, but expresses a caring attitude. This attitude fosters client compliance.[59] One factor to consider is that foods thought of as delicacies by one client may be rejected as totally inedible by another. A classic example is that corn, a favorite in the diet of many North Americans, is considered only fit for hogs in the Netherlands.

Religion. There are religious groups who maintain dietary laws and regulations as a part of their beliefs. The dietitian needs to be thoroughly informed about these laws so that, in working with a client, he does not offend the client by his insensitivity. Knowledge of the major denominations of the world, and of local religious groups with whom the dietitian might come in contact, is important. Clients are often offended when dietary recommendations are made that run counter to religious beliefs.

Recreation. Since physical activity and emotional health play a significant role in nutritional health, the availability of recreational resources may well affect the client's ability to maintain or achieve nutritional health.[60] If local recreational facilities are expensive, they may be prohibitive for many people. Some activities require expensive equipment. Other activities, such as dance classes, may be scheduled at inopportune times. The clinician will need to be aware of the impact of the recreational environment on the client. Small communities may offer little except spectator sports, which may be relaxing but certainly do not provide opportunities for the client's own program of energy expenditure.

Residence. An individual's place of residence gives an indication of possible environmental factors that influence food behaviors. The place of residence can give supportive evidence about income, social affiliation, material resources, and even personal responsibility for food preparation. A simple clue, such as distance from work, suggests the extra time commitment for the commuter, or the possibility of lunching at home.

A person whose usual place of residence is an institution will be dependent upon the stardards and rules of that institution as well as its good will in providing nourishment. That institution may be a nursing home, prison, hospital, school, or other such highly structured organizations.

Summary. For most of these environmental variables, there is no absolute predictability of the influence they will have on the client's behavior. Their value lies in the probability factor. Each hypothesis of probable influence will need to be substantiated in the interview, or by some other means, if it is considered relevant to the client's problem.

Analysis of behavioral data. The purpose of nutritional counseling is to assist the client in identifying needed behavior change, and facilitating that change. The process of change must begin with an analysis of present behaviors, the feelings and ideas attached to them, and the circumstances in which they occur. The basic elements of behavior have been described by psychologists, and comprise what is termed "learning theory." Learning theory attempts to explain why people do what they do, and why they change their behavior.

Behavioral incidents. Human behavior is extremely complex. Any attempt to illustrate it graphically will fall short of ideal. There is some value, however, in approximating the process of a behavioral incident. If the significant events[61,62] of a behavioral incident can be identified, then there is a road map for planning behavior change. The desired change may be facilitated by modifying one or more of these events.

Figure 10.5 is a description of a behavioral incident. The stimulus cue (A) is the initiator of a behavior. This cue can be an externally occurring event, such as the word sauerkraut on a restaurant menu, or an internal event such as a depressed blood glucose level.

The internal physiologic cue or the external environmental cue, once perceived, is followed by a thought (B). That thought may be conscious or subconscious, and often occurs with great speed. This thought also may be in the form of internal verbalizing or mental imagery.

Almost instantly following the thought is a feeling or emotion (C). The relevance of the thought to the person appears to affect the in-

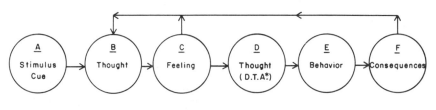

* Decision To Act

FIGURE 10.5   A model of a behavioral incident

tensity of the feeling. People seem to remember best those experiences which have intense emotion associated with them, both negative and positive. Extreme emotional trauma, however, can cause total repression (apparent inability to recall) of an experience.

At this point the feeling can stimulate another thought (B) which elicits another feeling (C). In other words, there may be alternating thoughts and feelings until one feeling prompts a decision to act (D).

This repetition is, perhaps, the reason for the disagreement among some behavioral scientists as to whether thoughts follow feelings or feelings follow thoughts.[63] This argument is akin to the chicken-egg dilemma and does not affect the use of the behavioral incident model. Thus, when the balance of feelings generated is adequately positive, the person decides to act or, if the feelings are adequately negative, he may choose to use avoidance behavior (D). Whatever that decision, the chosen behavior is emitted (E) either verbally or nonverbally.

When the behavior is emittted, a consequence (F) follows. The consequence is an external event that may be planned or incidental, an internal event such as appetite satiation, or even a nonevent. The decision not to provide a planned consequence is a consequence that is termed a nonevent, as is the absence of any significant incidental change in the environment following a behavior. When the consequence occurs, it acts as a new stimulus cue and the next behavioral incident begins.

In demonstration of the figure, the following example describes a sequence of behavioral events initiated by an internal stimulus cue. In the example, the letters relate to the behavioral events depicted in Figure 10.5.

A. Sally experiences hunger pangs.

B. Sally thinks she's hungry, imagines herself eating.

C. Sally feels pleasant anticipation of eating.

D. Sally decides to eat lunch.

E. Sally consumes her lunch.

F. Sally feels satiated.

This example describes the way most people who are able to maintain normal weight without great difficulty experience their eating behavior.[64] In contrast, it has been demonstrated that people with weight problems are responsive to external cues; for example, in place of hunger pangs, a glance at the clock may trigger the hunger thought. Such people also have more difficulty sensing the point of satiation.[64]

In the next example, the stimulus cue arises from the environment; thus it may be termed an external cue, as opposed to cues that arise from within the person.

A. Client works in a bakery and sees his favorite doughnuts.

B. Client thinks he's hungry, imagines taste of doughnut.

C. Client feels discomfort.

B. Client thinks of how doughnuts taste.

C. Client feels satisfaction doughnuts might bring.

D. Client decides he wants doughnuts.

E. Client eats six doughnuts.

F. Boss frowns.

B. Client thinks he might get fired.

C. Client feels fear.

D. Client decides to stop and go back to cleaning.

E. Client cleans counter.

F. Boss returns to office.

These phenomena may possibly be explained by the thought process going on during the behavior, much of it subconscious (just as driving an automobile and other habitual behaviors become subconscious). Somewhere in the past, conscious thoughts accompanied cues, feelings, and behaviors, which later were stored at the subconscious level. Although the thoughts appear to have been "forgotten," they remain to influence behavior for years afterwards, only to be recalled with great difficulty.[61] Thoughts or bits of information stored in the brain could be described as analogous to the storage and retrieval capacity of the computer. Once stored for the computer or the mind, the information remains "dormant" until a specific program request is made for retrieval of that information. For example, the behavior related to driving an automobile has been stored and is available on request long after the original behavior was learned. A program is entered in the computer and, once it works smoothly, is "lost" in storage until a specific effort is made to retrieve it. While the program is stored, however, a problem may be entered and manipulated by that program, and solved without the terminal operator ever seeing the process the computer follows to prepare that solution. In the same way, the subconscious mind may work to solve problems while the conscious mind is otherwise engaged.[65]

An example of another behavioral incident related to food intake might illustrate these ideas more clearly:

A. Bill's phone rings.

B. He thinks, "I haven't heard from Jan in a month. She doesn't care about me any more."

C. He feels lonely.

B. Bill thinks, "Mama always gave me a cookie when she said I was lovable, or when I was hurt, or sick."

C. He experiences warm feelings.

D. Bill thinks, "A cookie will make me feel better."

E. Bill eats a cookie.

F. He experiences physical comfort.

B. He thinks "I'm OK!"

C. He feels loved.

D. He decides to eat another cookie.

E. He eats a cookie.

F. He feels satiated and loved.

Maintenance of behavior. To further complicate behavior analysis, the value of the consequence (positive [+] or negative [−]) is determined primarily by the client.[66] Actual and perceived values are not always congruent. A client may actually prize a consequence that will be detrimental to him on a long range basis. There are extreme cases where some people view, as desirable, consequences that are painful for a large majority of the population, such as pain or incarceration. That means the clinician must not only analyze a behavioral incident, but needs to determine the value clients place on consequences. The client assigns value in the thinking and feeling events that immediately follow the consequence.

In addition to a consequence having a positive or negative connotation, it also has an intensity (e.g., 2+, 3+, etc.). A frown may be only a mild negative consequence, while a punch in the nose is a severe punishment.

Since human experience is seldom simple, there is the probability that more than one consequence is maintaining a behavior. Doubtless, many people would say they work at their jobs for more than one reason: to avoid abject poverty, to feel competent, to obtain material goods, to feel productive, to be with stimulating people, and so on. In addition, the consequences may be mixed, i.e. positive and negative.

In that case, the more powerful consequences probably control the decision to maintain or avoid the behavior. For example, a client may prefer to adhere to a nutritional care plan, as it helps him to feel healthy and energetic, which is more rewarding to him than the frustruation of saying "no" to inappropriate foods. In contrast, another client may choose to accept the consequences of inappropriate food intake in order to enjoy what he perceives to be the delights of eating.

Reconstructing behavioral incidents.   In the model of a behavioral incident (Figure 10.5), the importance of the acquisition and use of effective interviewing skills is demonstrated. Only the client can describe the stimulus cues in his environment that influence him, the thoughts and feelings he has, and the value of the consequences that he perceives to influence his behavior. Much of this, particularly food behaviors that have been established over a long period of time, occurs below his conscious awareness.

The extensive listening and attempt to label ambiguous feelings approximate a return journey to a once familiar city. The client is unable to reconstruct a map from sheer memory, but by driving slowly, paying attention to the landmarks, he recalls a familiar one at each corner in the road, remembering each turn one by one. Occasionally, when there is doubt, the client may venture down a strange road a short distance looking for familiar landmarks. When he realizes he is in unfamiliar territory, he retraces his steps and tries another route, finally reaching his destination. Although unfamiliar with that particular city, the clinician in the counseling setting acts as a fellow traveler, helping the client retrace his steps. In reconstructing the past events leading to current food behaviors, the clinical dietitian helps the client recall the stimulus cues for those behaviors. For example, following current food practices back to childhood for an obese client may help him to recall that he was always required to eat everything on his plate, whether at home or in a restaurant, so as not to "waste money." But the client may then recall that this is, in reality, "unfamiliar territory;" with the assistance of the clinical dietitian, the client may remember that his behavior originated not with the "cleanplate" attitude, but with food used as a "reward for being a good boy."

More specific food behavior data may be obtained on forms that the client uses to record his food intake and the circumstances in which he consumes that food. Forms for such assessment have been presented elsewhere.[5] These results are then discussed in a follow-up interview for further behavior analysis.

The implication of this analysis is that the better a clinician's understanding of the events of a client's behavior patterns, the more likely intervention strategies can be planned that will be effective in altering those patterns. Because of the complex etiology of a nutritional problem, it is easy to understand why a client does not always act in his own best interests. He behaves inappropriately because he does not know what to do or how to do it, because external circumstances seem insurmountable, or because he is not motivated. The primary task for the clinical dietitian is to ascertain exactly the client's concerns.

Synthesize Pertinent Data: Are They Adequate?

The four categories of nutritional care data are collected simultaneously during the phases of the assessment component, even though one phase may be emphasized more than another at any point in time. In other words, in the preliminary data collection phase, the focus is on biologic and environmental data from the medical record. During the first interview, food intake data and some behavioral data are the primary categories collected. Subsequent interviews may include discussions of the client's own records of his intake data and food practices.

Although the collection of data may be random, the final data interpretation is more effectively carried out in a step-wise fashion. The clinical dietitian may first determine if there are any physiologic indicators that are supportive of nutritional intervention. Any "abnormal" biologic data with nutritional implications will have significant impact on the determination of the criteria for adequate food intake. The lack of any abnormal biologic data, though, does not imply that all is well; such lack only eliminates the probability of current need for therapeutic prescriptions. The potential for future pathology remains.

Ultimately, the various data are synthesized in order to determine how they relate and interact. In an ecologic system, the related elements will be affected by a change in any one element.[67] Information about the client must be considered, not in isolation, but in relation to the effect it has on other aspects of the client's life and, conversely, the effects other aspects have on it.

As before, Figure 10.3 contains a decision step that asks if the data are adequate. At this stage in assessment, the clinician has greatly expanded on both the quality and quantity of client data. Now he must again judge whether or not he is ready to proceed to the next phase of assessment, identification of baseline data, or if he should return to the data collection step.

IDENTIFYING BASELINE DATA

The last step in assessment takes the totality of the synthesized data and then identifies those factors that indicate a need for intervention (Figure 10.6). Again, that intervention may be directed toward desirable or undesirable behaviors. When the baseline data are finally determined and found acceptable to the health team and to the client, they are recorded on an assessment worksheet and in the medical record, and the assessment process is concluded as the major focus. Assessment data, however, may be acquired during the subsequent phases and incorporated into the total counseling process at any time.

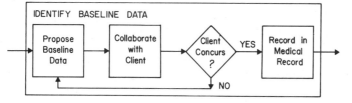

FIGURE 10.6   Assessment: Identifying baseline data

Propose Baseline Data

The conclusion of the analysis and synthesis of biologic data leads to decisions about whether or not there are any deviations that indicate a need for food and/or nutrient intake modification. If there is not, the next step is to examine the food intake data to see if there are patterns that would be a harbinger of future concerns. If there are deviations, then other types of data may give clues as to their relationship to the deviations in physical health. If the client is consuming adequate nutrients, the practitioner may reinforce her behavior by planning to acknowledge food intake practices.

Even though the client's food intake provides adequate nutrition, she may have questions and concerns with which the dietitian should deal. The concerns may relate to any aspect of the client's nutrition, but will manifest themselves most likely in relation to confusing or conflicting information the client has heard that she perceives to affect her. For example, the client may know she has experienced sudden deafness syndrome and wants to find out if what she had read in an organic food publication about the curative powers of several organic foods is true. This example illustrates that the determination of an adequate food intake may not be a cue for conclusion of the assessment process. Clients with need for counseling include those who do and do not have requirements for modified nutrient intakes. If the client is healthy and has adequate food intake but wishes to have information, she remains a client until she is satisfied that she has obtained and understood the information that she wanted. All other clients with inadequate food intakes and/or nutrition-related biologic deviations are potential clients for continued counseling, either until the deviations are corrected or until the client terminates the counseling.

The synthesis of environmental data may provide information about which of those factors play a significant role in client food practices. Some environmental factors are supportive; others are obstacles to desirable client behavior. If an obstacle is unalterable, then the client and clinician need to find ways to circumvent (legally) the obstacles. This may take ingenuity, as the client may well have exhausted the more obvious avenues of resolution. If there are removable obstacles, the client needs to remove them, assuming she has the capability. The clinical dietitian can make suggestions when the client seems stymied, or the clinician may arrange for resolution of the environmental problem when it is beyond the client's scope of skills or influence.

When all of the environmental data are related to inappropriate food intake, a determination must be made as to whether or not there are any that adversely affect dietary status. If factors are identified, they are recorded on the assessment worksheet to become a part of the baseline data.

The last step in identification of baseline data is based on an analysis of behavior (Figure 10.5). Lack of knowledge and skills are primarily centered in the thinking process, and manifested in a behavioral incident. The method of assessing intellectual ability is generally referred to, in learning design, as *pretesting*. That is, pretesting is the discovery of what the learner knows *before* the instruction is planned. If the client lacks required knowledge and skill, instruction in appropriate food behaviors should be considered.

A pretest also will identify those clients who know how to eat adequately, but do not do so. For such individuals, a plan for motivation is required. Some clients have no need for motivational support once they know how to proceed. If the initial interview determines lack of knowledge and/or skills, it is impossible to collect reliable data regarding the level of motivation at the same time. Obtaining motivational data may require a waiting period while the client has an opportunity to implement his newly acquired skill.

Motivational data also must be collected over a period of time in order to assess continuity of behavior. An analysis of food diary data that can be collected by the client while in his natural environment is examined in terms of the:

1. Actual stimulus cues that precipitate his food behaviors
2. Attitudinal thoughts (those accepted by the client as true, based on his experiences)
3. Subsequent feelings
4. Frequency of behaviors
5. Nature of the consequences and their value to the client

Such data can give the clinical dietitian clues as to which factors are contributing to behavior maintenance or inhibition. People tend to repeat behaviors that produce positive consequences (consequences that lead to positive feelings), and to avoid behaviors that produce negative consequences.[68]

An example of proposed baseline data appears in the next chapter, Planning. Recall, for a moment, Mrs. S. R. who was the client in the case study in Chapter 4. She is pregnant, has an undesirable hemoglobin level, and a limited food intake. We saw her through a cursory counseling process in the earlier chapter; next we will demonstrate, for Mrs. S. R., how identified baseline data lead sequentially to planning.

Collaboration with the Client

When the baseline data have been identified by the clinician, the next critical step is consultation with the client. The client is considered a member of the health care team and, consequently, participates in decisions about his own health care. Collaboration with the client to determine with which data the client wishes to work will increase the probability of compliance to the health care regimen.

The ultimate decision on the continuation of counseling occurs here. The only exceptions to making decisions at this point are the potential client who refuses to become involved, in spite of biologic indicators of his need to do so, or the client who has no biologic deviations and is convinced that his nutritional behavior is appropriate.

Record in the Medical Record

Under the assessment (analysis) segment (S-O-A-P) of the Problem-Oriented Record (or in the SOR progress notes), the clinical dietitian should briefly summarize the baseline data identified. The statements should be supported by a rationale drawn from both the subjective and objective data, and from the relevant scientific literature. As the medical record is viewed as a legal document, baseline data statements must have documentation in the subjective and objective notes. Having the baseline data recorded in the medical record also serves as a communication to other health care providers. Their concurrence is one of the clinician's goals.

SUMMARY

Assessment involves a three-step process: assessing preliminary data, assessing diet history data, and identifying baseline data. Four types of data are surveyed: biologic, food intake, environmental, and behavioral data. Careful attention to the process of assessment and to the data categories will provide the clinician with the keys to facilitating significant changes in a client's nutritional behavior.

CITED REFERENCES

1. Carnevali, D. Nursing process: A problem-oriented system. *In* Walter, J. B., Pardee, G. P., and Molbo, D. M., Eds. *Dynamics of Problem-Oriented Approaches: Patient Care and Documentation*. Philadelphia: J. B. Lippincott Co., 1976.
2. Becker, M. H., Drachman, R. H., and Kirscht, J. P. A new approach to explaining sick-role behavior in low-income people. *Am. J. Publ. Health* 64:205, 1974.
3. Wills, B. B. Food becomes fun for children. *Am. J. Nurs.* 78:2082, 1978.
4. Weed, L. L. *Medical Records, Medical Education, and Patient Care.* Cleveland: The Press of Case Western Reserve Univ., 1970.
5. Ferguson, J. M. *Learning to Eat: Behavior Modification for Weight Control. Leader Manual.* Palo Alto, CA: Bull Publ. Co., 1975.
6. Science and Education Administration. *Food. A Publication on Food and Nutrition by U.S. Department of Agriculture.* Home and Garden Bull. No. 228. Washington: U.S. Dept. Agric., 1979.
7. Ballantyne, R. M. Canada's Food Guide—revised. *J. Canad. Dietet. A.* 38:183, 1977.
8. Food and Nutr. Serv., Agric. Res. Serv. *A Daily Food Guide.* FNS-13. Rev., July, 1975. Washington: U.S. Dept. Agric., 1975.
9. King, J. C., Cohenour, S. H., Corruccini, C. G., and Schneeman, P. Eval-

uation and modification of the Basic Four Food Guide. *J. Nutr. Educ.* 10:27, 1978.

10. Hunscher, H. A., and Macy, I. G. Dietary study methods. I. Uses and abuses of dietary study methods. *J. Am. Dietet. A.* 27:558, 1951.

11. Adams, C. F. *Nutritive Value of American Foods in Common Units.* USDA Handbook No. 456. Washington: U.S. Dept. Agric., 1976.

12. Pennington, J. A. T., and Church, H. N., Eds. *Bowes and Church: Food Values of Portions Commonly Used.* 13th Ed. Philadelphia: J. B. Lippincott Co., 1980.

13. Consumer and Food Econ. Res. Div., Agric. Res. Serv. *Nutritive Value of Foods.* Sl. Rev. USDA Home and Garden Bull. No. 72 Washington: U.S. Dept. Agric., 1971.

14. Watt, B. K., and Merrill, A. L. *Composition of Foods—Raw, Processed, Prepared.* Rev. USDA Handbook No. 8. Washington: U.S. Dept. Agric., 1963.

15. Posati, L. P., and Orr, M. L. *Composition of Foods. Dairy and Egg Products, Raw-Processed-Prepared.* Rev. USDA Agric. Handbook No. 8-1. Washington: U.S. Dept. Agric., 1976.

16. Marsh, A. C., Moss, J. K., and Murphy, E. W. *Composition of Foods. Spices and Herbs, Raw—Processed—Prepared.* Rev. USDA Agric. Handbook No. 8-2. Washington: U.S. Dept. Agric., 1977.

17. Gebhardt, S. E., Cutrufelli, R., and Matthews, R. H. *Composition of Foods. Baby Foods, Raw—Processed—Prepared.* Rev. USDA Agric. Handbook No. 8-3. Washington: U.S. Dept. Agric., 1978.

18. Reeves, J. B., and Weihrouch, J. L. *Composition of Foods. Fats and Oils, Raw—Processed—Prepared.* Rev. USDA Agric. Handbook No. 8-4. Washington: U.S. Dept. Agric., 1979.

19. Posati, L. P. *Composition of Foods. Poultry Products, Raw—Processed— Prepared.* Rev. USDA Agric. Handbook No. 8-5. Washington: U.S. Dept. Agric., 1979.

20. Marsh, A. C. *Composition of Foods. Soups, Sauces, and Gravies, Raw— Processed—Prepared.* Rev. USDA Agric. Handbook No. 8-6. Washington: U.S. Dept. Agric., 1980.

21. Richardson, M., Posati, L. P., and Anderson, B. A. *Composition of Foods. Sausages and Luncheon Meats, Raw—Processed—Prepared.* Rev. USDA Agric. Handbook No. 8-7. Washington: U.S. Dept. Agric., 1980.

22. Food and Agric. Organ. of the United Nations, Food Policy and Food Science Service. *Amino Acid Content of Foods and Biological Data on Proteins.* Rome: FAO, 1970.

23. Orr, M. L. *Pantothenic Acid, Vitamin B_6 and Vitamin B_{12} in Food.* USDA Home Econ. Res. Rep't. No. 36. Washington: U.S. Dept. Agric., 1969.

24. Orr, M. L., and Watt, B. K. *Amino Acid Content of Foods.* USDA Home Econ. Res. Rep't. No. 4. Washington: U.S. Dept. Agric., 1957.

25. Toepfer, E. W., Zook, E. G., Orr, M. L., and Richardson, L. R. *Folic Acid Content of Foods*. USDA Handbook No. 29. Washington: U.S. Dept. Agric., 1951.

26. Mayer, J. Food composition tables: Basis, uses and limitations. *Postgrad. Med.* 28:295, 1960.

27. Whiting, M. G., and Leverton, R. M. Reliability of dietary appraisal: Comparisons between laboratory analysis and calculation from tables of food values. *Am. J. Pub. Health* 50:815, 1960.

28. Hertzler, A. A., and Hoover, L. W. Development of food tables and use with computers. Review of nutrient data bases. *J. Am. Dietet. A.* 70:20, 1977.

29. Watt, B. K., Gebhardt, S. E., Murphy, E. W., and Butrum, R. R. Food composition tables for the 70's. *J. Am. Dietet. A.* 64:257, 1974.

30. Hoover, L. W. Computers in dietetics: State-of-the-art, 1976. *J. Am. Dietet. A.* 68:39, 1976.

31. McConnell, F. G., and Wilson, A. Computerized nutritional analysis in the dietetic department of a teaching hospital. *J. Hum. Nutr.* 30:405, 1976.

32. Walsh, K. A. Computerized dietary calculations: An interactive approach. *J. Hum. Nutr.* 30:395, 1976.

33. Bell, L., Hatcher, J., Chan, L., and Fraser, D. Development of a computerized system for calculating nutrient intakes. *J. Canad. Dietet. A.* 40:30, 1979.

34. Sheehan, E. T., Kight, M. A., and Forcier, J. I. Computerized dietary analysis: Per cent *animal, plant,* and *mixed* items. *J. Am. Dietet. A.* 71:530, 1977.

35. Harper, A. E. Recommended Dietary Allowances: Are they what we think they are? *J. Am. Dietet. A.* 64:151, 1974.

36. Committee on Dietary Allowances, Food and Nutrition Board. *Recommended Dietary Allowances*. 9th Rev. Ed., 1980. Washington: Nat'l. Aca. Sci., 1980.

37. Committee for Revision of the Canadian Dietary Standard, Bureau of Nutritional Sciences, Health and Welfare Canada. *Dietary Standards for Canada*. Rev. 1975. Ottawa: Information Canada, 1975.

38. Sabry, Z. I. The Canadian dietary standard. *J. Am. Dietet. A.* 56:195, 1970.

39. Hegsted, D. M. Dietary standards. *J. Am. Dietet. A.* 66:13, 1975.

40. Robinson, C. H. The dietitian's use of the RDAs. *J. Am. Dietet. A.* 73:434, 1978.

41. Consumer and Food Econ. Res. Div., Agric. Res. Serv. *Food Intake and Nutritive Value of Diets of Men, Women and Children in the United States, Spring, 1965. A preliminary report.* Agric. Res. Serv. Rep't. 62–18. Washington: U.S. Dept. Agric., 1969.

42. Consumer and Food Econ. Res. Div., Agric. Res. Serv. *Dietary Levels of*

Households in the Northeast, Spring, 1965. Household Food Consumption Survey, 1965-66. Rep't. No. 7. Washington: U.S. Dept. Agric., 1970.

43. Inano, M., Pringle, D. J., and Little, L. Dietary survey of low-income, rural families in Iowa and North Carolina. I. Research procedures. *J. Am. Dietet. A.* 66:356, 1975.

44. *Ten-State Nutrition Survey, 1968–70.* V—Dietary. DHEW Publ. No. (HSM) 72-8133. Washington: U.S. Dept. Health, Educ., and Welfare, 1972.

45. Kohrs, M. B., O'Hanlon, P., and Eklund, D. Title VII-Nutrition Program for the elderly. I. Contribution to one day's dietary intake. *J. Am. Dietet. A.* 72:487, 1978.

46. Burke, B. S. The dietary history as a tool in research. *J. Am. Dietet. A.* 23:1041, 1947.

47. Clarke, M. and Wakefield, L. M. Food choices of institutionalized vs. independent-living elderly. *J. Am. Dietet. A.* 66:600, 1975.

48. Shapiro, L. R. Streamlining and implementing nutritional assessment: The dietary approach. *J. Am. Dietet. A.* 75:230, 1979.

49. Hegsted, D. M. On dietary standards. *Nutr. Rev.* 36:33, 1978.

50. Sorenson, A. W., Wyse, B. W., Wittwer, A. J., and Hansen, R. G. An index of nutritional quality for a balanced diet. *J. Am. Dietet. A.* 68:236, 1976.

51. Wyse, B. W., Sorenson, A. W., Wittwer, A. J., and Hansen, R. G. Nutritional quality index identifies consumer nutrient needs. *Food Tech.* 30:22, 1976.

52. Rose, M. S., Hessler, M. C., Stiebeling, H. K., and Taylor, C. M. Visualizing food values. *J. Home Econ.* 20:781, 1928.

53. Hansen, R. G. An index of food quality. *Nutr. Rev.* 31:1, 1973.

54. Hansen, R. G., Wyse, B. W., and Sorenson, A. W. *Nutritional Quality Index of Foods.* Westport, CO: AVI Publishing Company, Inc., 1979.

55. Hertzler, A. A., and Vaughan, C. E. The relationship of family structure and interaction to nutrition. A review. *J. Am. Dietet. A.* 74:23, 1979.

56. Taylor, R. B. Family: A systems approach. *Am. Fam. Phys.* 20:101, 1979.

57. Christensen, E. W., Wyse, B. W., Brown, G., Hansen, R. G., and Harding, D. J. Effects of food location on the tray and scheduling of playtime on food consumption. *Sch. Food Serv. Res. Rev.* 3:1:16, 1979.

58. Smith, L. K. Mexican-American views of Anglo medical and dietetic practices. *J. Am. Dietet. A.* 74:463, 1979.

59. Bonaparte, B. H. Ego-defensiveness, open-close mindedness, and nurses' attitude toward culturally different patients. *Nurs. Res.* 28:166, 1979.

60. Le Shan, E. J. *Winning the Losing Battle: Why I Will Never Be Fat Again.* New York: Bantam Books, 1981.

61. Harris, T. A. *I'm OK, You're OK. A Practical Guide to Transactional Analysis.* New York: Harper and Row Publ., Inc., 1969.

62. Kanfer, F. H., and Goldstein, A. P. Eds. *Helping People Change. A Textbook of Methods.* New York: Pergamon Press, Inc., 1975.

63. Johnson, D. W., and Mattross, R. P. Attitude modification methods. *In* Kanfer, F. H., and Goldstein, A. P., Eds. *Helping People Change. A Textbook of Methods.* New York: Pergamon Press, Inc., 1975.

64. Silverstone, J. T., Ed. *Obesity: Pathogenesis and Management.* Acton, MA: Publ. Sci. Group, Inc., 1975.

65. Welsch, P. K. *The Nurturance of Creative Behavior in Environments: A Comprehensive Curriculum Approach.* Unpublished Ph.D. dissertation, Michigan State University, 1980.

66. Krumboltz, J. D., and Krumboltz, H. B. *Changing Children's Behavior.* Englewood Cliffs, NJ: Prentice-Hall, Inc., 1972.

67. Rae, J., and Burke, A. L. Counselling the elderly on nutrition in a community health care system. *J. Am. Geria. Soc.* 26:130, 1978.

68. Smith, W. I., and Moore, J. W. *Conditioning and Instrumental Learning.* New York: McGraw-Hill Book Co., 1966.

SUGGESTED REFERENCES

Alfin-Slater, R. B., and Jelliffe, D. B. Evaluating diets—there is no perfect method. *Cajanus* 10:2:86, 1977.

Allport, G. W. *The Person in Psychology: Selected Essays.* Boston: Beacon Press, 1968.

Anderson, R. D., and Carter, I. E. *Human Behavior in the Social Environment: A Social Systems Approach.* Chicago: Aldine Publ. Co., 1974.

Baird, P. C., and Schutz, H. G. Life style correlates of dietary and biochemical measures of nutrition. *J. Am. Dietet. A.* 76:228, 1980.

Beaton, G. H., Milner, J., Corey, P., McGuire, V., Cousing, M., Stewart, E., deRamos, M., Hewitt, D., Grambsch, P. V., Kassim, N., and Little, J. A. Sources of variance in 24-hour dietary recall data: Implications for nutrition study design and interpretation. *Am. J. Clin. Nutr.* 32:2546, 1979.

Dietary standards. *N. Eng. J. Med.* 292:915, 1975.

FAO/WHO Handbook on Human Nutritional Requirements, 1974. *Nutr. Rev.* 33:147, 1975.

Gifft, H. H., Washbon, M. B., and Harrison, G. G. *Nutrition, Behavior, and Change.* Englewood Cliffs, NJ: Prentice-Hall, Inc., 1972.

Guthrie, H. A. The role of nutrition education in dietary improvement. *Food Tech.* 32:9:89, 1978.

Harper, A. E. Meeting recommended dietary allowances. *J. Fla. Med. A.* 66:419, 1979.

Harper, A. E. The recommended dietary allowances. Part III. Critique of the British prescription. *Nutr. Today.* 14:5:28, 1979.

Hertzler, A. A., and Owen, C. Sociologic study of food habits—a review. I. Diversity in diet and scalogram analysis. *J. Am. Dietet. A.* 69:377, 1976.

Hertzler, A. A., and Owen, C. Sociologic study of food habits—a review. II. Differentiation, accessibility and solidarity. *J. Am. Dietet. A.* 69:381, 1976.

Kee, B. L., and Kilby, M. E. Use of a programmable calculator for nutrient analysis. *J. Am. Dietet. A.* 72:629, 1978.

Koh, E. T., and Caples, V. Nutrient intake of low-income, black families in southwestern Mississippi. *J. Am. Dietet. A.* 75:665, 1979.

Leverton, R. M. The RDAs are not for amateurs. *J. Am. Dietet. A.* 66:9, 1975.

McMasters, V. History of food composition tables of the world. *J. Am. Dietet. A.* 43:442, 1963.

Monteith, M., and Nakagawa, A. A flow chart approach to nutritional screening and assessment in long-term care facilities. *J. Am. Dietet. A.* 75:684, 1979.

Munro, H. N. The ninth edition of Recommended Dietary Allowances, revised 1980. *Food & Nutr. News* 51:3:1, 1980.

Munro, H. N. How well recommended are the Recommended Dietary Allowances? *J. Am. Dietet. A.* 71:490, 1977.

Passmore, R., Hollingsworth, D. F., and Robertson, J. The recommended dietary allowances. Part II. Prescription for a better British diet. *Nutr. Today* 14:5:23, 1979.

Schafer, R. B. The self-concept as a factor in diet selection and quality. *J. Nutr. Ed.* 11:37, 1979.

The recommended dietary allowances. Part I. The new recommended dietary allowances *Nutr. Today* 14:5:10, 1979.

Watt, B. K. Concepts in developing a food composition table. *J. Am. Dietet. A.* 40:297, 1962.

Watt, B. K., and Murphy, E. W. Tables of food composition: Scope and needed research. *Food Tech.* 24:674, 1970.

Zacharewicz, F. A., and Coger, R. Educational needs assessment: A systematic approach. *J. All. Health.* 6:54, 1977.

11
Planning

> . . . *nutritional counseling is a growth-producing process in which the client begins with a diet or food consciousness and grows toward awareness of nutrition as a body of scientific knowledge and research. Nutrition plays too great a role in health to be a "hit or miss, one-shot affair" after a medical crisis. Nutrition professionals are now seeking to move nutrition education from the treatment of disease to health planning.*
>
> Judy Wylie and Jeanne Singer, **Growth process in nutrition counseling** (*J. Am. Dietet.* A. 69:505, 1976).

In the growth-producing process described by Wylie and Singer,[1] the second component of clinical practice, planning, is of vital importance in the sequential development of client independence. The appropriate sequel to the collection and analysis of comprehensive assessment data is the development of a plan for action.

In Chapter 1 we described the roles of clinical dietitians in client-centered nutritional care. Each role—provision of nutritional counseling and provision of nutrient sources—is related to well-defined levels of client independence in the food selection process. Clients are envisioned to be in one of three stages in the dependence–independence continuum. They may be dependent, incapable of both self-sufficiency and self-determination; they may be self-determined, yet not self-sufficient; or they may be both self-determined and self-sufficient, striving for independence in the food selection process.

For all stages in the continuum, the process of planning in nutritional care is essential. For those clients who are unable to enter into the decision-making process about their food choices, the planning component is managed by the clinical dietitian until such time as the client is able and/or willing to be a partner. We earlier described planning in a health crisis as practitioner-managed care.*

In primary prevention (illness prevention) or secondary prevention (disability prevention),† the efforts of the clinical dietitian are directed toward the achievement of client independence in a food selection process aimed towards the acquisition of healthful nutritional behaviors. These clients, as envisioned in Figure 1.1, are persons capable of self-determination and, as such, are those individuals for whom clinical dietitians have the greatest responsibility. Thus, the process of nutritional counseling is that aspect of nutritional care which is the focus of attention of practitioners in client-managed care.*

This chapter is devoted to the development of plans for nutritional counseling and not to the planning for provision of nutrient sources. Clinical dietitians working in practitioner-managed crises environments are directed to the abundant literature in basic nutritional science and nutritional pathology.

The responsibility of the clinical dietitian in the planning phase of nutritional counseling is the design of appropriate instruction for a client. Such instruction may have been prescribed by a primary care provider, but, if not, most certainly should be recommended or prescribed by the dietitian for any client assessed as having the need to alter food intake. Whether or not the client wishes to adhere to the prescription or even to partake of the counseling process is his own choice, but the clinician has the responsibility of informing the client of his dietary status so that he can make intelligent, thoughtful decisions about his own nutritional care.

As defined in Chapter 1, nutritional care is the creative act of translating the bodies of knowledge of nutrition and other scientific disciplines to resolve the food problems and concerns of humans. The blueprint for nutritional care is the nutritional care plan, and is both a *process* and a *tool*.

As a *process*, the nutritional care plan follows assessment and incorporates a series of dynamic management strategies designed to facilitate controlled change on the part of the client to realize optimal nutritional status. As a *tool*, the plan is a documentation communi-

---

* We are again in the debt of C. A. Johnson for highlighting these phrases.

† This was first discussed in Chapter 2.

cating those management strategies. Nutritional care planning is the logical thought process employed in generating the nutritional care plan. Planning begins with hypothesis of needs that translates to the statement of the goals to be achieved. The goals then direct the development of objectives.

WRITING GOALS AND OBJECTIVES

The keystone to instructional planning is the statement of objectives. Objectives are specifically designed to describe desired behavioral changes (learning) in the client.[2] Clearly stated objectives define the evaluation experience and guide the development of appropriate learning for achieving the goal, the end toward which effort is directed. The goal statement reflects the primary need of the client, usually in terms of altered food intake. The objectives are observable, verifiable steps to attainment of the goal. For example, Mrs. S. R., the pregnant client described in Chapter 4, needs to consume more meat, fruits, and vegetables in an effort to improve her nutritional status. The *goal of the nutritional care plan* is to improve Mrs. S. R.'s food intake. When adequate intake is achieved, the desirable consequence of increased hemoglobin level (primary care goal) may or may not be realized. If not, the primary care provider must try another solution. The goal of the nutritional care plan, however, is attained when the client begins to eat more appropriate foods.

From an analysis and synthesis of data we may determine that Mrs. S. R. has the following needs:

1. Biologic: increased weight and hemoglobin level
2. Food intake: increased consumption of meats, fruits, and vegetables
3. Environmental: financial assistance
4. Behavioral: improved food preparation skills; improved knowledge of budgeting/purchasing; improved knowledge of meal planning; improved attitude toward regular mealtimes

The behavioral needs may be identified using Figure 10.5. Mrs. S. R.'s limited food preparation skills, knowledge of budgeting and purchasing, and meal planning are all associated with the thought processes (Figure 10.5, event B), and thus will require the development of intellectual instructional plans. Mrs. S. R.'s preference for spontaneous snacking rather than formal mealtimes is a result of negative feelings associated with formal eating, and therefore, will require attention to motivational objectives and strategies.

Thus, from the goal of improved food intake the client goals are derived:

1. Improved food preparation skills
2. Better food budgeting and purchasing skills
3. Acquisition of food stamps
4. More formalized meal settings
5. Skill in planning appropriate food intake

The goal statements above are loosely constructed and require refinement for a format we shall term *behavioral objectives*. Behavioral objectives for Mrs. S. R. could be written as follows:

1. Using the Daily Food Guide, Mrs. S. R. will plan daily meals for a week that meet the minimum servings established for her.
2. Using the weekly meals she has planned, and cost information, Mrs. S. R. will revise the plan to keep within her established budget (including food stamps) and maintain the minimum servings criteria.
3. Mrs. S. R. will obtain food stamps from an available distribution site each month for 3 consecutive months.
4. Using the final weekly meal plan and appropriate recipes, Mrs. S. R. will prepare the foods with the product meeting her family's standards of acceptability, using all of the basic components of each recipe (seasonings can be varied).
5. For a period of 3 weeks, Mrs. S. R. will plan, prepare, and eat at least three formally presented meals providing adequate intake each day for 5 out of 7 days of each week.
6. Mrs. S. R. will eat half of her meals with her husband, using the meals she planned.

A thorough examination of these objectives shows that desired nutritional behaviors can be clearly formulated. Of the six objectives, 1, 2, and 4 are *competence* objectives; 3, 5, and 6 are *motivation* objectives. It is important to plan for both. A client may demonstrate great skill in planning her own food intake, but if she has difficulty adhering to it, the energy invested in teaching the skill is wasted. Furthermore, the client may be more frustrated by her unsuccessful attempts to follow through on the plan, thus feeling guilty or inadequate. Although providing motivational support is not a simple task, there are strategies the clinical dietitian can use to enhance the probability that the client will succeed and persist in her new behavior.

Components of Objectives

According to Mager,[3] a good learner objective has three distinct components: the terminal behavior, the conditions, and the criteria. The phrase terminal behavior describes an observable, verifiable behavior exhibited by the learner. The conditions state the circumstances in which the behavior occurs, and the criteria establish the level of achievement expected. Thus, the six objectives previously presented may be analyzed as follows:

1. Using the Daily Food Guide (condition), Mrs. S. R. will plan daily meals for a week (terminal behavior), which meet the minimum servings established for her (criteria).

2. Using the weekly meals she has planned, and cost information (condition), Mrs. S. R. will revise the plan (terminal behavior) to keep within her established budget (including food stamps) and maintain the minimum servings criterion (criteria).

3. Mrs. S. R. will obtain food stamps (terminal behavior) from an available distribution site (condition) each month for 3 consecutive months (criteria).

4. Using the final weekly meal plan and appropriate recipes (condition), Mrs. S. R. will prepare the foods (terminal behavior) with the product meeting her family's standards of acceptability, using all of the basic components of each recipe (seasonings can be varied) (criteria).

5. For a period of 3 weeks (criteria), Mrs. S. R. will plan, prepare, and eat (terminal behavior) at least three (criteria) formally presented meals providing adequate intake each day for 5 out of 7 days of each week (conditions).

6. Mrs. S. R. will eat (terminal behavior) half of her meals (criteria) with her husband, using the meals she planned (conditions).

Attributes of Quality Objectives

An objective, though, is more than a mechanical statement with the three component parts. The content of objectives is important in determining their value. There are several qualities that will render an objective both humanistic and functional. To determine whether or not a written objective has these qualities, the authors suggest the following guideline, an adaption of an acronym proposed by Connell.[4] The acronym, RHUMBA, represents:

Relevant: related to the assessed needs of the client and the real world in which he functions

High-fidelity: real or an approximation of reality to the extent ethics and resources permit

Unambiguous: easily understood by several different observers (interjudge reliability)

Measurable: describable in terms of time, duration, or number of responses

Behavioral: observable or audible action

Achievable: capable of being learned by the learner in a reasonable period of time

For a better understanding of the acronym, the following examples and nonexamples* of quality objectives are introduced here:

Assessment Data: Client (Mrs. M.) has an abnormally high blood glucose level that can be controlled by diet. She is now ready to acquire independence in meal planning.

Relevant:

Example: Using the appropriate instruction booklet, Mrs. M. will plan meals for 3 days for her family, designating the selection and amounts of each food she will eat for her calorie-controlled diet, with no error.

Nonexample: Without looking at any references, Mrs. M. will state the number of grams of carbohydrate in each of the fruits listed in USDA Handbook 456 without error.

Comment: The client doesn't need to have these memorized or even use USDA Handbook 456, because she won't use the information this way at home. The instruction booklet provides adequate information for meal planning at the beginning.

High-Fidelity:

Example: Using the grocery items stocked in the nutrition counseling office, Mrs. M. will point to those which

---

* In this context, nonexample is a term used to describe a situation, an idea, or an object that does not possess all the defined attributes of the designated concept. Thus, an *example* possesses all of the attributes of the concept; a *nonexample* lacks one or more attributes.

are acceptable on a calorie-controlled diet, with no error.

Nonexample: At the grocery store, Mrs. M. will point to those grocery items which are acceptable on a calorie-controlled diet, with no error.

Nonexample: At the grocery store, Mrs. M. will place a check mark on the label of every product which is acceptable on a calorie-controlled diet, with no error.

Comment: Since the clinical dietitian seldom has the time to go to the grocery with a client (excessive use of resources), the example is a high-fidelity simulation (real food items, simulated setting). In the second nonexample, a rather extreme example of unethical behavior is given.

Unambiguous:

Example: In a restaurant, Mrs. M. will order and consume meals that are acceptable on her calorie-controlled diet at least five times out of six.

Nonexample: At the restaurant, Mrs. M. will demonstrate her willingness to watch her caloric intake.

Comment: What will she do to demonstrate her willingness? Say "I'm willing"? Order a low-caloric meal, but also eat some of her husband's dessert? Say "I wish they'd brought me vinegar instead of salad dressing"?

Measurable:

Example: Using the food models, Mrs. M. will arrange three meals on placemats, representing an adequate daily nutritional intake and meeting the criteria of her calorie-controlled diet.

Nonexample: Using a recipe book, Mrs. M. will decide what to eat each day.

Comment: For how many days? Can the deciding be measured?

Behavioral:

Example: Using a pocket calculator, Mrs. M. will calculate the unit price of 10 grocery items with no error.

Nonexample: Mrs. M. will be aware of unit prices on grocery items.

Comment: What is Mrs. M. doing when she's *aware* . . .?

Achievable:

Example: From the hospital menu, Mrs. M. will circle the foods she wishes for each meal for a week. Each selection must be acceptable on her calorie-controlled diet.

Nonexample: Using Handbook 456, Mrs. M. will calculate the nutrient content of a week's meals for 37 nutrients, with no error.

Comment: Mrs. M. would need a minicourse in nutrition to learn how to calculate nutrients.

If these RHUMBA criteria are applied to the development of learner objectives, these objectives should contribute to more effective instruction and client compliance.

THE VALUE OF OBJECTIVES

While defining objectives for a client's nutritional care plan is a demanding exercise, it yields several rewards:

1. The client knows exactly what is expected of him before he begins to learn and when he has achieved his goals

2. The clinical dietitian has clear direction as to what she must do to help the client learn

3. The clinical dietitian has specified what method she will use to evaluate learner achievement

4. Other health professionals can understand the plans the client and dietitian have made together

5. The plan can be understood and followed by other dietitians who may need to substitute for the original planner, or those involved in peer review.*

To demonstrate the importance of stating objectives, Yelon and Scott relate the following anecdote:

After teachers had been complaining about the foul language of his children, Mr. Brown decided to do something to teach them to speak properly. At breakfast, he asked his oldest boy, "What will you have for breakfast?" The son replied, "Gimme some of those damn cornflakes." Immediately the father smashed an open hand across the boy's mouth. The boy's chair tumbled over and the child rolled up against the wall. The father then turned to his second oldest boy and inquired, "And what do YOU want for breakfast?" The son

* Peer review is discussed briefly in Chapter 15.

hesitated and then blurted out, "I sure as hell don't want any of those damn cornflakes."

Moral: If you want (people) to learn something, tell them your objectives.[5] (p. 5)

Notwithstanding the inappropriate, although effective, choice of instructional strategy, the lack of an explicit statement of the desired outcome led to the child's learning an unintended behavior; he refused to eat cornflakes. Although admittedly dramatic, this situation is replayed many times over in a variety of learning experiences. Unfortunately, the unintended learning often is either unnoticed by the instructor or not perceived as a consequence of the inappropriate instruction.

The lack of objectives often results in the use of ill-conceived evaluation techniques and may result in little or no correlation between learning outcomes, activities, and evaluation planned by the instructor. Without clear objectives, the learner may learn unnecessary trivia instead of focusing on the important points.

Another disadvantage of very general or nonexistent objectives is that unless the instructor has clarified to himself what he wants to teach, the selection of learning experiences can, at best, be incomplete or haphazard, and, at worst, nonexistent. Giving the client a printed pamphlet about calorie-restricted meal planning may be somewhat helpful, but the real problem may be the late-night snacks following the Friday night bowling league and during the Monday night football game. The pamphlet won't provide the needed learning.

One of the values of both client and dietitian recognizing the goals to be achieved lies in the clear communication of these goals to each other. It is also important to communicate to other health professionals what is being planned and executed on a client's behalf. There are, for example, instances where continuity of care is contingent upon clear communication of not only objectives but all aspects of care. All health team members should know what the client's goals and objectives are so that there may be better coordination of care.[6,7]

The selection of appropriate behavioral objectives is crucial to the success of the care plan. One element that often undermines a plan is an objective that requires the cooperation of another person. If the objective stated, "The client will eat lunch with a co-worker each day," the client would not meet the objective if the co-worker were unavailable. It is better to state that, "The client will *ask* a co-worker to lunch with her each day." In this instance, success is contingent only on the client's own behavior.

It is also inappropriate to state as an objective the resultant consequence instead of the desired behavior change. Consequences, such as weight loss or lowered blood glucose levels, are indicators of the success of the clinical dietitian in selecting appropriate behaviors to meet the desired goals. Such consequences, however, are not always reliable indicators that the client has adhered to his nutritional care plan. The client needs to view his adherence as his objective so that his compliance is worthy of reinforcement. If the compliance does not result in lowered glucose levels or weight loss, the client is not at fault—the plan is! This is a crucial point as feelings of failure heaped on the client may well cause him to give up. It is important to convey the message that "the plan isn't working and needs revision," not "you've failed." This is particularly significant for those clients who have struggled with food restriction in the past without achieving their desired goals.

CLASSIFYING OBJECTIVES

It has been accepted that learning is not merely the acquisition of knowledge, but any change in thoughts and feelings that manifests in behavior. That behavior will emphasize cognitive, affective, or psychomotor skills, and thus will be located in one of three learning domains:[8-10]

1. *Cognitive domain*, with objectives dealing with recognition or recall of knowledge, and the development of intellectual abilities and skills
2. *Psychomotor domain*, with objectives describing manipulative or motor skills
3. *Affective domain*, with objectives describing change in interest, attitudes, and feelings, and the development of appreciation and values

As a means of assuring that care plan objectives comprehensively address the client's problem, and to aid in sequencing the presentation of learning experiences, a classification system of behavioral objectives is useful. Objectives are usually categorized by the domains. Learning theorists have also classified the behaviors within the domains by levels of complexity or commitment. This has been done for cognitive,[8] affective,[9] and psychomotor[10] objectives. An adapted version of the classification of objectives is appropriate for the purposes of nutritional counseling. Such an adapted version is illustrated in Table 11.1. In this text, the cognitive and psychomotor domains are considered together (*competence*), while the affective domain remains separate (*motivation*). Competence implies both intellectual and physical "know-how" expressed in some behavioral form. Motivation, also expressed behaviorally, is related to feelings, attitudes, and values. Very simply, clinical dietitians need to be concerned with the client behaviors that are evidence of "*know-how*" and "*want-to.*" There must be some caution exercised in viewing these components separately, as they are inextricably intertwined and do not function in isolation. All behavior is motivated by perceived needs, processed through both thoughts and feelings.

TABLE 11.1.   CLASSIFICATION OF OBJECTIVES

	LEARNING DOMAINS		
	Competence		Motivation
HIERARCHY	Cognitive	Psychomotor	Affective
Simple to Complex	Recall Concepts Principles	Manipulative skills	Awareness Attention Approach Acquisition Assimilation

Competence Objectives

The first and lowest level of cognitive learning is *recall* or memorization. The second is *concept* or definition learning (classification), and the third and highest in this format is *principle* or rule learning. The three levels of cognitive learning provide for sequential development of *competence* or "know-how." *Manipulative skill* learning may also be required by clients engaged in the counseling process.

Recall learning.   An example of a recall objective is:

Without referring to the instruction booklet, the client will list the foods and serving sizes of at least ten items in each food listing, with no error.

The condition phrase, "without referring to the instruction booklet," is the primary clue that this behavior is a recall task.[11,12] Although there are situations in which it is important to have committed to memory some knowledge, there are limitations to the value of memorizing information. Unless memorized facts are applied to a higher level of thinking, they are usually forgotten within a day or two. Retention requires much repetition, preferably in an application task. The important questions in deciding whether or not something should be memorized are: Is there any reason the learner will need to remember the information? Will an information source be available? For recall purposes, most people can easily post a chart on a kitchen cabinet door and carry a folder in their pocket.

Concept learning. The next level of cognitive learning is concept learning.[11,12] An example of an objective follows:

> *Given a list of food items not previously categorized, the client will identify in which group of the Daily Food Guide each item belongs, with no more than two errors.*

Here again the clues are seen in the condition, the words "not previously categorized," and in the terminal behavior, "identify in which groups." This learning requires *defining* the nature of each group and then, on the basis of the definition, placing examples in the appropriate groups.

A concept is defined by a description of its attributes. For example, a concept of "food" may be described as follows: It can be ingested by the organism and digested in the gastrointestinal tract; it provides nutrients and/or energy; and it can be natural or synthetic.

The learning of concepts is extremely important in the acquisition of adequate nutritional behaviors. Each of the attributes of a concept are concepts in themselves. A client must know the concepts of nutrients, energy, digestion, and so on before he is able to understand the concept of food. Even though food is a more commonly used word than nutrient, it is probably an ill-defined concept for most people. Among dietitians, it is more important for the concept to be defined and applied correctly.

Principle learning. The learning and memorization of concepts is also important in the learning of principles or rules.[11,12] Principles are guides to solving problems and making decisions. An example of an objective at the principle learning level is:

> *Given a calorie restriction and the exchange list booklet,* the client will plan, in writing, 1 day's food intake, with no errors.*

---

* We refer here to the publication of The American Diabetes Association and The American Dietetic Association, *Exchange Lists for Meal Planning*, rev. 1976.

In order to perform this behavior, the client must know at least the following concepts: Calories, food, intake, meat, bread, vegetable, fruit, exchange lists, and so on. In addition, there is a list of rules or principles for planning. For the example above, the list of rules may include:

1. The total energy intake per day must be restricted to 1200 calories.
2. The plan must contain seven meat exchanges, two milk exchanges, four fruit exchanges, three vegetable exchanges, four bread exchanges, and three fat exchanges.
3. The exchanges must be distributed among at least three meal times and several may be used at snack time instead of regular meal times.
4. There are some foods that are to be avoided.

Many of the nutritional behaviors needed by clients require the cognitive skill of problem solving[13] or decision making.[14,15] There should be concerted attention given to planning nutritional instruction which includes these important skills as well as the lower level skill objectives.

Manipulative skill learning.   There are some objectives that require manipulative skills[16] in order to demonstrate competence. An example follows:

Using a high-calorie food supplement powder and a standard eggbeater, the client will prepare the supplement in a liquid form, using the prescribed portions and following the directions correctly.

Assume that, for some reason, the client does not have a mixer or a blender, and has never seen an eggbeater. To master this objective, the client requires some prerequisite knowledge of the *concepts*, high-calorie food supplements and eggbeaters, as well as *recall* of a tablespoon and other measures. There are prerequisite *rules*, such as how to measure an exact tablespoon and operate the eggbeater. In addition to knowing the rules, he needs to have practiced the manual (psychomotor) skill of operating the eggbeater. Then he is ready to learn to prepare his own supplement.

Motivation Objectives

To aid in understanding levels of motivation development, the following singular descriptions of affective behavior may be helpful. The descriptions (Table 11.1), presented in sequential order, are:

1. Awareness
2. Attention
3. Approach
4. Acquisition
5. Assimilation

These descriptions, or categories, compare roughly with levels two through six of client needs awareness presented in Table 3.1.

The category of *awareness* suggests that a client knows he behaves in a certain way and the consequences of that behavior. *Attention* means that the client not only is aware of his behavior, but is willing to discuss it and see it as a problem. *Approach* goes beyond attention to emitting the desired behavior at least once or twice. *Acquisition* means the behavior is present often enough to assure the motivation to continue, although it is usually at a lower priority than other behaviors. *Assimilation* is the level at which the behavior is highly valued and consistently performed. This is the level to which clinical dietitians should strive to bring their clients. To help the client achieve assimilation requires a sophisticated, but accessible, set of skills.

The following example is provided as a means to illustrate, in a clinical context, the levels of motivation behavior:

Mr. G. has a back injury treated by a spinal fusion and has been hospitalized for 4 months in the local chronic care community hospital. Currently, he expresses total disinterest in the food served to him. Following a conversation with a member of the nursing staff, the clinical dietitian stops by to see Mr. G. In the course of the conversation, the dietitian discovers that Mr. G. is not particularly concerned with his inadequate food intake because he's afraid of putting on weight and he doesn't see any relationship between his food intake and the healing process. The dietitian discusses the value of improving his food intake and the role counseling could play in helping him. Mr. G. replies that he didn't know that before now (awareness). He agreed to work with the dietitian to better understand his nutritional needs (attention). After instruction, Mr. G. made an effort to eat an appropriate selection of foods at least several times a week (approach). The dietitian continued to work with him, and by the time he was discharged, he was eating meals that met the criteria established in his care plan objective (acquisition). When Mr. G. returned a year later for follow-up, he told

*the dietitian that he was feeling so much better, now understood
the relationship between food intake and his own nutritional needs,
and had been following the guidelines he had been given* (assimilation).

SEQUENCING OBJECTIVES

In the sequencing of objectives[17] in a care plan, it is recommended that
the *key* objective be stated first. The key objective is the motivation
objective that describes the *end results* of the counseling process. The
implication is that a client who performs a behavior over a given period
of time has demonstrated not only motivation but competence in that
behavior. The converse is not true: Demonstration of competence does
not assure the needed motivation.

The key objective is usually a rather complex or advanced task that
requires the completion of a number of subtasks of a simpler nature.
The prerequisite objectives that are *steps to success* are as important
to define clearly as is the key objective. In the last pages of this chapter,
examples of both kinds of objectives are shown in the client care plan.

When the subtasks are defined, those requiring sequential learning
will need to be listed in chronologic order. The others may be listed
randomly.

There are many proponents of the idea that each objective should
be accompanied by a statement of relevance or a rationale for the
selection of the objective. Whether this rationale is explicit or implicit,
any health professional should be able to justify his decisions on the
basis of optimal client care.

PLANNING LEARNING EXPERIENCES

The process of selecting appropriate instructional strategies for providing learning experiences is based on the nature of the behavioral
objectives. As a guide to planning, the model of a behavioral incident
(Figure 10.5) may be used for reference. The planning of learning
experiences involves describing the instructional strategies and resources, the environment, and the management strategies employed.
The instructional strategies are based on educational theory. The resources are selected to correlate with the appropriate strategies and
are discussed in Chapter 8 in detail. Management strategies deal with
time, sequence, and so on.

Strategies for Competency Objectives

The clinical dietitian's facilitation of a client's competence requires attention to all aspects of a behavioral incident in order to produce change in behavior. For example, in the analysis of an incident, the assessment may reveal that the client lacks certain verbal and/or non-verbal behaviors (knowledge or skill). The plan must propose alterations in the behavioral events that will ultimately result in a change in behavior.

The conventional approach, still viable, is to provide new thoughts and ideas that, hopefully, will result in new behavior.[18] As conventional classroom instruction has so aptly demonstrated, that is often not enough. The clinician must help the client identify new cues that will stimulate the appropriate responses, and consequences that reinforce the correctness of the behavior. Appropriate stimulus cues include correct examples, directions, demonstrations, and so on. The consequences should be in the form of feedback on the correctness of the learner's intellectual or manipulative behavior. If a learner knows he is correct, he will feel pleased and it will increase his ability to remember what he has learned, particularly if the feedback immediately follows his behavior.[19]

Strategies for Motivational Objectives

If the client requires motivation, plans may be designed to alter the events in a behavioral incident. The clinical dietitian and client can examine the stimulus cues in the environment and decide which ones can be altered.[20] Keeping certain prohibited food items out of sight, or obtaining only those which require effort and time to prepare can interfere with the usual "grab a quick bite" behavior.

A change in the stimulus cue to make desirable behavior easier is also a good strategy, as a positive stimulus cue can be used to trigger the more desirable behavior. For example, tacking a form for recording weekly body weight next to the refrigerator can serve as a cue to select acceptable foods from the refrigerator.

Another influence related to stimulus cues is the process of *modeling*.[21] This occurs when a person with whom the learner identifies emits a behavior, and is then either reinforced or punished for that behavior. The learner integrates into his thinking the possibility that the behavior might work the same way for him and thus emits the same behavior (remember the "cornflakes" story?). The clinical dietitian may need to identify and instruct a suitable model.

A second approach is to "reprogram" the habitual thinking (cognitive) processes.[22] If a client has the practice of saying he is addicted to coffee, he will truly believe that. He can begin to influence his own behavior, when this is pointed out to him, by thinking and overtly declaring, "I don't want to be and I don't have to be addicted to coffee." Another way to influence motivation is to discuss and analyze consequences of the present behavior (the relevance statement).

Since feelings can arise from associations with concurrent incidents, the clinical dietitian must be alert to other stimuli that are producing thoughts and feelings that may interfere with desired attitudes, or reinforce undesirable attitudes.[23] If the client is uncomfortable, he may associate the discomfort with the newly acquired knowledge and choose to avoid the behavior. The client's general feelings about counseling will also affect his feelings about the specific learning occurring at any given point.

An analysis of the feeling reactions that accompany thoughts can often bring about a change in the attitudes that influence behavior. This analysis should evolve from appropriate interview techniques, which help the client uncover his attitudes toward his food practices. When the feelings are clarified,[24] the dietitian can help the client arrange more pleasant *associations*[25] with the new thoughts and behaviors, and to remove undesirable ones. If the client dislikes eating because the atmosphere is unpleasant, he should arrange a more desirable place to eat. An example is eating with friends instead of alone.

A client can even help change his behavior by agreeing to try a new behavior in an environment where the odds are that he will be reinforced for the behavior. Another way of altering behavior is to plan desirable behaviors that compete with undesirable ones, such as swimming instead of snacking.[26]

Behaviors are also influenced by the *consequences* that follow them.[27] "Approach" behavior results when a stimulus cue encourages the client to respond in a manner that produces positive consequences. "Avoidance" behavior occurs when the client perceives a cue as a sign to avoid a behavior that usually receives a negative consequence.[26,28]

An example of approach behavior is when someone who has learned that, when the clock shows 11:30 AM (stimulus cue), the cafeteria will be open, and, when he goes there (approach behavior), he can satisfy his hunger (consequence). In contrast, if a teenager comes in the house and smells liver cooking (stimulus cue), he may slip out, call home saying he can't make it for dinner, and then grab a hamburger (avoidance behavior). As a result, he avoids eating something he detests (consequence).

The client and clinical dietitian can arrange external consequences if needed, but if the selected behaviors themselves are personally beneficial (reinforcing), external reinforcements may not be needed.[29] If Mrs. S. R. learns to cook, she may well enjoy eating appropriately without anyone verbally rewarding her behavior. There is often a need, however, for temporary external reinforcement to stimulate a behavior until it is perceived by the client as intrinsically valuable.

DESIGNING EVALUATION INSTRUMENTS

The statement of objectives is the guide for designing appropriate evaluation instruments. The instrument is a "tool" used for evaluating, and varies with the type of evaluation conducted. The instruments should be prepared during planning, prior to the implementation of the plan, rather than at its conclusion. If the development of the instrument is delayed, a clinician may tend to design it on the basis of what was actually implemented rather than on what was originally planned. The latter enhances the possibility that the evaluation will not relate to the objectives.[30] The basic types of instruments fall in the categories of pencil-and-paper tests,[30] recording forms, and checklists,[31] to be discussed in Chapter 13.

A CLIENT CARE PLAN

The following is a proposed format of a nutritional care plan designed for an ideal weight achievement program. The plan can be personalized easily to meet the needs of an individual client. By designing a standard format, the clinician can be relieved of the need to begin anew with every plan. The standard format is individualized by checking those components that are assessed as relevant to a given client.

In the example to follow, the terms key and prerequisite objectives have been replaced by terms that can be more easily understood by the client. Thus, the key objective is labeled "end result" and the prerequisite objectives are labeled "steps to success."

NUTRITIONAL CARE PLAN FOR _____
Prepared for you by _____
    The following care plan has been devised for persons with weight control problems. The plan has been personalized for you by checks marking those portions specifically designed for you.
    I. Primary care provider's clearance _____ (date)
    II. Prescription _____

III. Instructional plan:
   Goal: Attain a weight of _____ pounds.
   End result: _____ will adhere to the individualized diet and exercise plan, recording his/her daily food intake and exercise on the record sheet, until the weight goal is reached.

   Steps to success: _____ will do the following (only those steps checked):

   _____ Using the instruction plan, _____ will plan 7 days' meals, including correct portion sizes to equal _____ calories with no error.

   _____ Using an exercise guide, _____ will plan 7 days' exercise activities that utilize at least _____ calories/day.

   _____ Identify problem foods (e.g., high calorie foods).

   _____ When the diet/exercise plan is in effect, _____ will do the following at least 90% of the time:

   _____ Eat in only one place at home, while not engaged in any other activity except socializing.

   _____ Shop for groceries within 1 hour after meals, purchasing only items on the grocery list.

   _____ Refrain from placing high-calorie problem foods on the table or within view.

   _____ Purchase only problem foods that require at least moderate preparation time (minimum of 15 minutes).

   _____ Limit exposure to excessive food to only those special occasions that are unavoidable.

   _____ Serve own food on small size plates and in smaller containers.

   _____ Eat every meal (at least three a day).

   _____ Sleep at least 7 hours a night.

   _____ Engage in three enjoyable activities per week.

   _____ Plan for and prepare a wide variety of attractive and acceptable foods.

   _____ Eat each bite with a utensil, laid on the plate between each bite.

   _____ _____
         _____

Evaluation:
   _____ 1. Record the steps to success on the forms provided.
   _____ 2. Have another person at home or at work (or _____) record the steps to success.
   _____ 3. Share the steps with a group.

_____ 4. Share the steps with the clinical dietitian at each individual session.

_____ 5. Record weight _____/day/week/month.

_____ 6. Record measurements _____/day/week/month.

Learning experiences:

_____ 1. Read _____

_____ 2. Work through the self-instructional package on weight control:

    _____ Unit 1. Calculating the caloric value of food using the Daily Food Guide

    _____ Unit 2. Planning caloric restricted menus using the Daily Food Guide

    _____ Unit 3. Calculating caloric intake using the exchange list booklet

    _____ Unit 4. Planning calorie restricted menus using the exchange list booklet

    _____ Unit 5. Calculating energy output by exercise

    _____ Unit 6. Planning exercise routine for weight loss

_____ 3. Join a group of people with weight control problems.

_____ 4. Continue individual counseling sessions.

_____ 5. Obtain other literature of interest from the dietitian, or titles of printed material available in the local library.

_____ 6. _____

Motivation plan:

_____ Select a material or activity reward from a prepared list (prepared by you) and obtain or engage in it upon completion of each day's food requirement and each day's exercise requirement.

_____ _____

Referrals:

Special instructions:

SUMMARY

A nutritional care plan is a carefully thought out design for helping a client meet his assessed needs as independently as possible. The plan includes immediate attention to the provision of nutrient sources in practitioner-managed crises environments. In nutritional counseling, the plan is a systematic design for eventual achievement of client independence in the food selection process (client-managed care).

Nutritional counseling plans are composites of competence and motivation objectives, human and material resources, and learning and evaluation strategies.

The competence and motivation objectives should be written behaviorally, and the learning strategies should be based on the theoretical foundations of educational psychology. The time invested in learning to write good objectives and in selecting optimal resources will be recompensed in the personal satisfaction of client success and the feelings, on the part of the practitioner, of a job well done.

The conclusion of the planning phase is the documentation of the plan in the medical record. A brief summary of salient points in the plan is to be transferred to the narrative notes (S-O-A-P notes) prior to implementation.

CITED REFERENCES

1. Wylie, J., and Singer, J. Growth process in nutrition counseling, *J. Am. Dietet. A.* 69:505, 1976.

2. Tyler, R. W. Some persistent questions on the defining of objectives. *In* Lindvall, C. M., Ed. *Defining Educational Objectives*. Pittsburgh: Univ. Pitt. Press, 1964.

3. Mager, R. F. *Preparing Instructional Objectives*. 2nd Ed. Palo Alto: Fearon Publ., Inc., 1975.

4. Connell, K. J. Workshop Workbook. Dietetic Internship Council, The American Dietetic Association Midyear Meeting, Feb. 18–20, 1974. Chicago: Am. Dietet. Assoc., 1974.

5. Yelon, S. L., and Scott, R. O. *A Strategy for Writing Objectives*. Dubuque: Kendall/Hunt Publ. Co., 1970.

6. Douglass, L. M., and Bevis, E. O. *Nursing Management and Leadership in Action: Principles and Applications to Staff Situations*. 3rd Ed. St. Louis: C. V. Mosby Co., 1979.

7. Parker, A. W. *The Team Approach to Primary Health Care*. Neighborhood Center Seminar Program. Monograph Series No. 3. Berkeley: Univ. Extension, Univ. Calif., 1972.

8. Bloom, B. S., and Krathwohl, D. R. *Taxonomy of Educational Objectives. Handbook 1: Cognitive Domain*. New York: Longman, Inc., 1977.

9. Krathwohl, D. R., Bloom, B. S., and Masia, B. B. *Taxonomy of Educational Objectives. Handbook 2: Affective Domain*. New York: Longman, Inc., 1964.

10. Simpson, E. J. The classification of educational objectives in the psychomotor domain. *In Contributions of Behavioral Science to Instructional Technology: The Psychomotor Domain.* Washington: Gryphon Press, 1972.

11. Davis, R. H., Alexander, L. T., and Yelon, S. L. *Learning System Design.* New York: McGraw-Hill Book Co., 1974.

12. Gagné, R. *The Conditions of Learning.* 3rd Ed. New York: Holt, Rinehart and Winston, Inc., 1977.

13. Carkhuff, R. R. *The Art of Problem Solving.* Amherst, MA: Human Res. Dev. Press, 1974.

14. Paolucci, B. A., Hall, O., and Axinn, N. W. *Family Decision-Making: An Ecosystem Approach.* New York: John Wiley and Sons, Inc., 1977.

15. Peck, E. B. The "professional self" and its relation to change processes. *J. Am. Dietet. A.* 69:534, 1976.

16. Redman, B. K. *The Process of Patient Teaching in Nursing.* 4th Ed. St. Louis: C. V. Mosby Co., 1980.

17. Popham, W. J., and Baker, E. L. *Planning an Instructional Sequence.* Englewood Cliffs, NJ: Prentice-Hall, Inc., 1970.

18. Goldfried, M. R., and Goldfried, A. P. Cognitive change methods. *In* Kanfer, F. H., and Goldstein, A. P., *Helping People Change: A Textbook of Methods.* New York: Pergamon Press, Inc., 1975.

19. Bruner, J. S. *Toward a Theory of Instruction.* Cambridge: The Belknap Press of Harvard Univ. Press, 1971.

20. Karoly, P. Operant methods. *In* Kanfer, F. H., and Goldstein, A. P., Eds. *Helping People Change: A Textbook of Methods.* New York: Pergamon Press, Inc., 1975.

21. Marlatt, G. A., and Perry, M. A. Modeling methods. *In* Kanfer, F. H., and Goldstein, A. P., Eds. *Helping People Change: A Textbook of Methods.* New York: Pergamon Press, Inc., 1975.

22. Ellis, A., and Harper, R. A. *A New Guide to Rational Living.* No. Hollywood, CA: Wilshire Book Co., 1976.

23. Bem, D. J. *Beliefs, Attitudes and Human Affairs.* Belmont, CA: Brooks/Cole Publ. Co., 1970.

24. Hackney, H., and Cormier, S. N. *Counseling Strategies and Objectives.* 2nd Ed. Englewood Cliffs, NJ: Prentice-Hall, Inc., 1979.

25. Krumboltz, J. D., and Thoreson, C. *Behavioral Counseling: Cases and Techniques.* New York: Holt, Rinehart and Winston, Inc., 1969.

26. Watson, D. L., and Tharp, R. G. *Self-Directed Behavior: Self-Modification for Personal Adjustment.* Monterey, CA: Brooks/Cole Publ., 1972.

27. Hosford, R. D., and deVisser, L. A. J. M. *Behavioral Approaches to Counseling: An Introduction.* Washington: APGA Press, 1974.

28. Bandura, A. *Principles of Behavior Modification.* New York: Holt, Rinehart and Winston, Inc., 1969.

29. Krumboltz, J. D., and Krumboltz, H. B. *Changing Children's Behavior.* Englewood Cliffs, NJ: Prentice-Hall, Inc., 1972.

30. Mager, R. F. *Measuring Instructional Intent or Got a Match?* Belmont, CA: Fearon Publ., 1973.

31. Irby, D. M., and Morgan, M. K., Eds. *Clinical Evaluation: Alternatives for Health Related Educators.* Gainesville: Center for Allied Health Instructional Personnel, Univ. Florida, 1975.

12

Implementation

> . . . words are only as good as the flexibility and skill with which the teacher adapts her own vocabulary and her methods to the needs of each learner. . . . Patients whose learning abilities and preferences are severely limited often prefer only to talk about their own familiar foods. In such cases, the dietitian will evaluate the nutrient intake and ultimately make only those minor modifications required to match the . . . goals. Here lie the unique skills of a good educator.
> **What is an exchange?** (*J. Am. Dietet. A.* 69:609, 1976.)

With a nutritional care plan designed on the basis of sound educational theory, the clinical dietitian is ready to implement the plan. Although the plan has been prepared by the expert, it is by no means a final document. In fact, the inclusion of alternatives from which the client may make choices can make the initial step of implementation an effective motivating experience.

CLIENT CONCURRENCE ON THE PLAN

A key strategy for client motivation is his participation in the decision-making process, which includes agreement on the content of the nutritional care plan. Concurrence comes in a discussion with the client of the components and rationale of the plan in terms the client can understand. Commitment to any regimen is most effective when the client has[2]:

1. Accepted the dietitian as someone whose recommendations are based on expertise
2. Selected the objectives toward which he will work
3. Chosen the strategies which he feels will help him learn most effectively

The most effective relationship, then, is one of joint participation, the professional having knowledge in technical areas and the client knowledge of his own personal preferences. This relationship is far more effective than the authoritarian relationship where the professional takes a coercive and patronizing role, or the more recent laissez-faire role of letting the client generate his own solutions without guidance. Few clients have adequate knowledge of foods or nutrition. A preferred approach is a presentation to the client of suggested options, their consequences, and their rationales. The client then decides which to accept and which to reject. When experiences are imposed on clients, they often demonstrate passive resistance by failing, and then blaming the imposer for the failure. In some instances, a client selected experience may not be effective either, but the client is more likely to consider it "our failure" or the "plan's failure" and return to reconsider other alternatives. Such an approach is an integral part of client-centered health care.

COORDINATION OF CARE PLANS

In many instances of health care provision, the client is involved with several professionals simultaneously.[3] Certainly this is true in acute or chronic care settings. The ambulatory setting will also have more than one professional providing care. Whenever multiple-care provision exists, it is of the utmost importance to consult with other health professionals to assure that care plans do not conflict in objectives, strategies, or implementation.

Without coordination, for example, the clinical dietitian could suggest exercise for weight control while the physical therapist has recommended limited activity because of balance problems. The client may not feel he can challenge this conflict and be thoroughly frustrated or confused. In another situation, the nursing staff may plan a half-hour teaching session at the same time the dietetic assistant delivers a supplemental snack. Clients are seldom appreciative of this scheduling fiasco, losing confidence in the professional, the care, and the plan.

PROVISION OF COGNITIVE LEARNING EXPERIENCES

After the plan has been tentatively agreed upon, the clinical dietitian arranges the learning experiences, and gives the client clear directions regarding how he is to proceed. Unless there is reason to believe it will be a stumbling block to accomplishment, the client should arrange as many experiences as possible. He may go to the library to check out a book or an audiovisual unit so long as the information is adequate to tell him how, where, and when to do so. A trip to the library only to find it closed may turn into the last trip he makes there.

Another set of directions necessitating clarity is the plan for the succeeding client-clinician contact, and preferably for the pattern of contacts proposed throughout the counseling experience.

One tendency instructors have is presenting information and then evaluating the learner for his ability to learn it and to apply it, leaving a significant portion of the learning to the client without any guidance. The result is learner frustration levels high enough to provoke lack of involvement in the learning experiences. In order to avoid this frustration, the provision of learning experiences should be viewed as a two-step process.[4] The first is called *presentation*, the second, *practice*. Instructional strategies and learning experiences* are complete only when they include both steps *and* the participation of the clinician.

The *presentation* step can be considered to have four components: a statement of the objective, a relevance statement, knowledge transmission, and learning aids. Each component plays an essential part in this initial phase.

The value of stating the objective in the presentation phase is in the role it plays in directing the learner toward the mutually agreed upon behaviors. A reminder of the "cornflakes" episode (Chapter 11) should be adequate to emphasize this role.

The relevance of each objective chosen should be understood by the client. A cognitive awareness of the importance of a behavior is the

---

* An instructional strategy is a systematically designed *plan* intended to facilitate learning. A learning experience is any actual set of circumstances, planned or unplanned, that influence learning.

second step in achieving attitude change (the first is an awareness that the behavior is absent or present). This relevance is described in terms of both the short- and long-range consequences the behavior has, not only for the client, but for significant others as well.

When the objectives and their relevance have been clarified, the next step is to provide the client with the knowledge he needs to proceed with his learning. This may be done in a variety of ways, such as in writing, films, tapes, or clinician presentation.[5,6] The means by which the client obtains the knowledge must be tailored to his learning level and preferred style.[7,8] Some people prefer to learn by reading the printed word, others by listening to the spoken word, still others in a discussion where they can ask questions as they listen. Some of the variables that influence knowledge acquisition are reading ability, language fluency, mathematical skills, vocabulary level, emotional and interpersonal skills, perception, and physical capability.[9] Learning experiences have to be designed to optimize the client's growth, using whatever skills he has.

To facilitate learning, it is helpful to provide the learner with aids to help him remember and/or understand the material. The use of concrete (real) objects, which the learner can manipulate, enhance learning. Therefore, concrete objects should be used whenever possible. Real food items or food models can help a client retain the knowledge he must have for planning portion sizes.

There are also mental techniques that aid in learning. Associating a person's name with a visual image or a personal characteristic can help in remembering his name the next time; e.g., Mr. Lowman can be visualized as 2 feet tall. Memory aids (mnemonics) generated by the client or clinician can serve as an aid in learning.

When the presentation step has been completed, the client and clinician move to the *practice* step. This step also has four basic components: display or stimulus, directions, response, and feedback. In fact, the process (learning experiences) and the product (behavioral outcome) in the practice step are almost indistinguishable from the evaluation step, except that, in the former, the learner is given periodic feedback at increasing levels of difficulty. In practice this may be self-evaluation against stated criteria and is particularly possible at the recall and concept levels, where learner responses can be compared to feedback previously prepared by the clinician. In principle learning, because of the complexity of behavior and the variability of some outcomes, it may be difficult to provide feedback that is succinct enough for the learner to make decisions regarding his level of achievement. More complex behavioral expressions usually call for observer feedback.

Recall Learning

In the learning of recall level knowledge, the *presentation* step is one of illustrating the labels that are applied to objectives, events, or symbols. Since this is primarily memory work, a helpful device used to facilitate memory is called a mnemonic.[4] An example of a mnemonic link is "HOMES," representing the Great Lakes, **H**uron, **O**ntario, **M**ichigan, **E**rie, and **S**uperior. When there is a need to memorize facts, the clinical dietitian can help create mnemonic links as an aid to learning.

The *practice* of recall learning requires repetition for mastery. Since there is seldom a need to memorize something for its own sake, early application of this information at a higher level can be a more effective way of learning than repetition alone. In other words, repetition by usage, rather than rote repetition, can be beneficial both in aiding actual learning and in motivating the client by demonstrating relevance through usage.

Even before the knowledge is firmly committed to memory, the client can move to learning higher level skills; for example, using recall knowledge cue cards that are withdrawn periodically until the learner has no further need for them.[10] Another help for the learner is to break any large quantities of material into manageable segments, working on mastery of one segment at a time and building on it.[11] There is evidence to suggest that learning a sequence of steps (chaining) can be facilitated by learning the last segment first, then adding on segments in reverse order as each one is mastered. This technique is called *backward chaining* and has been used in such diverse tasks as memorizing poetry and teaching children to dress.[12]

Another useful technique is to provide some framework for recall of sequential material. For example, to learn the tasks in nutritional counseling, it is helpful to remember the master design of assessment, planning, implementation, and evaluation. Even within these components, major subdivisions serve as guides. If the sequence is complex, it is also helpful for the clinician to ask questions of the learner about the segment he has just learned.

Concept Learning

At the concept level, the *presentation* step follows the same format of objective, relevance statement, demonstration, and learning aids. Demonstration (knowledge transmission) should point out examples and nonexamples, including the attributes or characteristics. To provide *practice*, it is most helpful to first present example–nonexample pairs and have the learner identify each, explaining as did the clinician in the demonstration, the present and absent attributes. The first pairs should be distinctly different, then become increasingly more similar. The second phase is to present example–example pairs which appear different, but in reality have similar characteristics. As a third phase, it is helpful to mix these two kinds of pairs, and then finally present single instances of examples and nonexamples in random order. The final evaluation of the client should be comparable to the last phase. As with any practice, the learner should receive immediate feedback on each response to facilitate learning.

Principle Learning

When the material to be learned is application of principles or rules, there are some specific strategies that must be included in the *presentation*. The criteria by which the outcome of the application of rules will be evaluated should be made clear to the client. If these criteria are in the form of a checklist,* the list should be given to him together with clarification of any questions he has. Not all performance criteria on the checklist will have meaning for the client until he has practiced the skill, but a preliminary overview permits him to have some understanding of what he's doing. If a general rule or principle is stated, then specific examples should be demonstrated as well. Feedback can be given at points along the way, including comments on why the step would receive a check.

Prior to practice, it is important to ascertain that the client has mastered knowledge of the concepts which are integral parts of the principle. Neglecting to do so is often the cause of failure to learn the principle, because the client may have learned inaccurate or ambiguous definitions. The client frequently incorporates these misconceptions into his procedure.

During the *practice* session, as the client is attempting to work a problem or produce a product, feedback should be given at each step. When he successfully completes a step, he should know it immediately. If he is faltering at a step, it is often helpful to not only demonstrate again the correct procedure, but to describe the common errors made at that point. The learner also needs adequate numbers of problems as well as variation. More complex problems require more practice.

As the lower level skills require less time and resources to teach and to learn, clinicians may tend to focus on them at the expense of prin-

---

* A checklist is an evaluation instrument (to be discussed in Chapter 13).

ciple learning. Reality, however, is an endless process of problem solving, and the ability to function at the principle level has the most relevance to increased competence in living. The value of the lower level skills exists in their support of the problem solving skills.

Manipulative Skill Learning

The *presentation* of a psychomotor skill is quite similar to that of principle learning, but with greater emphasis on performance of a physical rather than a verbal behavior. A demonstration of the skill, e.g., the operation of certain equipment, is performed from beginning to end. When the clinician is demonstrating, he should describe to the learner the important characteristics of each step. Using a checklist, the client's skill is compared with the clinician's demonstration of the skill. Again, the clinician should be alert for tasks that exceed the client's developmental level and prerequisite skills. These variables also affect the amount of instruction the learner can handle in any given unit.

For some psychomotor skills, drawings and diagrams as well as verbal directions may be used; the former may be adequate if well written or sketched, and well tested. The advantages to using prepared information sources for enhancement of manipulative skill learning lie in the consistency of information given to each client, the opportunity for other clinical dietitians to evaluate the material, and the avoidance of repeating comparable material over and over again to clients. Other advantages include the convenience for the client in being able to practice at any time, the availability of the instructional material to more than one dietitian, and the opportunity to get learner feedback on the content, permitting improvement of instructional materials.

In the *practice* sessions, the client should be provided ample opportunity to practice the behavior. Simple tasks may only require a brief practice session, more complicated ones extensive practice time. The clinician should provide feedback both by continued demonstration, and by descriptions of appropriate and inappropriate movements immediately after each performance or segment of performance if the behavior is complex. The same technique employed in recall of sequential events (backward chaining) is suitable for the learning of manipulative skills. If speed and accuracy are important, accuracy should be mastered first, then speed. Unless speed is absolutely necessary in the application of the skill in real life, it should not be stressed in the learning environment. It is best for the clinician to emphasize practice for confidence so that the skill becomes almost automatic.

PROVISION OF AFFECTIVE LEARNING
EXPERIENCES

The area of motivation (affective domain) demands a somewhat different approach than that used to facilitate competence. The process of *presentation* for motivation behavior requires an interview approach, with the client examining his perceptions of the need for changing his behavior. This discussion is an opportunity to bring the client to at least the attention level (Table 11.1), which is necessary for the continuation of counseling. Once agreeing that he probably does need counseling, then his perception of consequences at the awareness level needs clarifying. This initial period of the interview is an appropriate time to do so.

The client who agrees to counseling, and understands why, is ready to move into the approach level if it is a new behavior, or he may already be either in that level or possibly into the acquisition level. If the latter is the case, the behavior is already in the behavioral repertoire, and only requires strengthening by strategies suggested in Chapter 11. If the client is at the assimilation level and values the behavior, he should no longer require the support of the clinical dietitian for the problem.

The *practice* for motivation behavior occurs in both simulated and real settings, and is based on a group of principles drawn from learning psychology (Chapter 11). These principles provide the framework for developing strategies that are known to influence human behavior.

For strategies requiring modification of external events—for example, consequences and cues (Figure 10.5)—a definite plan and time schedule are established to implement them. If the strategies are based on positive reinforcement (i.e., consequences that increase behavior), a schedule is established which first provides reinforcement for each time the desired behavior is performed. The schedule then moves to intermittent reinforcement to allow for strengthening the behavior, and later withdrawal of external reinforcement.[13]

Implementation of behavioral strategies requires a rather constant surveillance of client behavior, in order to ensure that rewards and other events are appropriately scheduled and take place. The plan may be implemented and monitored by a layperson as well as a professional. If the plan is to be monitored by the former, the design of the plan must be in great detail; each task the change agent* performs must be clearly defined.[14,15] A significant other who is viewed as not manipulating the client selfishly will usually be most helpful. The draw-

---

* A change agent is a person who functions as a catalyst.

back associated with asking significant others to serve as change agents is that any serious motivational problem is often associated with interpersonal relationships and communication breakdown among intimates. Difficulty in one relationship, however, does not imply that the client has problems in all relationships. Thus, a supportive friend may provide needed help in the face of negative factors elsewhere, such as a spouse who refuses to stop behavior that undermines the client's progress.

Not all practice for behavior modification needs to occur in the natural environment. There can be simulation and role playing to help the client practice the new behaviors, particularly in group counseling where other counselees may provide initial reinforcement. Experiences can be set up in a "laboratory" environment to structure new associations or desensitize old ones. Modeled behavior is particularly functional as a strategy in a group counseling environment. The client can observe other clients performing new behaviors and receiving the natural reinforcement of improved interpersonal responses, or planned reinforcement by the clinician.[16-18]

There are a number of ways to implement strategies directed toward modifying internal events, for example, thinking and feeling (Figure 10.5). Implementation of the strategies discussed in Chapter 11 can be accomplished in ways that motivate the learning of new behaviors. There is some evidence that since attitudes are of an intense, personal, and interpersonal nature, interaction with other human beings can speed the process of change.[19] The immediate feedback a client can receive from his peers, or the intensity of meaning associated with actual experiences shared by others is more readily perceived[20] and valued.

Role playing is a simulation of reality in which the client acts out his chosen behaviors before confronting the real, perhaps more threatening experience. Role reversal is also a valuable tool in helping a client understand the other person's point of view and reaction to him. In this simulation, the client's role is assumed by a group member or the clinician, and the client takes the role of spouse, parent, child, or friend.

The clinical dietitian is most helpful when he works to facilitate the client's understanding of his own behavior. In this way, the client can make informed choices about what he wants to change. This is far superior to manipulation of the client, who is unaware of the forces influencing him. The greatest service clinicians can provide is an environment in which the client achieves independence in healthful nutritional behaviors through self-understanding.[21]

If behavior change is unsuccessful over a period of time, the client (with the clinician) may need to reexamine his environment in an effort to determine which, if any, related factors are influencing his failure.[22] Human components of the environment are most resistant to change, as they have a vested interest in retaining the status quo. If a human factor (other than the client) is identified as the major block to learning, role playing, perhaps coupled with referral, is probably the most helpful tool. In rare instances, the client may be temporarily removed from his natural environment. The distinct disadvantage to such a plan is that the client will probably have to return to that environment later. Unless he has developed extensive strength in his new behaviors, the client may return to his old ways. If he must return to the hostile environment, the client should be referred to an appropriate professional for ongoing support in his coping behavior.

SUMMARY

Implementation of nutritional counseling plans requires that the clinical dietitian be flexible, continually monitoring progress, making decisions about priorities, creating novel approaches to seemingly insolvable problems, calling on a variety of human and institutional support systems, and managing these many resources for clients. These activities of the clinician are such that they promote the client's acquisition of healthful behaviors and an increase in his self-confidence in his ability to do so. Along the way, a satisfying professional experience for the practitioner occurs.

CITED REFERENCES

1. What is an exchange? *J. Am. Dietet. A.* 69:609, 1976.
2. Haynes, R. B. A critical review of the "determinants" of patient compliance with therapeutic regimens. *In* Sackett, D. L., and Haynes, R. B., Eds. *Compliance with Therapeutic Regimens.* Baltimore: The Johns Hopkins Univ. Press, 1976.
3. Parker, A. W. *The Team Approach to Primary Health Care. Neighborhood Center Seminar Program.* Monograph Series No. 3. Berkeley: Univ. Extension, Univ. Calif., 1972.
4. Merrill, M. D., and Goodman, R. K. *Selecting Instructional Strategies and Media: A Place to Begin.* Washington: Nat'l. Special Media Inst., 1972.
5. Moore, W. Increasing learning among developmental education students. *In* Lenning, O. T., Ed. *Improving Educational Outcomes.* San Francisco: Jossey-Bass, Inc., Publ., 1976.

6. Hassell, J., and Medved, E. Group/audiovisual instruction for patients with diabetes. Learning achievements and time economics. *J. Am. Dietet. A.* 66:465, 1975.

7. Kolb, D. A., Rubin, I. M., and McIntryel, J. M. *Organizational Psychology: An Experiential Approach.* 3rd Ed. Englewood Cliffs, NJ: Prentice-Hall, Inc., 1979.

8. Abrahamson, S. Helping individual students to learn. *J. Med. Educ.* 51:1025, 1976.

9. Cole, M., Gay, J., Glick, J. A., and Sharp, D. W. *The Cultural Context of Learning and Thinking: An Exploration in Experimental Anthropology.* New York: Basic Books, Inc., 1971.

10. Karoly, P. Operant methods. *In* Kanfer, F. H., and Goldstein, A. P., Eds. *Helping People Change: A Textbook of Methods.* New York: Pergamon Press, Inc., 1975.

11. Mager, R. F. *Developing Attitude Toward Learning.* Belmont, CA: Fearon Publ., 1968.

12. DeCecco, J. P. *The Psychology of Learning and Instruction: Educational Psychology.* Englewood Cliffs, NJ: Prentice-Hall, Inc., 1968.

13. Krumboltz, J. D., and Krumboltz, H. B. *Changing Children's Behavior.* Englewood Cliffs, NJ: Prentice-Hall, Inc., 1972.

14. Berman, L. M. *New Priorities in the Curriculum.* Columbus: Charles E. Merrill Publ. Co., 1968.

15. Peck, E. B. The "professional self" and its relation to change processes. *J. Am. Dietet. A.* 69:534, 1976.

16. Ohlsen, M. *Group Counseling.* 2nd Ed. New York: Holt, Rinehart and Winston, Inc., 1977.

17. Gazda, G. M. *Group Counseling: A Developmental Approach.* 2nd Ed. Boston: Allyn and Bacon, 1978.

18. Lieberman, M. A. Group methods. *In* Kanfer, F. H., and Goldstein, A. P., Eds. *Helping People Change: A Textbook of Methods.* New York: Pergamon Press, Inc., 1975.

19. Johnson, D. W., and Matross, R. P. Attitude modification methods. *In* Kanfer, F. H., and Goldstein, A. P., Eds. *Helping People Change: A Textbook of Methods.* New York: Pergamon Press, Inc., 1975.

20. Flowers, J. V. Simulation and role playing methods. *In* Kanfer, F. H., and Goldstein, A. P., Eds. *Helping People Change: A Textbook of Methods.* New York: Pergamon Press, Inc., 1975.

21. Evans, R. I., and Hall, Y. Social-psychologic perspective in motivating changes in eating behavior. *J. Am. Dietet. A.* 72:378, 1978.

22. Mahoney, M. J., and Caggiula, A. W. Applying behavioral methods to nutritional counseling. *J. Am. Dietet. A.* 72:372, 1978.

13
Evaluation

Health is no halfway thing, it is absolute and complete.

Doris M. Molbo, in *Dynamics of Problem-
Oriented Approaches: Patient Care and
Documentation* (Philadelphia: J. B.
Lippincott Co., 1976).

Perhaps the most painful part of the counseling process is evaluation: It is very difficult for humans to confront their own success or failure. Evaluation as it is carried on in learning environments is a poorly understood process. The common practice, if any evaluation is done at all, is to evaluate the client for her acquisition of knowledge. This is, however, only part of the evaluation process. A client's behavior change is a far better indicator of true learning. A thorough evaluation of the counseling process is also required, the success or failure of which depends on both the clinical dietitian and the client.

Effective evaluation is best understood as a complex process that looks at the who, what, when, where, how, and why of intervention and change. Worthen and Sanders[2] define evaluation as a procedure designed to determine the worth of something. Bloom and co-workers describe evaluation as ". . . . a method of acquiring and processing the evidence needed to improve the student's learning and the teaching"[3] (p. 7). Essentially the same thought is expressed by Stufflebeam et al.: "Evaluation is the process of delineating, obtaining and providing useful information for judging decision alternatives"[4] (p. xxv). They initiate their work with the declaration that the purpose of evaluation is not to prove but to improve. Worthen and Sanders describe the purpose as assisting decisionmakers in choosing among decision alternatives.[2]

THE SUBJECTS OF EVALUATION

The most obvious subject of evaluation is, of course, the client. The clinician seeks to discover if the client has learned anything (changed her behavior) and if that change appears to be relatively permanent (changed her attitudes). At the very least, the ultimate goal of nutritional counseling is improved nutrition behaviors. Thus, the client is the most important focus of the evaluative efforts.

Since the client lives in an ecologic system that involves her interaction with her environment, the human beings that impact on her behavior also may be subjects for evaluation of their own behavior change. These persons may be considered secondary clients if the clinician also chooses to work with them.

Although it has been common practice to lay success and failure at the feet of the consumer, the Contractual Model of health care, defined in Chapter 5 and accepted by the authors, places responsibility in the hands of both the client and the clinician. Thus, the clinician as counselor is also a subject of evaluation. In addition, when a health care team shares the delivery of services, the team members are evaluated likewise on their impact on the outcomes of counseling and health care.

THE EVALUATORS

The client, again, is the most important person in this process of evaluation. The client needs to be capable of monitoring her own progress, because self-evaluation is motivating. In addition, as she is independent, she will spend most of her time without the professional looking over her shoulder. The client must not depend on the clinician for continual feedback.

The practitioner needs to be a competent and persistent evaluator. Using the systems approach, new evaluation data are the basis for adjustments in the system when it is not working or working only minimally. As the assessor of needs and designer of plans, the clinician implicitly accepts the responsibility for determining the appropriateness of his decisions.

The client and clinician, therefore, will evaluate both themselves and each other. This dynamic allows for assessing the accuracy of each person's perceptions.

In addition to these primary participants in the counseling relationship evaluating themselves and each other, the clinician's peers should be involved. This process is known as "peer review."* Peers may be other clinical dietitians or members of the health care team. Periodically, outside evaluators are brought in to audit medical records. Information recorded in records is used by the auditors as a means of determining the effectiveness of health care delivery within a practice or institution.

THE OBJECTS OF EVALUATION

When the client is evaluated, the four basic categories of data are examined again (Figure 9.2). The evaluator looks for any changes in biologic, food intake, environmental, and behavioral baseline data.

An evaluation of the clinician is similar to that of the client. Data about the clinician are examined only as they influence the client's learning. The outcome of evaluation of the clinician may well indicate a need to learn new behaviors or to determine the value of a new behavior. The clinician's teaching and personal behaviors, as well, are considered as factors in effective instruction and need to be identified as such. The practitioner should serve as a credible model.

The specialized environment of the instructional setting is also evaluated. Physical elements, such as heat, light, and comfort, are considered. The nature and impact of the instructional resources discussed in Chapter 8 are identified and an effort made to determine their contribution to the client's learning. A synthesis of all of these evaluation data is used to determine the need for revision of the selected instructional strategies and objectives or the continuation of effective ones.

A working committee of the American Public Health Association summarized the foci of evaluation as (1) appropriateness, (2) effectiveness, (3) efficiency, (4) adequacy, and (5) side effects.[5] Appropriateness is based on the degree to which the selected outcomes and strategies are designed to meet learner needs and abilities, and societal needs. Effectiveness describes whether or not the intervention worked. Efficiency examines the cost in time, money, and other resources as

* Discussed in Chapter 15.

they relate to extent of achievement of outcomes. Adequacy is the measure of the degree of impact on bringing about needed change. The last focus is on side effects, sometimes referred to as unintended outcomes. These side effects may be so detrimental as to offset the benefits of the intended change. Thus they deserve careful consideration.

THE EVALUATION SCHEDULE

Although evaluation is usually considered an examination of the end results of counseling, that is not adequate to maintain a systems approach to learning. A final evaluation, made when the client is terminating his care, has been labeled *summative* evaluation to differentiate it from the continuous process of *formative* evaluation that is done during the many individual steps of behavior change designed to reach the final goal.[3] Formative evaluation looks at achievement of the prerequisite objectives whereas summative evaluation looks at the key objective. For example, the key objective for a client might be a 25 pound weight loss, whereas the prerequisite objectives may address effective meal planning, daily exercise, new food choices, and a 5 pound initial weight loss. Each of the intermediate steps are formatively evaluated. There is also a need for follow-up evaluation to determine the effectiveness of maintenance of the newly learned behavior.[6] Long-term compliance is what is sought as the preferred goal of health care.[6] Follow-up is the means to determine that compliance.

Although individual client and counselor evaluation is continuous, more formalized evaluations of total practice may be periodic. Audit teams and peer review activities may only spot check the activities of health care providers. While these groups monitor the general effectiveness of a total practice, it is not enough. Each client must be evaluated for his progress as well as increased motivation, and each counselor for his effectiveness.

EVALUATION SITES

The most frequent and easiest place to evaluate clients is in the learning environment. The clinician is present and generally has resources that can be used to evaluate client knowledge acquisition. The drawback is that this environment is least likely to represent the real world in which the client must function, so there may be little transfer of acquired information to his ongoing behavior. To moderate this effect, the use of simulations, as opposed to pencil-and-paper, academic type tests, are recommended for evaluation strategies as well as for instructional strategies.

The next most available opportunity for client evaluation is in the regular routine of the institutional setting. As in assessment, observations can be made of client menu choices, food consumption, and related food behaviors during a mealtime visit by the clinician or recorded by a technician collecting menus or trays.

The most effective and most difficult location for evaluation is in the client's natural environment. Here he will be trying his newly learned behaviors in a familiar context with the usual environmental pressures and cues that stimulate habitual behavior patterns. Any efforts that can be made to acquire evaluation data in the natural environment will yield large dividends in most cases when the clinician earnestly wishes to facilitate client behavior change. The clinician need not be the only person involved in the collection of evaluation data. A reliable family member, a community health nurse, or even an acceptable friend chosen with the client's approval may serve as the recorder of data. Note that we did not say "evaluator." The evaluator not only observes and records, but must have the skills to analyze and synthesize the data to provide the basis for decision making.

THE PROCESS OF EVALUATION

The major task of evaluation is to compare the post intervention data with the baseline data. The first principle an evaluator should apply is that achievement of the objectives is confirmed if, and only if, the behaviors are demonstrated by the learner.[7] Subjective reporting by the client that he knows how to do something may be considered only an indicator of achievement, not proof of it; i.e., the results of the evaluation are only tentative. If the evaluation must be subjective, it is again important to remember the absolute necessity of providing the client an atmosphere of acceptance and trust. If the client expects judgmental responses, indications that his behavior is "good" or "bad," he will rationalize his responses as much as he can to avoid receiving negative feedback.

In the cognitive and psychomotor domains (*competence*), it is mandatory that the client actually perform the desired behavior to assure competence. In the affective or *motivation* domain, monitoring of performance may not be feasible, at least by the clinical dietitian, as it involves performance over time. Therefore, other means of evaluating motivation will need to be planned, with as much objectivity as possible.

A second important principle in the systems approach to learning is that in order to determine achievement, it is necessary to compare performance after instruction (posttest) with performance assessed prior to instruction (pretest).[3] The most obvious reason for pre- and posttesting, i.e., obtaining "before-after" information, is to verify that an observed behavior is the result of planned intervention and not one the client performed in the past. Since learning is behavior *change,* the pretest provides a yardstick against which to measure change.

A corollary principle is that, to be valid indicators of change, the pre- and posttests should be "parallel." Each item or observation on the pretest should have a comparable item on the posttest. The wording can be changed, items reordered, different values inserted, but the responses should demonstrate the same cognitive skill. In this text, pre- and posttesting implies any kind of evaluation of competence, such as observation of performance and written or oral quizzes.

In evaluation there is a basic process that should be used to provide enhanced results.[8] Using the objective as the statement of the evaluation strategy, the clinician selects or develops some form of *stimulus.* This can be a display of objects, written or spoken words, or human behaviors. The stimulus must be accompanied by *directions* for the learner (and, in some cases, for the person who is acting as a stimulus or manipulating the stimulus). Depending on the nature of the objective, one stimulus may form the complete evaluation or a number of stimuli may be grouped together for evaluation purposes. The nature of the stimulus will vary according to the complexity of the objective. The next step is *presentation* to the learner of the stimuli to which he is to *respond,* as requested in the directions. These responses are compared to previously established *criteria* stated in the objective, and then scored according to a predetermined procedure. Even in summative (final) evaluation, the client should be informed immediately of results (feedback).[9]

Specific evaluation strategies are selected according to the kind of objective being evaluated. These can be grouped according to the learning domains discussed earlier in Chapter 11.

Competence Evaluation

For *recall* strategies, the purpose is to evaluate rote learning or memory. If what is learned by recall is relevant to client needs, it is important for the learner to have immediate recall; that is, there should be a time limit on the response. If there is a significant delay in response, the memorization is not thorough. A "live" evaluator can identify this more effectively than a paper-and-pencil tool, although a timed test may be used. The implication of the relevancy statement is that what is important to memorize must be known well and what is not relevant to client needs should not be memorized at all.

It is also necessary to scramble the order of the stimuli so that they are not learned by artificial associations. A purposeful association, as in a sequential task, is relevant and not artificial. In addition, whether the facts are singular or serial, performance should be 100 percent for all responses. In testing for this knowledge, the clinician can use short-answer or essay-type questions, or, at an even less demanding level, can provide cues in a multiple-choice, matching, or true-false format.

Memory is important in recalling concept attributes and rules, but they should be memorized during practical application rather than as a separate exercise. Clients recall best those facts which have meaning for them by association with other important skills.

Concept learning is a different process than recall learning. The purpose is to classify novel objectives, processes, or ideas into labeled categories; this implies recognizing examples and nonexamples. To facilitate the evaluation of concept acquisition, a selection of examples and nonexamples should be presented in random order.

In many instances, nonexamples of a concept lie on a continuum from obviously different to barely different. For example, suppose the concept is *fish:* A house is quite unlike a fish, a dog not much, a frog comes closer (it swims), an eel is very close, and a porpoise is indistinguishable except to the trained eye. In evaluating nonexamples, the criterion of expected correct responses in measuring the recognition of nonexamples that are distinctly different from the concept can be more stringent than for those nonexamples that are quite similar.

A helpful evaluation technique for those difficult examples is to ask the learner to identify the attributes that render it an example or nonexample. He may well know the attribute, yet not label it as such (a result of failure to teach prerequisite concepts). For example, a student identifying examples of "trees" might say pines are not trees because they have needles instead of leaves. He had not learned that a pine needle has the attributes of the concept "leaf," yet he did know the concept definition of tree.

The test format for concept learning is relatively simple, since it involves identification or classification. The display may be pictures, objects, living beings, written characters, and the like. The display may be on paper, in a real world or simulated setting, on a video screen or computer terminal screen or printout, or any other imaginative method that fits the problem. Then the learner responds orally, in writting, on the computer, or in some other way to indicate his selection of examples. Multiple-choice or matching tests are the simplest, but not always the most effective methods of evaluating concept learning.

Attention must be given in instrument preparation to arranging the items so as to avoid giving clues or permitting such techniques as the process of elimination. These may be acceptable on a history test, but when a client with cardiovascular disease has to classify foods according to their sodium content, the potential consequences of error require more assurance that he really knows what he is identifying.

The highest level addressed in the cognitive domain (in this text) is *principle* or rule learning. The purpose of this behavior is to produce a product, render a decision, or solve a problem by applying rules. As in concept learning, the learner will be evaluated according to his ability to apply the rules to novel problems or situations. Asking him to list the rules is not adequate. When the learner responds with a product, solution, or decision for which there is no predetermined answer, the response should be judged primarily by the process (steps) used to achieve the outcome. For example, a client's solution to his problem is judged on whether or not he used effective problem solving skills.

If criteria for the outcome have been stated ahead of time, the outcome may also be evaluated. In these situations, the outcome may be evaluated on the basis of whether it works or meets a stated need.

Since principle learning may involve several rules, each containing concepts, the client must have learned the prerequisite knowledge before he proceeds to the final application of principles. The prerequisite levels of learning are stated in the objectives that prepare the learner for the key objective.

The instrument often used in evaluating principle learning is a checklist.[10-13] A checklist may contain descriptions of each step of a process and criteria for the product. Even in the simplest form of problem solving (e.g., mathematics), an instructor may not have a written checklist, but if he evaluates appropriately, he checks off each step of the solution to determine whether it was solved correctly. A right answer is not a guarantee—it could be a lucky guess.

If a distinct and new *manipulative* skill is involved, the skill must be taught as a prerequisite objective. For example, the ability to use a computer terminal, pocket calculator, or food preparation appliance might be a prerequisite objective. For this type of objective, a checklist developed from a task analysis is the most effective means of evaluation. The evaluation should require the actual manipulation of the object, not just a verbal description of its use.

Motivation Evaluation

The real challenge to the clinical dietitian is the evaluation of affective behavior.[14] Any measure of motivation must look at more than a single point in time. Even the baseline data on affective behavior must take into account the frequency with which a behavior is emitted by the learner over a stated period of time before instruction. This might be expressed as the number of meals per week, or days per week, that caloric intake met the prescribed level, or the length of time spent eating each meal for a 3 day period. The initial tally is crucial because the purpose of affective learning is to establish a new behavior or to increase, decrease, or extinguish an existing behavior. Success is measured against the baseline data.

After a motivational strategy has been implemented, another tally is done for an equivalent period to determine whether the change stated in the objective has occurred. Such tallies may be done periodically or continuously until either the criteria are achieved or there is an indication that success is unlikely, at which time alterations should be made in the plan.

The very presence of the clinical dietitian presents problems in the evaluation of client motivation. Since the ultimate goal of nutritional counseling is independence, the client must be motivated to adhere to the mutually agreed upon nutritional care plan. Such adherence must eventually occur without the reinforcement and support of the clinician which occurs in the learning phase. Thus, any evaluation of affective behavior should be designed so that the client does not perform *for* the clinical dietitian. Such a plan will require that clinicians develop some innovative approaches.

Some evaluators suggest that clients not be told the nature of the affective objective.[15] Such a perspective, however, is directed to formal educational settings in which students perform for grades, which provide strong external rewards. It is more appropriate that the clinical dietitian be open with the client about the nature of the evaluation. The client in nutritional counseling may want to please the clinician, but the extrinsic reward is probably far less powerful than grades. A significant amount of evidence describing successful evaluation techniques for compliance* to health regimens has not yet been acquired,[16] although there is presently a surge of interest in this research area.[17]

---

* Compliance is defined as "... *the extent to which the patient's behavior (in terms of taking medications, following diets or executing other life-style changes) coincides with the clinical prescription.*"[17] (p. xi)

Motivation evaluation will probably require both the involvement of a trusted, significant other selected by the client, and the client's own self-reporting. To facilitate the tally of behavior, a checklist or tally sheet is a useful tool. In addition, graphs, diaries, and other such records are helpful and may be employed as they were in the assessment process.

Summing Up

Evaluation of the client is a most important facet of counseling. The purpose is to determine behavioral change from the period prior to intervention to a post-intervention event. The evaluation should look at both competence and motivation, and include a determination of the *value* for the client of performing the behavior (a statement of relevance). Assurance that the client has in fact acquired or improved a desirable behavior, or eliminated a destructive one, is the first step in validating professional intervention.

Evaluating the client's success is only part of an effective evaluation program. Evaluation is also a means of gathering information that is used to make decisions about the effectiveness of the counseling process.[18] The data regarding client success or failure are the primary information with which to begin evaluating the counseling process.

If the client has successfully met the criteria of the objective, the process of counseling can be considered relatively successful. There is, however, usually room for improvement even in good plans.[9] The client may have helpful suggestions that will assist the clinical dietitian in developing later plans with increasing skill. Indeed, the practitioner should also perform a self-evaluation for the same purpose. In other words, evaluation is clinical research (as opposed to laboratory research) that enhances a clinican's knowledge and skill.

When the client has not met the criteria, there is an urgent need to evaluate the process. The model for the provision of nutritional care (Figure 9.1) demonstrates the routes for recycling the learning process. When the objectives are not met, the problem is usually the plan, not the client. The appropriate professional response is a revision of the plan based on identification of the nonfunctional components of the system. The decision to revise and continue is, of course, made in consultation with the client, who may choose instead to leave counseling. Revising the process may mean collecting additional assessment data, revising objectives, revising or adding learning strategies, or creating new or revised forms of evaluation. Decisions to begin anew at any point in the learning process are based on a thorough evaluation.

THE RATIONALE FOR EVALUATION

Evaluating the counseling process is a necessary component of a systems approach to nutritional care. It is done for several reasons. The first and foremost reason is to help clinicians make decisions that will increase the facilitation of client success in achieving personal goals. This is the ultimate goal of client-centered health care. A secondary reason is to give the clinician feedback that will reward his efforts and direct him toward the continuing learning experiences that will allow him to grow professionally. The third major reason to evaluate is to provide professional accountability to those who underwrite the services, whether taxpayers or management.[19]

SUMMARY

The major purpose of evaluation is to determine the *value* of counseling. Value is based not only on the fact that something works, but that it is an asset to the client, his significant others, and his natural environment.[2,20] Consequently, evaluation is a serious responsibility. It requires thorough comparison of the observed results with standards of competent professional practice. The results of implementation and the contributing factors are documented in the medical record in order to bring closure to the counseling process. The result can be truly effective client-centered nutritional care.

CITED REFERENCES

1. Molbo, D. M. Participative health care. *In* Walter, J. B., Pardee, G. P., and Molbo, D. M., Eds. *Dynamics of Problem-Oriented Approaches: Patient Care and Documentation.* Philadelphia: J. B. Lippincott Co., 1976.
2. Worthen, B. R., and Sanders, J. R. *Educational Evaluation: Theory and Practice.* Worthington, OH: Jones Publ. Co., 1973.
3. Bloom, B. S., Hastings, J. T., and Madaus, G. F. *Handbook on Formative and Summative Evaluation of Student Learning.* New York: McGraw-Hill Book Co., 1971.
4. Stufflebeam, D. L., Foley, W. J., Gephart, W. J., Guba, E. G., Hammond, R. L., Merriman, H. O., and Provus, M. M. *Educational Evaluation & Decision Making.* Itasca, IL: F. E. Peacock Publ., 1971.
5. Committee on Evaluation and Standards. Glossary of evaluating terms in public health. *Am. J. Publ. Health* 60:1546, 1970.

6. Glanz, K. Dietitians' effectiveness and patient compliance with dietary regimens. *J. Am. Dietet. A.* 75:631, 1979.

7. Redman, B. K. *The Process of Patient Teaching in Nursing.* 4th Ed. St. Louis: C. V. Mosby Co., 1980.

8. Nelson, F. *Evaluation for Instructional Development.* Washington: Nat'l. Special Media Inst., undated.

9. Shortridge, R. C. Learner success or failure? *J. Nutr. Educ.* 8:18, 1976.

10. Wandelt, M. A., and Ager, J. W. *Quality Patient Care Scale.* New York: Appleton-Century-Crofts, 1974.

11. Irby, D. M., and Morgan, M. K., Eds. *Clinical Evaluation: Alternatives for Health Related Educators.* Gainesville: Center for Allied Health Instructional Personnel, Univ. Florida, 1975.

12. Tower, J. B., and Vosburgh, P. M. Development of a rating scale to measure learning in clinical dietetics. I. Theoretical considerations and method of construction. *J. Am. Dietet. A.* 68:440, 1976.

13. Vosburgh, P. M., Tower, J. B., Peckos, P. M., and Mason, M. Development of a rating scale to measure learning in clinical dietetics. II. Pilot test. *J. Am. Dietet. A.* 68:446, 1976.

14. Mager, R. F. *Goal Analysis.* Belmont, CA: Fearon Publ., 1972.

15. Merrill, M. D., and Goodman, R. K. *Selecting Instructional Strategies and Media: A Place to Begin.* Washington: Nat'l. Special Media Inst., 1972.

16. Haynes, R. B. Strategies for improving compliance: A methodological analysis and review. *In* Sackett, D. L., and Haynes, R. B., Eds. *Compliance with Therapeutic Regimens.* Baltimore: The Johns Hopkins Press, 1976.

17. Sackett, D. L., and Haynes, R. B., Eds. *Compliance with Therapeutic Regimens.* Baltimore: The Johns Hopkins Press, 1976.

18. Kaufman, R. A. *Educational System Planning.* Englewood Cliffs, NJ: Prentice-Hall, Inc., 1972.

19. Payne, D. A., Ed. *Curriculum Evaluation: Commentaries on Purpose, Process, Product.* Lexington, MA: Heath and Co., 1974.

20. Sabine, C. D., Ed. *Accountability: Systems Planning in Education.* Homewood, IL: ETC Publ., 1973.

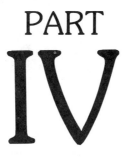

PART

IV

Management of Nutritional Counseling

14
Managing Client-Centered Care*

Management is not a general, rigid set of rules and actions, but is a set of flexible responses to a particular situation. Managerial actions are goal oriented and are related to available or obtainable resources. A single action is not isolated in time, but is related to the past and the future. Comprehending the wholeness or totality of given situations is important to understanding them in terms of management.

Ruth E. Deacon and Francille M Firebaugh,
Family Resource Management: Principles and Applications (Boston: Allyn and Bacon, Inc., 1981).

The terms flexibility, situation, action, goal oriented, resources, past, future, and even management are ones the reader has encountered many times. The statement, "Comprehending the wholeness or totality of given situations is important to understanding them in terms of management"[1] (p. 29), is a mandate to clinical dietitians if their practice is to be personally and professionally successful. Thus far, the discussions of the previous chapters have focused on a system with the goal of providing nutritional care to a client. The management of time, personnel, and other resources has not been specifically addressed in the process of proceeding through the system; however, the clinical dietitian's "real world" of practice is *multiple* clients.

* We acknowledge the contributions of Faye Fuentes, Deon Gines-Schweitzer, Audrey C. McCool, Sara C. Parks, and Mary Wenberg, all Registered Dietitians, in the formulation of concepts presented in this chapter.

Management of resources was a topic noted in the first chapter with the admonition, "The clinician who delivers quality care is also the effective manager of the resources available to him." Figure 3.1, Relationships of Knowledge and Role Skills to Nutritional Counseling, presents Manager as one of the necessary role skills. In the discussion of that topic, the conclusion was that, "Unless the clinical dietitian has an operative system and can serve as an effective manager, less than optimal nutritional counseling will be provided to clients." The purpose of this chapter is to address the fusion of the goal of quality nutritional care with the goals of the dietetic team, the health care team, the employing institution, and the profession. Discussion will focus first on a theoretical base for management, followed by application of management theory and functions of management for clinical dietetic practice.

THEORY OF MANAGEMENT

Definition of Management

There are various definitions of management, but most describe the concept in a similar manner. Longest defines management as ". . . a process, with both inter-personal and technical aspects, through which the objectives of an organization, or that part of it being managed, are accomplished by utilizing human and physical resources and technology"[2] (p. 40). Hersey and Blanchard define it as ". . . working with and through individuals and groups to accomplish organizational goals"[3] (p. 3). Sabine describes management as ". . . a technology of achieving organizational purposes efficiently and effectively"[4] (p. 11). The theme that comes through these definitions and others is that management is a *process* or activity that is applied to *meet* established *goals,* particularly those of an organization. It requires competence in a variety of functions and skills in the utilization of resources to achieve those goals.

A Theoretical Base for Management

The way a person approaches her professional role will be founded upon her acceptance of a selected theoretical position. There have been various theories of management through the years, many of which worked in some contexts. In response to the realization that there is no one best way to manage, a newer theory, Contingency or Situational Theory of Management, has been proposed.[5,6] The Contingency Theory is in concert with the systems approach. The basic functions of assessment, planning, implementation, and evaluation are addressed. The means by which these functions are accomplished, however, should be individualized for each organization. The final decisions as to a choice of action are based on what works to achieve the stated objectives of the organizations, i.e., the way a manager chooses to behave depends upon each individual situation.

THEORY INTO PRACTICE

The translation of theory into practice is an essential activity when the theory is management and the application is to clinical dietetic practice. Longest described it quite graphically in the first edition of his book (1976):

> . . . there has not been a systematic program for equipping health professionals with the knowledge and skills they need in order to manage. One thing is absolutely certain—being a good physician, nurse, or technologist does not make one an effective manager.[2] (p. x)

The Contingency Theory of Management,[5] in concert with the systems approach, is an excellent response to Longest's conclusion that health professionals must be prepared to be managers. The model for the provision of nutritional care (Figure 9.1) is a system identifying four components, but clearly illustrates the interdependence of each component. If our goal is the provision of nutritional care utilizing a system, the management activities that result in achieving that goal should also be circumscribed in a system. The Contingency Theory allows the choice of management activities to be based on those that will best achieve the goal. Since this management theory and our model appear to be congruent, they will be used as a basis for our discussion of the application of management theory to clinical dietetic practice.

The client as the focus of the process of nutritional counseling has been a continuing theme of this book. Figure 14.1 provides an illustration identifying this theme:

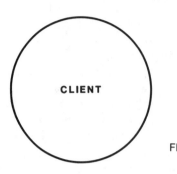

FIGURE 14.1   Nutritional counseling: Focus of client-
centered care

When the client is identified as the focus of nutritional counseling, it is in primary relationship to the provider of that care, the clinical dietitian. Figure 14.2 shows the relationship of the client to the clinical dietitian and underscores the client as the focus of her activities.

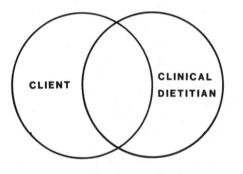

FIGURE 14.2   Nutritional counseling:
Identification of the primary
relationship in client-centered care

From the simplistic concepts in Figures 14.1 and 14.2, we move to the more complex, as demonstrated in Figure 14.3. To assist the client in achievement of jointly established goals, the clinical dietitian must consider the goals of other groups and ensure that all goals are congruent.

Two different teams, the dietetic team and the health care team, are identified in Figure 14.3, as the clinical dietitian is an active member of both. The goal concept of the health care team has been thoroughly discussed, but the goal concept of the dietetic team is relatively new. The clinical dietitian employed in a health care facility will no doubt be placed in the middle of the team between a dietetic technician and the director of dietetic services.*

In one study of dietitians' perceptions of goals, 240 questionnaires

* There appears to be a trend toward relabeling "dietetic services" as "nutrition services."[7]

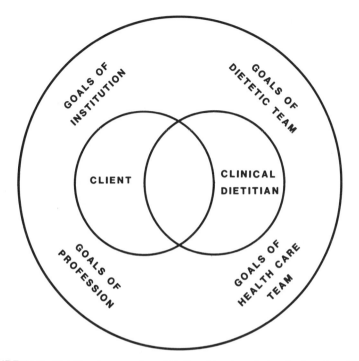

FIGURE 14.3 Nutritional counseling: Relationship of goals to client-centered care

were mailed to acute care facilities.[8] The respondents (74%) reported that dietitians perceive the patients' well-being and satisfaction as the foremost goal of a dietetic department. The next highest goal was serving nutritionally adequate food to patients and personnel. The latter goal served as a means of achieving the first goal. Furthermore, the study revealed that high morale in a dietetic department is associated with group decision making in addition to the director's concern that all dietitians are satisfied with the decision. This study is one documentation that dietetic departments of health care facilities identify goals that are client-centered with emphasis on what the department is uniquely qualified to provide: nutritionally adequate food to ensure clients' well-being and satisfaction, which easily translates into quality nutritional care.[8]

If high morale and hence satisfaction are derived when decisions are reached through group consensus, the dietetic team must then truly perform as a team. Who are members of the team? In the American Dietetic Association's Role Delineation Study, "clinical dietetic personnel" were defined to encompass ". . . all levels of dietetic personnel providing nutrition care to individual clients/patients in acute, ambulatory, and long-term facilities, in private practice, and in community service programs"[9] (p. 1). The methodology of the study clarified the interpretation of "clinical dietetic personnel":

> After the "actual" role was delineated, the Working Committee was instructed to delineate "appropriate" responsibilities for the entire field of clinical dietetics at the entry-level.* The commonly used three-position classification scheme for dietetic practitioners (i.e., dietitian, dietetic technician, and dietetic assistant) was disregarded. The question of the number of practice levels reflected in the delineated responsibilities for the field was addressed only after the supporting skill and knowledge requirements were identified. On this basis, . . . it was determined that there were but two levels of practice in the entry "appropriate" role of clinical dietetics, i.e., the professional dietitian level and the dietetic technician level.[10] (p. 1)

In the Association's last published glossary, the latter dietetic practitioner was defined as:

> Dietetic Technician: A technically skilled person who has successfully completed an associate degree program which meets the educational standards established by The American Dietetic Association. The dietetic technician, working under the guidance of an R.D. or an A.D.A. dietitian, has responsibilities in assigned areas in food service management; in teaching foods and nutrition principles; and in dietary counseling.[11] (p. 664)

With members of the dietetic team identified, what are the responsibilities of the clinical dietitian to the other team members? Longest,[2] in his discussion of the interpersonal aspect of management, identified a very large component he called the "human factor." He expanded on this concept by stating "There is no such thing as the average human being; human beings work to satisfy their own needs; and human beings respond to leadership"[2] (p. 135). In Longest's opinion, managers who fail to recognize these factors of human behavior will be unsuccessful in their practice.

Drucker[12] labels the person who has had specialized schooling and served some period of apprenticeship learning the practice role as the "knowledge worker." In Drucker's estimation, the key to deriving pro-

---

* "Entry-level" was defined as ". . . meaning minimum-basic, includes those practicing one year or less"[9] (p. 1).

ductivity from the knowledge worker is to demand responsibility from her. To achieve this result, each knowledge worker (from the lowliest and youngest to the highest officer) should be asked at least once a year:

What do you contribute that justifies you being on the payroll? What should this company, this hospital, this government agency, this university, hold you accountable for, by way of contributions and results? Do you know what your goals and objectives are? And what do you plan to do to attain them?[12] *(p. 75)*

Longest provides a further recommendation:

In applying the modern approach to directing subordinates the manager's central task is to show the subordinate that his objectives and the objectives of the health care facility are essentially compatible. It is doubtful whether organizational objectives can be identical to those of the individual. However, the similarity is often greater than some managers assume. Even when the worker's objectives are not identical to those of the health care facility, it does not mean that they must be mutually exclusive.[2] *(p. 137)*

Having clarified the clinical dietitian's managerial responsibilities to the supportive personnel of the dietetic team, it is critical to remember that the team has vertical relationships. Considering the upward direction of a manager's responsibilities, a recent paper has been aptly entitled "Managing Your Boss."[13] The authors' advice is comprehensive:

Managing your boss requires that you gain an understanding of both the boss and his context as well as your own situation and needs. All managers do this to some degree, but many are not thorough enough.

At a minimum, you need to appreciate your boss's goals and pressures, his or her strengths and weaknesses. What are your boss's organizational and personal objectives, and what are the pressures on him, especially those from his boss and others at his level? What are your boss's long suits and blind spots? What is his or her preferred style of working? Does he or she like to get information through memos, formal meetings, or phone calls? Does your boss thrive on conflict or try to minimize it?

Without this information, a manager is flying blind when dealing with his boss, and unnecessary conflicts, misunderstandings, and problems are inevitable.[13] *(p. 94)*

In summary, the clinical dietitian must ensure that the goals of each member of the dietetic team are not only compatible but are well understood by each member. High morale and productivity are dependent on that understanding being achieved through participative decision making to reach concensus.[8]

In addition to the goals of the dietetic team, Figure 14.3 documents the need also to work with and through the goals of the health care team, the goals of the institution, and the goals of the profession. Each of these groups were identified in the professional society's Role Delineation Study.[14] The Study's first technical report was a comprehensive review of the literature resulting in the identification of the clinical dietitian's responsibilities. These responsibilities were further categorized and summarized:

Responsibilities (of the clinical dietitian) to the health care team:

Provides nutrition education programs for staff
Meets and consults with health team regarding nutrition care
Participates in grand rounds
Coordinates client/patient care with dietetic team members
Coordinates nutrition service program activities

Responsibilities to the institution (strategic direction and personnel management):

Coordinates work and communicates effectively
Designs/implements/evaluates programs in conformance with policies and procedures
Formulates and monitors budgets
Monitors quality of care
Administers personnel functions/supervises staff
Develops staff
Plans and provides training experiences for dietetic students

Responsibilities to the profession (identification and management of extraneous influences on nutrition care):

Interprets professional guidelines and legislation/regulation
Develops/implements plans and/or procedures in conformance with laws, regulations, and guidelines
Identifies role of dietetic practitioner in the legislative process
Identifies/contacts appropriate government agencies and personnel
Identifies/solicits sources of outside funding for nutrition care services.[14] *(p. 38)*

The subtitle of Figure 14.3, "Relationship of Goals to Client-Centered Care," describes the broad spectrum of groups for whom the clinical

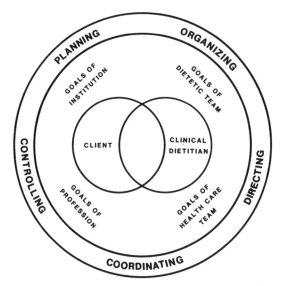

FIGURE 14.4   Nutritional counseling: Relationships of management functions to the goals of client-centered care

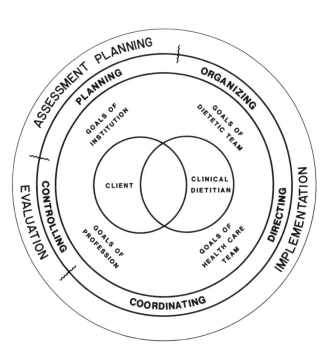

FIGURE 14.5   Nutritional counseling: Relationships of the nutritional care model to management functions focusing on client-centered care

dietitian has a range of responsibilities if the overall goal, quality nutritional care, is to be delivered. Figure 14.4 displays a set of managerial functions that can be utilized by the clinical dietitian in meeting those responsibilities.

The essential managerial functions identified in Figure 14.4 have been derived from a review of the literature that is resplendent with models, theories, and terminology. Planning, organizing, directing, coordinating, and controlling are management functions[2] derived as basic and reflective of the managerial needs of the clinical dietitian. To take the concept one step further, Figure 14.5 proposes a graphic way in which the identified management functions relate to the overall systems model of providing nutritional care.

With the clinical dietitian's overall goal of providing client-centered quality nutritional care, reference to Figure 14.5 can serve as a tool in ensuring that the skills of management are applied at all levels.

FUNCTIONS OF MANAGEMENT

When clinicians are managing dietetic practice, they must deal with a variety of resources; the primary one is personnel. Although there are other resources to be managed, for example, time, money, information, facilities, hardware, and software, they are secondary because they exist only as an extension of the human use of them.

Each of these resources is managed with the use of various tools. This section will highlight a number of those tools used for each of the functions described in the paragraphs to follow. There will be only a cursory presentation of management concepts, however, as they are the subject of both courses and curricula. This chapter alone will not serve to prepare clinical dietitians to be effective managers; it will only suggest the scope of management expertise needed by all health care professionals.

Management specialists identify the basic management functions in various ways. For the purposes of this text, the authors prefer to use those functions proposed and defined by Longest[2]: (1) Planning, (2) Organizing, (3) Directing, (4) Coordinating, and (5) Controlling. These were illustrated in the model presented in Figures 14.4 and 14.5.

Planning

Management literature, by and large, tends to collapse assessment and planning under the label of planning. The process is basically the same as used in counseling a single client. The types of data sought, tools used, and decisions made are just more comprehensive. Planning is the process of gathering and analyzing data, setting objectives, developing strategies, establishing criteria, and interfacing these objectives and activities with those of the institution.

When there are many demands and objectives proposed, it is necessary to set priorities; this should not be an arbitrary process. There are several techniques available to facilitate setting priorities. These include "nominal group process"[15] and the Delphi technique.[16]

When the clinician is responsible for the management of personnel, she is involved in planning for staffing. This process involves such activities as job and task analysis, and writing of job descriptions. One approach utilized in many personnel management environs is a technique called Management by Objectives, MBO.[17] This technique is the same as that used in planning nutritional care, but rather than defining client expectations, it defines employee expectations.

Another major responsibility of a manager is to be a change agent. An organization can be managed in such a way that the status quo is maintained. The world is rapidly changing, however, and organizations must not only respond to change by changing themselves, but also must assume leadership in that change. The planning in any one department must be done in coordination with the rest of the institution. Two tools that are or can be used to plan for change are forecasting[18] and future problem solving.[19]

Planning also involves the resources of time, information, and money. As time management has become a very high priority skill in today's breakneck world, various methods and tools are available to help clinicians cope. Lakein[20] has developed a method of prioritizing demands on time by an "A, B, C" filing system. Other professionals and managers use a time-line method, as demonstrated in Figure 14.6. A more sophisticated method is called PERT or Program Evaluation and Review Technique.[21] This technique is a flow system design specifying task completion dates.

Information planning is also a necessary component of management. A descriptive method for examining planned information flow is called network analysis.[22] This technique examines the destinations and directions of information in the organization. Plans also need to be made for required and requested communications, including newsletters, brochures, memos, agendas, minutes, and other standard forms of conveying information.

The process of planning must be applied to financial resources as well. A well known and commonly accepted method of planning is the budget. As there are clarion calls for accountability[4] in today's insti-

Objectives

1. Increase nutritional services by dietetic technician
   a. Job description written
   b. Job description approved
   c. In—service topics developed and published
   d. Lessons designed

2. Expand nutritional education by closed circuit TV system
   a. Daily Food Guide script written
   b. Visuals produced
   c. Taping completed
   d. Scheduling completed
   e. Weight reduction script written
   f. Taping completed
   g. Scheduling completed

3. _____

Year _____

Month	June	July	Aug.	Sept.	Oct.	Nov.	Dec.	Jan.	Feb.	Mar.	April	May
Week	1234	1234	1234	1234	1234	1234	1234	1234	1234	1234	1234	1234

#1 #2 #3 #4 #5

tutions, sophisticated methods of financial planning have been developed. One method is the Planning-Programming-Budgeting System (PPBS). Sabine defines PPBS as "A conceptual approach to decision-making: emphasizes output, program activities, and accomplishment relative to predetermined objectives, long-range planning, economic rationality, and systems analysis for decision-making"[4] (p. 237). Although PPBS has been used mostly in educational institutions, it has applicability to any institution or unit within an institution delivering services. The purpose of more sophisticated approaches is not just to allocate dollars, but to do so with cost/effectiveness* as the goal.

Other resources for which planning must be done are in the area of hardware, software, and facilities. Hardware refers to the equipment used in the professional setting. In counseling, examples of hardware to consider are tape recorders, interactive computers, and video-tape units, discussed at length in Chapter 8. Planning for equipment is based on an assessment of the instructional strategies employed by clinicians and resources available in the organization. Software is a collection of books, tapes, records, food models, and so on. In addition, planning must be done to accommodate personnel, material resources, and the activities of the health care providers. Office assignments, traffic flow, access for handicapped persons, and designated counseling space are all in the purview of a manager.

Organizing

Once resources have been planned, they need to be structured in a system that defines their relationships. Organizational charts are one means to illustrate hierarchical and lateral relationships. In the area of personnel, the concepts of responsibility and authority are emphasized. Each unit of the organizational chart has its designated responsibilities. Effective management provides the employee with concomitant authority.[23] When appropriate authority is withheld, an employee is constrained from effectively meeting his responsibilities. A significant element in authority involves the privilege of delegation. Although delegation *is* a privilege, it is frequently difficult for managers to effect. An effective manager will delegate as much as possible, leaving time to deal with responsibilities that cannot be delegated.

The organizing of information is frequently referred to as Management of Information Systems, MIS.[4] The plethora of knowledge and data mandates the need for computer technology in management. Stor-

---

* Cost/effectiveness will be discussed in more detail in Chapter 15.

age and retrieval systems are capable of organizing and maintaining information on budget and expenditures, inventory, cataloging of resources and staffing.

Directing

The function of directing involves communicating, supervising, leading, and motivating. This function is comparable to teaching, in that information is communicated about expected outcomes (MBO), then the activity is supervised to determine that the objectives are met. Constant observation of an employee is not required (unless he is learning a skill), but ensuring that defined deadlines are met is necessary.

Leadership is the ability to inspire and motivate personnel. This quality is difficult to define, but may be at the least a mixture of serving as a credible model and being respected as a competent person. Leadership is particularly effective when the leader takes a personal interest in nurturing employees to work toward greater professional growth.

Motivation is another necessary skill of the manager. There are a variety of theories on motivation of employees, such as Theory X and Theory Y,[3] behavior modification,[24] and Maslow's hierarchy of needs.[25] The discussion of behavior and learning in Chapter 10 provided a brief overview of some basic concepts of behavior analysis.

Communication was addressed at length in the interview chapter (Chapter 5), and those basic principles certainly apply to managerial communication. In addition, the ability to write and speak clearly will enhance the attainment of intended outcomes.

One facet of directing is the initiation and continuing education of self and employees. This specialized form of directing requires the assurance that learning has occurred. The process spelled out in counseling is applicable to employee education.

Coordinating

The function of coordination involves the orchestration of all personnel and their responsibilities to achieve the established objectives. To accomplish coordination, a manager must be capable of facilitating team development. Team development is a process that groups undergo in order to become a functioning unit. It includes group decision making about role definition, role negotiation, and role conflict. The manager needs good communication skills, an understanding of the way teams develop, and the ability to deal with conflicts.

Subsumed under coordination of personnel is the coordination of time, often called "scheduling." Work schedules and client contact schedules prevent crisis management and conflicts in carrying out responsibilities such as the physical therapist and dietitian arriving at the bedside simultaneously. Coordination of care plans includes coordinated scheduling.

One of the more difficult tasks is the coordination of information. More frequently than not, "the right hand knows not what the left hand is doing." This phenomenon is responsible for such clichés as "reinventing the wheel" and "it slipped through the crack." One common means to confront this problem is the committee or staff meeting. Meetings can either be effective or useless in achieving coordination of information; the burden of facilitation is on the person in charge. There is now a selection of treatises on planning and conducting effective meetings that aid professionals in managerial roles with this task.[26]

Coordination of information with the outside world is also useful in achieving organizational goals. Public relations activities can pay real dividends. The use of an advisory council in facilities where community nutrition goals exist can benefit both the community and the institution.

Controlling

The controlling function in management is essentially the same as the evaluation component. Like the link between evaluation and assessment, control is linked to planning. According to Longest,[2] control is based on four steps: (1) establishing standards, (2) measuring performance, (3) comparing actual results with standards, and (4) correcting deviations from standards.

One type of evaluation or controlling is called performance appraisal.[27] This periodic activity is designed to give employees feedback on the performance of their responsibilities. In addition to evaluation of individuals, there is program evaluation. Planning done using PPBS is the basis for decisions concerning achievement of institutional goals (effectiveness and efficiency). In health care settings, another form of controlling is referred to as audit.* Teams of peers, either internal or

* Also to be discussed in Chapter 15.

external, review medical records to determine effectiveness of health care.

Controlling involves comparing all activities with the original plans. Client achievement is compared to nutritional care plans; employee progress is measured against original objectives (MBO). Completion of activities is compared to the original PERT or time-line. Expenditures are held up to budget figures. Communication effectiveness is examined in the light of the network analysis. The use of hardware and software is measured against the systems design in which they are utilized.

SKILLS OF MANAGEMENT

There are a number of subsidiary skills that help a clinician serve as a more effective manager. Several of these have been presented earlier in the text, for example, communication, motivation, instruction, assessment, planning, evaluation, and leadership. Three skills that are particularly useful and have not been given more than a mention heretofore are worth presenting at this point. They are decision making, problem solving, and creativity.

Decision making is a process that professionals in all roles must use, whether with one client or several, in other practice responsibilities or as a manager of a unit. Decision making follows the basic steps of:

1. Gathering facts
2. Identifying objectives and criteria
3. Examining given alternatives
4. Comparing alternatives to established objectives and criteria
5. Selecting the best alternative.

Decision making implies that the objectives, criteria, and alternatives have been presented to the decisionmaker(s). Their role is to decide which alternatives would be most effective in achieving the objective.

Problem solving is an extension of decision making. In addition, however, the problem solvers define the problem, and list their own alternative solutions. Thus the process of problem solving is:

1. Identifying the problem
2. Gathering the facts
3. Defining the problem

4. Identifying objectives and criteria

5. Listing known alternative solutions

6. Comparing the alternatives to objectives and criteria

7. Selecting the best alternative

Steps 2, 4, 6, and 7 are the same as the decision making process. Step 5 differs in that the problem solvers generally seek their own alternative solutions. Steps 1 and 3, problem identification and problem definition, are the major variations. The act of problem identification is the discovery of what the felt difficulty is, whereas problem definition is the process of pinpointing what the true problem is.

Creativity or creative problem solving is an even more specialized approach to problem solving.[28] This approach is used when there are not ready-made solutions available that satisfy the problem solvers. When the problem solvers reach an impasse, then it is time to implement the skill of creative problem solving. The steps of the process are as follows:

1. Identifying the problem

2. Gathering facts

3. Defining the problem

4. Brainstorming alternative solutions

5. Establishing criteria

6. Selecting a preferred solution(s)

7. Planning implementation and selling of the idea.

Once again, the components of both decision making and problem solving are included. There are, however, basic differences. The first major difference is that the selection of criteria is delayed until after solutions are generated. The purpose of this delay is to encourage the generation of creative ideas as creativity frequently is repressed by preconceived ideas of acceptability. The fourth step is included because there are no known effective solutions; thus, the purpose is to create novel solutions. The last major difference is in Step 7. Since the process of change usually confronts major efforts at resistance, the problem solvers must be prepared to tell the ultimate decision makers how (implementation) and why (selling) the solution works.

Each of these three skills can be learned by clinicians. The ability to use the skills can be a powerful tool for anyone in a managerial capacity.

SUMMARY

The practice of clinical dietetics is more than a collection of individual counseling experiences. A systematic approach to successful professional practice is required. The management functions a clinician needs to utilize are (1) planning, (2) organizing, (3) directing, (4) coordinating, and (5) controlling. These functions are comparable to the nutritional counseling components of assessment, planning, implementation, and evaluation. The clinician must manage a variety of resources including personnel, time, money, information, hardware, software, facilities, and the external environment to facilitate client growth toward independence and to achieve dietetic team, health care team, institutional, and professional goals. There are a variety of tools* and skills available to help the clinician develop managerial qualities. The clinician must avail herself of all opportunities to understand the theories of management and to acquire the capabilities needed to be an effective manager.

CITED REFERENCES

1. Deacon, R. E., and Firebaugh, F. M. *Family Resource Management: Principles and Application.* Boston: Allyn and Bacon, Inc., 1981.

2. Longest, B. B., Jr. *Management Practices for the Health Professional.* 2nd Ed. Reston, VA: Reston Publ. Co., 1980.

3. Hersey, P., and Blanchard, K. H. *Management of Organizational Behavior: Utilizing Human Resources.* 3rd Ed. Englewood Cliffs, NJ: Prentice-Hall, Inc., 1977.

4. Sabine, C. D., Ed. *Accountability: Systems Planning in Education.* Homewood, IL: ETC Publ., 1973.

5. Hellrigel, D., and Slocum, J. W. *Management: Contingency Approaches.* 2nd Ed. Reading, MA: Addison-Wesley Publ. Co., 1978.

6. Carlisle, H. M. *Situational Management: A Contingency Approach to Management.* New York: AMA COM, 1973.

7. Schiller, R. Improving Nutritional Care: Reader Response. *Dietetic Currents* 7:5: Oct.–Dec., 1980. Columbus: Ross Laboratories, 1980.

8. Jevnikar, G. A. *Dietitians' Perceptions of Goals, Organizational Cohesiveness, and Formality of the Decision-Making Procedures in Hospital Dietetic Departments.* Unpublished M.S. thesis, University of Washington, 1972.

9. Baird, S. C., and Armstrong, R. V. Role Delineation for the Field of Clinical Dietetics. Technical Report #3—*Survey Design and Sampling Procedure.* Chicago: The American Dietetic Association, December, 1980.

* One such tool is shown in Appendix K.

10. Baird, S. C., and Armstrong, R. V. Role Delineation for the Field of Clinical Dietetics. Technical Report #6—*Policy and Planning Implications.* Chicago: The American Dietetic Association, December, 1980.

11. Committee to Develop a Glossary on Terminology for the Association and Profession, American Dietetic Association. Titles, definitions and responsibilities for the profession of dietetics, 1974. *J. Am. Dietet. A.* 64:661, 1974.

12. Drucker, P. F. Managing the knowledge worker. *In* Beyers, M., Ed. *Leadership in Nursing.* Wakefield, MA: Nurs. Res., Inc., 1979.

13. Gabarro, J. J., and Kotter, J. P. Managing your boss. *Harvard Bus. Rev.,* Jan.–Feb., 1980.

14. Baird, S. C., and Armstrong, R. V. Role Delineation for the Field of Clinical Dietetics. Technical Report #1—*Literature Review and Annotated Bibliography.* Chicago: The American Dietetic Association, December, 1980.

15. Delbecq, A. L., Van de Ven, A. H., and Gustafson, D. H. *Group Techniques for Program Planning: A Guide to Nominal Group and Delphi Processes.* Glenview, IL: Scott Foresman Co., 1975.

16. Linstone, H. A., and Turoff, M., Eds. *The Delphi Method: Techniques and Applications.* Reading, MA: Addison-Wesley Publ. Co., 1975.

17. Odiorne, G. *Management by Objectives.* New York: Pitman Publ. Corp., 1965.

18. Makidakis, S. G., and Wheelwright, S. C. *Forecasting: Methods and Applications.* Santa Barbara, CA: John Wiley & Sons, Inc., Publ., 1978.

19. Mars, D. The role of the middle manager in nurturing creativity. *J. Creative Beh.* 5:270, 1977.

20. Lakein, A. *How to Get Control of Your Time and Your Life.* New York: Peter H. Wyden, Inc., 1973.

21. Kaufman, R. A. *Educational System Planning.* Englewood Cliffs, NJ: Prentice-Hall, Inc., 1972.

22. Boissevein, J., and Mitchell, J. C. *Network Analysis: Studies in Human Interaction.* The Hague: Mouton, 1973.

23. Gordon, T. *Leader Effectiveness Training: The No-Lose Way to Release the Productive Potential of People.* New York: Peter H. Wyden, Inc., 1978.

24. Bandura, A. *Principles of Behavior Modification.* New York: Holt, Rinehart and Winston, Inc., 1969.

25. Maslow, A. H. *Toward a Psychology of Being.* Princeton, NJ: Van Nostrand Reinhold Co., 1962.

26. McDougle, L. G. Conducting a successful meeting. *Pers. J.* 60:49, 1981.

27. McGregor, D. Performance evaluation. *In* Stone, S., Berger, M. S., Elhart, D., Forsich, S. C., and Gordon, S. B., Eds. *Management for Nurses: A Multidisciplinary Approach.* St. Louis: C. V. Mosby Co., 1976.

28. Parnes, S. J. *Creative Behavior Guidebook.* New York: Charles Scribner's Sons, 1967.

15

Measuring the Success of Practice

MANAGEMENT OF NUTRITIONAL COUNSELING
Managing Client-Centered Care
Measuring the Success of Practice

*A successful professional is an independent **decision-maker** and **change-agent,** able to apply to a variety of problems and settings the unique body of technical knowledge which distinguishes his/her profession from others. Therefore, if dietitians are to assume their responsibility to improve the nutritional status of the population by providing adequate nutritional care to all segments of society, they must become independent decision-makers and change-agents—"actors" determining their own roles, rather than "reactors" to the demands of others.*

Eileen B. Peck, *The "professional self" and its relation to change processes.* (*J. Am Dietet.* A. 69:534, 1976).

In the beginning of this text, the question, "What does a dietitian do?" was posed. One set of answers has been hypothesized in the model for a systems approach to the provision of nutritional care (Figure 9.1). The system supports Robinson's thesis[2] that dietitians must address nutrition as one of the preventive measures that assure good health and quality of life for the population. The proposed model also supports Galbraith's[3] prediction for the year 2000; that the expertise of the dietitian will be required beyond the acute episodic encounter to that of providing continuity of nutritional care in large numbers of increasing varieties of ambulatory settings. Peck[1] reaffirms the authors' proposal by emphasizing the dietitian's responsibility to all segments of society.

The model and processes set forth in the previous chapters demonstrate, for clinical dietitians, a pathway for the assumption of the role that will ensure concern for nutritional care for all segments of society. In this chapter we shall examine some of the ways in which practice may be evaluated.

First, however, to ascertain how clinical dietitians can best approach the future, an assessment of past practice seems in order. A limited number of research studies have been reported that focus on role performance of clinical dietitians. A review of these studies provides some guidance to future practice and its evaluation.

ROLE PERFORMANCE EVALUATION

Sociologically, "role" designates those tasks, responsibilities, and qualities that identify a specific relationship. . . . A dietitian is expected to act in a certain way and to assume a well defined pattern of activities, recognized and accepted by patients, physicians, directors of dietary departments, and hospital administrators. Each of these "role partners" has certain expectations of the dietitian, who also has personal convictions about her responsibilities.[4] *(p. 284)*

The last sentence of the quotation above should imply to clinical dietitians that there are a number of serious issues facing them as they go about their daily practice. Some of these issues may be expressed as follows: Are clinical dietitians able to identify their professional role and then practice accordingly? How well do they perform the role? Do others (e.g., clients, physicians, nurses, social workers, administrators) identify the role of clinical dietitians as readily or as clearly as the clinicians themselves? These questions—and others— have only recently begun to receive the attention they deserve.

The Study Commission on Dietetics, in the course of their work, assembled the views of other health professionals and administrators about the roles of dietitians. These opinions were gathered in numerous interviews. So far as physicians were concerned, the Commission reported, "It can be said that the physician's perception of the role of the dietitian is highly dependent on the physician's own interests and clinical practice"[5] (p. 11). Other health professionals, described as having limited contact with dietitians, saw them as "either consultants to those who render direct services to patients or as food management employees"[5] (p. 11). Administrators, according to the Study Commission, see dietitians as employees rather than fellow workers. These opinions may seem harsh to many, but have served to generate a number of investigations in the years that followed the publication of the report (1972). Prior to that time, the prevailing opinions on roles and role performance were primarily supported by "armchair" data. An exception to this statement is the work of Spangler and others[6,7] begun in 1969 and first reported in 1970.

For a study sponsored by the state hospital association and the state land grant university, a questionnaire was designed and sent to a variety of health professionals affiliated with 236 hospitals within the state of Michigan.[6,7]* The purposes of the study were twofold: (1) to identify physicians' attitudes about the contributions of clinical dietitians to health teams, their clinical responsibilities, and their prescribing of nutritional care plans; and (2) to determine the frequency of communication between physicians and clinical dietitians, and the use of nutrition therapy in client care by physicians. The surveyed sample included physicians (chiefs of staff), hospital administrators, dietetic department directors, nursing service directors, and dietitians.[7] Of the original 236 hospitals, 169 institutions returned one or more completed questionnaires (from the group named above). Among the 830 respondents, there were 231 dietitians and 135 chiefs of staff.

In response to the section of the questionnaire schedule designed to elicit opinions about the role of clinical dietitians in health care teams, Spangler *et al.* report that:

> *The dietitians expressed an overwhelming interest (80% +) in being recognized as decision-making members of the health team. On the other hand less than half of the physicians expressed an interest in including the dietitian in this capacity.*[6] *(p. 3)*

From this work, it is apparent that physicians and dietitians have quite differing views on the latter's role in client-centered care. In the second paper, Spangler remarks that "the largest percentage of chiefs of staff (57 percent) believed that the dietary department is at an auxiliary level, primarily implementing the orders of others"[7] (p. 647).

In a more recent paper, Jacobson described the results of a statewide survey of 50 teaching hospitals in New Jersey.[8] The survey was designed to solicit information regarding dietetic practices, services, and trends from four distinct groups of professionals affiliated with the teaching sites. The four groups were administrators (chief executive officers), dietetic services (clinical dietitians), medical services (chiefs

---

* Clinical dietitians are encouraged to read the reports of this and other studies in the original literature.

of staff), and nursing services (head nurses or nursing supervisors). Amazingly, of the 50 sets of questionnaires distributed, 100 percent were eventually returned!

The survey tool was a questionnaire schedule designed and distributed by a committee of the Medical Society of New Jersey. The questions were asked in the belief that the responses could provide information for two distinct planning purposes: patient services (current) and future planning. Some of the questions asked, and the responses they evoked, are revealing in terms of dietetic practice. For example, in all questions related to dietetic practice, less than half of the clinical dietitians responded positively. To the query "Is the recording of a diet history a part of therapeutic consultations?", only 20 percent of the respondents answered "always" or "yes." Twice that number, or only 40 percent, declared that they work with clients *not* on modified diets (indicating a lack of involvement in primary prevention). In Jacobson's words, "The most striking finding in the responses of dietitians is the minimal level of responsibility for dietary services assumed by (or assigned to) the dietary department; . . . only a small minority have significant patient contact"[8] (p. 17).

Even more interesting are what Jacobson describes as the "salient responses from chief of staff questionnaires." For those questions designed to elicit information about interdisciplinary communications, less than half of the responses fell into the "always" or "yes" category. The range of positive responses was from 40 percent ("Is the dietitian encouraged to record observations in the physicians' progress notes?") to 6 percent ("Do physicians and dietitians jointly discuss laboratory findings and their interpretations as they relate to dietary management?"). Jacobson describes these as "disturbing findings," but wisely does not render a verdict of guilt for any particular group among the four surveyed.

Some of the ideas about interdisciplinary communication generated from the New Jersey survey were earlier examined in a paper by Schiller. Reporting on role autonomy, Schiller wrote:

> *The role of physicians demands that they be decisive, authoritative, and assertive. They resist the health team movement and other developments which may require them to relinquish authority. Physicians have not accorded any allied health group the status or the occupational autonomy allied health professionals claim for themselves. Basically, the very concept of a health care "team" is unrealistic because to function as a team, all of the members must agree on their own specific roles, the roles of others on the team, and how all of the roles relate.*

Thus, isolationism and stratification among professions often prevent physicians and dietitians from communicating. The interaction of dietitians and physicians is seldom close or truly reciprocal. Although dietitians seem to have few problems consulting with nurses, they are not satisfied with their degree of participation on the medical team.[9] (p. 97)

Schiller's comments are appropriate in light of the findings of Jacobson, and Spangler and co-workers.

An extensive study on the role of clinical dietitians was reported in 1974 by Schiller and Vivian.[4,10] The research technique employed was again a questionnaire schedule, mailed to 2000 physicians and 1000 clinical dietitians. The purposes of the study were described as:

. . . to determine: (a) the level of agreement (role consensus) among physicians and dietitians on the activities, responsibilities, and qualities which compose the role of the dietitian; (b) the extent to which physicians and dietitians perceive differences between the ideal (role expectations) and actual performance of the dietitian; and (c) the common deterrents, which dietitians perceive as basic to dichotomies between ideal and actual role performance.[4] (p. 285)

The questionnaire contained 34 inventory statements about what Schiller and Vivian describe as "five conventional activities"* and "eight activities connoting high-level (decision-making) responsibility" of clinical dietitians. Of the sample surveyed, 728 (36.4%) physicians and 701 (70.1%) dietitians responded.

For the first purpose of the study, Schiller and Vivian found that physicians agreed that clinical dietitians should contribute to health team activities, but also found that there was a lack of agreement on the particular activities by which such participation is accomplished. Further,

. . . there was a lack of consensus on those activities implying a direct role for the dietitian in decision-making or in assessing, planning or evaluating nutritional care.[4] (p. 285)

As a group, the sampled dietitians were in high agreement for only three of the eight activities pertaining to "high-level responsibility." Consensus was high among clinical dietitians for general statements about high levels of responsibility, but it was lower for specific statements about the assumption of tasks basic to health team participation.

---

* These are: "knows food composition, follows dietary orders, takes nutritional histories, checks trays, and gives dietary instructions."[4] (p. 285).

... there was high consensus for "charts dietary information," a task generally practiced in some hospitals and for which specific procedures have been established and published. This finding supports the widely held concept that dietitians are insecure and reluctant to assume new responsibilities but are self-confident when following specific guidelines or performing traditional functions approved by other professionals.[4] (p. 286)

In the final paper of this series, Schiller and Vivian report the results pertaining to the second and third purposes of the study.[10] For the second, the investigators found that dietitians and physicians differed considerably in their evaluations of the actual and ideal role of clinical dietitians. This finding is in accordance with that of Spangler and co-workers,[6] and is called "role disparity" by Schiller and Vivian. The reported sources of conflict in role disparity are varied and include the inventory items of "initiates dietary prescriptions" and "recommends diets." In the analysis of these two items alone, almost half of the physicians believed that clinical dietitians should "recommend diets;" only a quarter believed that clinicians should "initiate dietary prescriptions." In contrast, 58 percent of the dietitians believed that they should "recommend" while 67 percent believed that they should "initiate!"

What are the deterrents to role performance? For the last purpose of the study, Schiller and Vivian examined the responses of the dietitians to a list of seven statements that they believed would account for the dichotomy between ideal and actual role performance:[10]

1. Lack of education
2. Hospital policy
3. Lack of time
4. Shortage of personnel
5. Physician prohibits
6. Not interested
7. Not relevant

As the reader may guess, "lack of time" was cited as the primary barrier to actual role performance for 88 percent of the inventory items. "Lack of education" was cited as a deterrent for 38 percent of the items, and "hospital policies" for 26 percent. In response to the inventory item "attends medical rounds," 45 percent of the participating dietitians cited lack of time as the major deterrent; 20 percent cited hospital policy. However, 79.8 percent of the dietitians agreed that attending medical rounds should be a part of the clinician's function! (But only 20.9 percent of the physicians agreed.) The authors conclude that:

> Since 45 percent of the dietitians listed lack of time and 20 percent, restriction of hospital policy as reasons for not attending rounds— an activity for which greatest role disparity was observed—it is an evasion to designate the physician as a primary deterrent to an expanded role for the dietitian.[10] (p. 289)

The general results of this significant study indicate that clinical dietitians have not fulfilled, to either their satisfaction or to the satisfaction of physicians, their responsibilities for basic, conventional activities associated with the practice of clinical dietetics. Schiller and Vivian[10] warn that until the practitioner adequately fulfills the lesser role, he should not attempt to seek the assumption of the greater role, that of high-level decision making.

The next major study to be reviewed in this section was reported by Johnson in 1975,[11] and was planned to evaluate views of dietitians and their practice held by the consumers of their services and by dietetic professionals. In this study, consumers were defined as clients, physicians, and administrators; dietetic professionals were educators and practitioners. The basic purpose of the study was to provide data for assessing and planning of educational objectives for learning programs in Dietetics.

Two sets of questionnaires were prepared and mailed to the surveyed population. The client sample, randomly selected from the lay members of a voluntary health interest group, were asked to respond to a "Client Perception Questionnaire." Preselected physician members of the same group, hospital administrators, dietetic educators, and randomly selected clinical dietitians were mailed the "Professional Perception Questionnaire." Of the schedules released, usable returns were received from 174 clients, 183 educators, 57 employers (physicians and administrators), and 140 practitioners. Interestingly, twice as many sampled clients (72.4%) responded as did dietitians (36.2%).

The data were assembled and elaborately evaluated. In the words of Johnson:

> . . . there is statistical evidence that these clients and professionals agree on the primacy of the planning, teaching, and counseling functions inherent in the delivery of client-mediated nutritional care.[11] (p. 262)

How this is true is borne out by an examination of the relative ranking of dietetic functions by the entire sample. For example, at the top of the rank ordered list is "explains dietary plans" and "listens and answers client's questions." These responsibilities are inherent in what Johnson describes as "client-mediated nutritional care."

In 1979, the Medical Research Bureau of Ross Laboratories revealed the results of a study conducted "To provide research information to the American Dietetic Association on the perception dietitians, directors of nursing and hospital administrators have of the Dietetic Profession"[12] (p. 1). Personal interviews were held with 106 "chief" dietitians, 95 "staff position" dietitians, and 51 directors of nursing; 25 hospital administrators responded to a mailed questionnaire. The subjects interviewed represented over 100 short term general hospitals (for the dietitians and nurses) and 25 large hospitals (for the administrators).

The findings of the Ross study are consistent with those of Schiller and Vivian[10] five years earlier: The major perceived obstacles to in-depth involvement in client care are time ("staff position" dietitians), physician resistance (dietitians and nurses), and lack of funds (administrators).[12] Even more disheartening, verifying one observation of the Study Commission on Dietetics, is the identification by directors of nursing and hospital administrators of dietitians as primarily supervisors of "food preparation."

Helping dietitians develop attitudes enabling them to more effectively "listen" and "explain" was the purpose of a continuing learning program conducted by Biltz and Derelian.[13] They worked with 30 practitioners in eight weekly 2 hr. sessions (and used 90 nonparticipants as controls in their evaluation). Attitude measures were taken before and after the sessions, which were devoted to the development of skills enabling dietitians to plan and implement successful client counseling strategies. Comparison of the pretest and posttest results showed that participation in formal sessions was significant in terms of development of client oriented attitudes and, interestingly, confidence in ability to document exactly the results of counseling. Perhaps one way to achieve Johnson's goal of client-mediated nutritional care is through formal continuing learning programs like that constructed by Biltz and Derelian.

In Summary

In this section on role performance evaluation, the available objective evidence is presented. The data suggest that clinical dietitians are not perceived as they may wish to be. Why is this so? History leads us to the conclusion that role delineation* is a problem of considerable mag-

---

* To be discussed in Chapter 16.

nitude. One issue related to this problem is succinctly summarized by Johnson:

> . . . *clinical dietitians will be limited in providing adequate nutritional care because of the numbers of people making independent judgments related to the dietitians' primary professional role, namely, providing client-managed nutritional care. Can it be that clinical dietitians, their educators, and employees each expect something different?*[14] *(p. 220)*

To Johnson's list of significant groups we would add clients, health care providers, and administrators.

In an extensive study of role definition in ambulatory care settings, Scialabba reported that roles and role performances have changed and will continue to change with the introduction of newer health care delivery systems. In light of the extension of clinical dietetic practice sites, Scialabba writes that:

> *The traditional role of dietitians in medical care has required that they view themselves as part of the medical team and, therefore, in a sense subservient to the physician in taking any initiative in the nutritional care of the patient. This medical model is still the model in the newer systems. If, however, this develops as envisioned and health care rather than medical care becomes the focus, one can speculate on the need for dietitians to seek approval or wait for suggestions from physicians before initiating programs. In the realm of therapy, the physician's direction is appropriate, but is it in the realm of nutrition education?*[15] *(p. 549)*

We shall now review some of the ways in which clinical dietitians find credibility for their role and the performance of that role, at least in the eyes of their peers and colleagues.

EVALUATION OF PRACTICE

There are a number of ways in which clinicians may evaluate their performance in their own practice sites. Two of these, "peer review" and "audit" are evaluation mechanisms that focus on quality of care as defined by the profession. The remaining concepts to be examined are cost/benefit and cost/effectiveness analyses that, in contrast to the first two, assess the benefits of practice in relation to its costs from a systems perspective.

Professional Standards Review and Peer Review

In 1972, the United States Congress' enactment of Public Law 92–603 included provisions regarding the establishment of Professional Standards Review Organizations (PSROs),* which were directed predominantly toward physicians.[16] Since that time many nonphysician health care professionals have investigated the implications of the possibilities of similar legislation for their own professional practice.

As the health care delivery system has grown in size and complexity, it has become increasingly difficult to control both quality and cost of care. The PSRO legislation is one response to society and its growing concern about health care.

Professional Standards Review (PSR) has often been incorrectly interpreted as peer review. Peer review is defined as:

> . . . the formal assessment by health care practitioners of the quality and efficiency of services ordered or provided by other members of their profession.[16] (p. 7)

Reporting on current activities of dietitians in PSR, Winterfeldt has lucidly described peer review:

> Peer review becomes a process of review of performance rather than a review of the person. "Review" means to look again, and "peer review" denotes re-examination by one's equals.[17] (p. 655)

A set of guidelines for peer review† (of performance—not the person) for dietitians first appeared in 1973.[19] The concept has continued to be studied and further defined with the publication of two documents in 1976.[16,20] One of these states the objectives for the dietitian's involvement in PSR:

> The primary goal of dietitians in their involvement in PSROs is the accountability of the profession to patients/clients for the quality of dietary services and appropriate utilization of resources. The following objectives are directed toward the attainment of this goal:
>
> 1. Establish a review system whereby appropriate utilization of dietitians' professional services are assured.

---

* PSROs are the organizations empowered by federal law to monitor health care services paid for wholly or partially under certain sections of the Social Security Act. PSR is the term used to describe the review and evaluation of the quality of those health care services.[16]

† Houle[18] suggests that the term peer review is inadequate to describe the process of practice evaluation. In his opinion, peer review too often means the procedures by which financial and other scarce resources are allocated. Hence, the term "peer appraisal," which more clearly suggests quality assessment.

2. Establish criteria by which dietetic practices can be evaluated.

3. Establish norms and standards by which dietetic practices can be evaluated.

4. Establish a system whereby a review of dietetic practices shall be conducted by professional peers who are engaged in similar practice.

5. Correct deficiencies in dietetic care and services identified by the review process through the use of problem-solving techniques, continuing education, and systematic study designed to improve patterns of dietetic care and services.

6. Establish a mechanism which will assure that issues related to the practice of dietetics will be decided by Registered Dietitians.[16] *(p. 10)*

These guidelines, specifically statement 4, indicate that peer review is but one objective to be met by dietitians as they work toward the goal of their involvement in PSR. Three of the others (statements 2, 3, and 5) describe activities that are now incorporated in a process known as "dietetic audit." The first and last statements remain areas of concern to the profession of Dietetics and shall be addressed in the last chapter of this text.

In the last of a series of four papers,[21-24] Schiller and Behm remark that the dietetic audit is one form of peer review. There is a difference between the two processes, however: In dietetic audit, individual practitioner performance is *not* identified, whereas in peer review the performance of an individual clinician is assessed.[24]

The Dietetic Audit

An audit has been defined as a ". . . two-part process in which the quality of care is first assessed and steps are (subsequently) taken to ensure improvement (of that care)"[21] (p. 122). The first part of the process requires selection of the audit topic, development of standards and criteria for evaluating the topic, and collection and evaluation of data. The second part involves the development and implementation of solutions to identified problems.

According to Schiller and Behm,[22] a variety of benefits accrue to practitioners involved in the audit process. Dietitians are able to evaluate their own performance as they assess their abilities to act as change-agents. They also increase their visibility as effective team members while frequently documenting the need for additional personnel to deliver services.

In 1978, an American Dietetic Association committee published an extensive document that sets forth nine steps in the audit process.[25] The steps provide a logical sequence for assessment of care:

Step 1. *Select a topic.* The topic may be limited or broad in scope. An audit topic may deal with process (assessment of procedures) or outcome (effect of care) or both. The topic selected must be amenable to change (treatable) and occur with some frequency in the practice site.

Step 2. *Develop criteria.* The criteria should consist of statements about process and/or outcome against which actual practice is measured. The criteria should contain three elements that describe the desirable level of care, the frequency with which the standard should be achieved, and any exceptions to the achievement of the standard.[26]*

Step 3. *Ratify the criteria.* The criteria are presented to the entire group participating in the audit process for their review and suggestions. This step should serve the purposes of gaining commitment to the audit and providing a learning experience for all concerned.

Step 4. *Review client records and identify problems.* Records, representing the written documentation of practice, are selected at random by medical record librarians or by the auditors themselves and then compared to the ratified criteria. Problems can be identified by comparing what is expected by what actually happened; problem identification occurs when recorded information does not meet one or more criteria.

Step 5. *Analyze the problem.* A list of possible explanations for deviations from the criteria is developed by peer groups or by the audit committee.

Step 6. *Develop solutions.* From the list of explanations, possible remedial actions may be identified. Such actions should reflect a recognition of cost effective strategies.[21]

Step 7. *Implement the solutions.* As soon as possible, the new strategies should be put into action. Monitoring progress of the solutions should occur.

Step 8. *Document and communicate the audit results.* At this stage, the results of the audit are made available to appropriate administrative officers of the health care facility. Included in the report is a documentation of solution strategies.

---

* Exceptions are normally considered only in cases where the standard is set at 100% or 0%. When the standard is otherwise set, exceptions are not included.[25]

Step 9. *When necessary, reaudit.* A reevaluation at this stage is beneficial to determine whether or not the problems identified in step 4 have been corrected. Reaudit should be conducted only after solution implementation has occurred.

Thoughtful readers will recognize that the nine steps of the audit process closely resemble our model for the provision of nutritional care, as depicted in Figure 9.1.

Audits are not limited to dietetic practice. El-Beheri[26] has identified three approaches to the audit process that encompass a wide variety of practitioners:

1. The *interdisciplinary* approach, in which all members of a team develop and agree upon a single set of criteria

2. The *multidisciplinary* approach, in which audit topics and client records are the same, but each discipline has the task of developing its own set of criteria

3. The *monodisciplinary* approach, in which each discipline acts independently of the other disciplines (as in the dietetic audit).

According to Walters and Crumley,[25] the first approach is the most efficient, and has the additional benefit of providing an environment where health professionals may learn from one another. From this effort, enhanced client-centered care is realized.

Cost/Benefit and Cost/Effectiveness Analyses

In addition to their responsibility to document and evaluate the quality of nutritional care through peer review and audit, clinical dietitians are also being asked to demonstrate the benefits of their services in relation to the costs of providing those services. Demonstration of the benefits of dietetic services in terms of health outcome is particularly difficult because of the multiplicity of factors that affect the achievement and/or maintenance of health. For example, many risk factors may be associated with a particular disease process or physiologic stress, not all of which are related to a specific health behavior (such as food intake) that is affected by dietetic services (such as nutritional counseling). In demonstrating the health outcome benefits of dietetic services it is necessary first to identify and then to quantify the linkages between dietetic services, intermediate target variables (risk factors), and ultimate health outcomes (morbidity and mortality). Determining ways to establish and quantify the linkages between ambulatory nutritional care services (e.g., nutritional counseling) and positive health outcomes (e.g., reduction in incidence and severity of atherosclerotic disease) was the goal of an American Dietetic Association committee.[27]

In every professional effort, either in individual client care or in large scale programs designed to meet the needs of many persons, there is a goal—an outcome toward which effort is directed. Cost/benefit analysis evaluates a program by comparing its benefits (measured in dollars) with its costs. The costs of a program are both direct and indirect, and both must be enumerated as fully as possible. Direct costs are the actual expenditures for resources used in the program. Indirect costs may include the value of the time lost from work by the clients, the value of undesirable side effects of the program, and other equally difficult factors to measure. Benefits are also direct and indirect, and must be enumerated and quantified.[28] Direct benefits are direct costs averted because of the program (e.g., dollars saved by reduced hospitalization). Indirect benefits are reduced morbidity and/or mortality due to the program.

In cost/benefit research, a program is judged worthwhile if the dollar value of the program's benefits is greater than or equal to the program's costs. Few examples of cost/benefit research of nutrition-related problems are reported in the literature[29]; the reason is that there is serious controversy about the exact nature of the linkages between nutrition and health.[28] One such report appeared in the 1980 scientific literature[30]; the economic analysis in this case showed that participation in a food assistance program yielded a cost/benefit ratio of 3.1:1 (the benefit of the program outweighed the cost of the program by a factor of 3 to 1). Without question, in this particular case, the program was proven to be worthwhile.

In contrast, cost/effectiveness research assumes that the program goal is legitimate. In this type of analysis, the problem is to determine which of several alternative methods is the most cost/effective in goal achievement; thus, for each alternative, both effectiveness and cost are considered. Cost/effectiveness research, for example, may determine which of several methods, available to achieve the goal of dental caries reduction in a specific school age population, should be adopted. A variety of approaches may be studied; that approach which demonstrates the greatest reduction in caries incidence per dollar of resources consumed (e.g., personnel, equipment) is the most cost/effective one. In a practice site, a clinician may wish to know which is the most cost/effective method to reach the goal of attaining and/or maintaining ideal body weight by elderly clients. The goal, achievement and/or maintenance of ideal body weight, is assumed to be valid. The question is how "best" to achieve that goal.

Most clinical dietitians are unprepared to assume the responsibilities of such evaluations alone; they need the assistance of a variety of professionals, including health care economists, research methodologists, and statisticians. Nonetheless, such evaluative activities are required to demonstrate the value of clinical dietetic services to the variety of individuals and groups who make decisions about reimbursement (payment) for such services and funding for dietetic programs. Tolpin said it well:

> That nutritional factors are significantly and positively related to health status appears a relatively uncontroversial assertion. However, what remains is a lack of evidence to demonstrate both qualitatively and quantitatively the exact nature of the linkages between nutritional services and improving and/or maintaining health status. The time is ripe for the careful design of prospective studies aimed at demonstrating such linkages. A need exists for adequate, standardized, and objective evaluation of nutrition intervention programs and simultaneously for rigorous development of relevant outcome definition and measurement. Until it is shown that nutrition services per se have an impact on health outcomes, one cannot begin to enumerate or quantify the benefits of such services to individuals and to society.[28] (p. 221)

SUMMARY

Measuring the success of practice, albeit difficult, is possible. History, in the form of role performance evaluation studies, has shown us that clinical dietitians and their significant others (clients, administrators, physicians, nurses, other therapists) often disagree on the dietitian's role. Indeed, dietitians disagree among themselves about their role. Resolution of the problem of role delineation is currently underway in a variety of settings; whether or not practitioners agree with the resolution remains to be seen.

In individual practice sites, role performance evaluation may be accomplished in a variety of ways. One of these, peer review, involves an examination of the performance of a practitioner by his peers, as measured against established criteria and standards. Dietetic audit, in contrast, deals not with the professional performance of an individual, but rather with the achievement of quality nutritional care in a given setting. The dietetic audit strives to rectify shortcomings in practice by implementing solutions to identified problems.

Cost/benefit and cost/effectiveness analyses are essentially research methodologies that are designed to provide objective data about the economic value of intervention strategies. Such research is difficult, particularly for clinical dietitians, since the nature of the links between nutritional care and positive health outcomes has yet to be definitively demonstrated. Clinical dietetic practitioners, however, have an important role in collecting the types of data necessary to identify and quantify such links.

CITED REFERENCES

1. Peck, E. B. The "professional self" and its relation to change processes. *J. Am. Dietet. A.* 69:534, 1976.

2. Robinson, C. H. Nutrition education—what comes next? *J. Am. Dietet. A.* 69:126, 1976.

3. Galbraith, A. L. The President's Page. *J. Am. Dietet. A.* 69:69, 1976.

4. Schiller, M. R., and Vivian, V. M. Role of the clinical dietitian. I. Ideal role perceived by dietitians and physicians. *J. Am. Dietet. A.* 65:284, 1974.

5. Study Commission on Dietetics. *The Profession of Dietetics.* Chicago: The American Dietetic Association, 1972.

6. Spangler, A. A., Florencio, C., and Giuliani, B. The role and responsibility of the hospital dietitian. A preliminary report. *Mich. Hosp.* 6:4:2, 1970.

7. Spangler, A. A., Cederquist, D. C., and Blackman, C. A. Physicians' attitudes on dietitians' contributions to health team care. *J. Am. Dietet. A.* 65:646, 1974.

8. Jacobson, H. N. Dietary practices, services and trends in the teaching hospitals in New Jersey. *Nutr. Today* 10:5 and 6:14, 1975.

9. Schiller, M. R. The dietitian's changing role. Increased responsibilities place dietitian on health care team. *Hosp.* 47:23:97, 1973.

10. Schiller, M. R., and Vivian, V. M. Role of the clinical dietitian. II. Ideal vs. actual role. *J. Am. Dietet. A.* 65:287, 1974.

11. Johnson, C. A. Entry-level clinical practice as viewed by clients and allied professionals. A pilot study. *J. Am. Dietet. A.* 66:261, 1975.

12. Martinez, G. A. *The Dietetic Profession—1979.* Columbus: Ross Laboratories, 1979.

13. Biltz, P. A., and Derelian, D. V. Changing dietitians' attitudes toward client counseling. *J. Am. Dietet. A.* 73:239, 1978.

14. Johnson, C. A. The need for better nutritional care. Who's responsible? *J. Am. Dietet. A.* 67:219, 1975.

15. Scialabba, M. A. Functions of dietetic personnel in ambulatory care. *J. Am. Dietet. A.* 67:545, 1975.

16. *Professional Standards Review Procedure Manual.* Chicago: The American Dietetic Association, 1976.

17. Winterfeldt, E. Professional Standards Review Organizations (PSROs). I. Professional standards and peer review. *J. Am. Dietet. A.* 65:654, 1974.

18. Houle, C. O. *Continuing Learning in the Professions.* San Francisco: Jossey-Bass Inc., Publ., 1980.

19. Winterfeldt, E. Current concerns of the consultant dietitian. IV. A dietetic association's Peer Review Committee. *J. Am. Dietet. A.* 63:47, 1973.

20. Professional Standards Review Committee. *Guidelines for Evaluating Dietetic Practice.* Chicago: The American Dietetic Association, 1976.

21. Schiller, R., and Behm, V. Auditing dietetic services. (First of a series). *Hosp.* 53:8:122, 1979.

22. Schiller, R., and Behm, V. Auditing dietetic services. (Second of a series). *Hosp.* 53:9:105, 1979.

23. Schiller, R., and Bartlett, B. Auditing dietetic services. (Third of a series). *Hosp.* 53:10:118, 1979.

24. Schiller, R., and Behm, V. Auditing dietetic services. (Fourth of a series). *Hosp.* 53:12, 113, 1979.

25. Walters, F. M., and Crumley, S. J., Eds. *Patient Care Audit. A Quality Assurance Procedure Manual for Dietitians.* Chicago: The American Dietetic Association, 1978.

26. El-Beheri, B. B. Dietetic audit—a giant step for nutritional care. The approach at Brooke Army Medical Center. *J. Am. Dietet. A.* 74:321, 1979.

27. Mason, M. Purple serendipity. *J. Am. Dietet. A.* 76:215, 1980.

28. Tolpin, H. G. Economics of health care. The necessity of a cost/benefit approach. *J. Am. Dietet. A.* 76:217, 1980.

29. Mason, M., et al. *Costs and Benefits of Nutritional Care: Phase 1.* Chicago: The American Dietetic Association, 1979.

30. Berkenfield, J., and Schwartz, J. B. Nutrition intervention in the community—the "WIC" program. *N. Eng. J. Med.* 302:579, 1980.

SUGGESTED REFERENCES

Drexler, L., and Caliendo, M. A. Developing and implementing a nutritional care audit. *J. Am. Dietet. A.* 76:374, 1980.

Farrington, J. F., Felch, W. C., and Hare, R. L. Quality assessment and quality assurance. The performance-review alternative. *N. Eng. J. Med.* 303:154, 1980.

Heywood, P. On planning and evaluating the activities of dietitians and nutritionists. *Food and Nutr. Notes and Rev.* 34:184, 1977.

Janke, T. A. Cost accounting: The vital link to cost effectiveness. *J. Am. Dietet. A.* 77:167, 1980.

Krejici, C. B. Quality assurance audit. *J. Am. Dietet. A.* 76:378, 1980.

Moore, K. R. What nurses learn from nursing audit. *Nurs. Out.* 27:254, 1979.

Ometer, J. L. An intradepartmental process audit to measure quality of care. *J. Am. Dietet. A.* 75:566, 1979.

Ometer, J. L. Documentation of nutritional care. *J. Am. Dietet. A.* 76:35, 1980.

Sadin, R. R. Impact on dietetics of PSROs (Professional Standards Review Organizations). *J. Am. Dietet. A.* 72:292, 1978.

Weed, J. E., and Molleson, A. L. Establishing guidelines for peer review of the clinical dietitian. *J. Am. Dietet. A.* 70:157:1977.

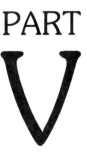

PART V

Clinical Dietetic Practice Revisited

16
In Prospect

At the point of admission to a professional school, the student may have a hazy, perhaps even romanticized notion of what the professional role entails. Thus an important function of professional training is to initiate trainees into the "culture" of the profession and to develop in them a more realistic expectation of the role to be played.

Alex J. Ducanis and Anne K. Golin, **The Interdisciplinary Health Care Team** (Germantown, MD: Aspen Systems Corp., 1979).

The preceding sections of this text have addressed the components of clinical dietetic practice with the primary purpose of presenting a rationale for the "culture" of the role of the clinical dietitian. By now the reader should have laid to rest any "romanticized notions" and have gained instead some "realistic expectations" of practice. Our final discussion will focus on some hypotheses about current societal trends and research findings that have impact on future practice.

One way to begin to address the future is to examine the results of a study conducted by Ducanis and Golin.[1] These workers sampled the codes of ethics of 20 associations representing health professionals and concluded that ethics statements could be organized into five major categories: professional competence, responsibilities to clients, responsibilities to colleagues, legal responsibilities, and responsibilities to society. As the practice of clinical dietetics is interwoven with the profession and the professional society (and, thus, its code of ethics), we shall focus this chapter on the findings of Ducanis and Golin.

PROFESSIONAL COMPETENCE

Professional competence encompasses education, research, standards, and performance. In 1978, a Task Force on Competencies of the American Dietetic Association[2] described a system for promoting the development of quality practitioners. Based on societal and practitioner needs, the system includes standards of practice that serve as the basis for standards of education. The latter includes standards for both entry-level education as well as standards for programs designed to ensure that practitioners maintain competence. The Task Force postulated that utilization of the system would ensure quality practitioners who are professionally competent.

The relationship of practice to education was the basis of a report published early in 1980 by the National Commission on Allied Health.[3] The report was a landmark as it was the first comprehensive study of health science professionals (including dietitians) and their educational preparation. The Commission made 15 primary recommendations; the first two are especially germane to our discussion:

1. *Alliance in service and education should be strengthened, based on an appreciation of the interdependence of all health occupations and understanding of their roles, functions, and special contributions.*

2. *Education should be linked to practice through role delineation.*[3]
   (p. 161)

Later that same year, the American Dietetic Association published a series of technical reports entitled "Role Delineation for the Field of Clinical Dietetics."[4] This study, conducted over a period of 15 months, parallels the Commission's description of step 1 in role delineation. A series of statements describing the "actual role" of the clinical dietitian was generated; a companion series of statements describing the "appropriate role" of the clinical dietitian was formulated. Technical Report #6[4] indicated that continuing with the successive steps of the role delineation process is in the future.

The concept of continuing education, one of the components of the total system of ensuring professional competence, is graphically displayed in Figure 16.1 Houle[5] has conceived the preparation and practice of the professional as a continuum. "General Education" includes the person's early years and the formal educational patterns of our society. "Selection" describes that point when the person decides which particular profession to pursue. "Pre-Service Specialized Education" follows, and when completed, is documented by "Certification of Competence" (our "entry-level" certification). When the new professional enters the practice setting for the first time, Houle describes the associated activities as "Induction." Once the practitioner is past that phase and practicing comfortably, the Classic Model describes the remainder of the continuum as "Continuing Education."

Professional competence and continuing education have been his-

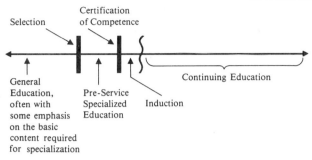

FIGURE 16.1   The Classic Model of Professional Education
Reproduced with permission from Houle, C.O. *Continuing Learning in The Professions.* San Francisco: Jossey-Bass Inc., Publ., 1980.

torically viewed as interdependent and interwoven. From his comprehensive study of the subject, Houle[5] concluded that there were a variety of approaches to ensuring professional competence, and identified at least three trends that have contributed to a change in the traditional approach. First, many people are entering professions later in their lives. Second, an increasing number of persons are shifting to second professions requiring a different pattern of preservice education and induction to practice. Last, the insatiable desire to learn may come somewhat later in life than has been historically assumed. In response, Houle designed a more contemporary model of professional education (Figure 16.2). The Emerging Model includes the components of the Classic Model, but goes beyond the latter in reflecting the influence of the needs of both the professional and society. A distinctive difference in the Emerging Model is the change in label from Continuing Education to Continuing Learning. The Emerging Model succinctly describes how the professional takes responsibility for his own learning by indicating those points (preparation for change) when new content or new directions will be pursued.

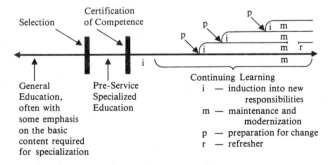

FIGURE 16.2   An Emerging Model of Professional Education
Adapted with permission from Houle, C.O. *Continuing Learning in The Professions.* San Francisco: Jossey-Bass Inc., Publ., 1980.

We initiated the discussion of professional competence by noting that the concept encompassed education, research, standards, and performance. In the 1980s, clinical dietitians, both entry-level and in established practices, are in improved positions, reasonably able to substantiate their role based on widely accepted documents.[1-7] Continued research will assist in refining the role and developing tools to assess continuing competence.

RESPONSIBILITIES TO CLIENTS

Health professionals have frequently viewed their clients in terms of morbidity, and often held that the determination of treatment modalities lies solely within the realm of professional practice. Such attitudes are being increasingly challenged with efforts now directed toward maintenance of health. In addition, our citizenry has increasingly insisted on a greater share of the decision making process as it affects them. Factors that have been identified as contributing to this trend are an increased general awareness of health care, a result of the influence of various media; the effect of the "consumer movement" on health care and human services; and a general rise in the educational level of the population.[1]

Perhaps the most significant influence on the trend toward joint provider and client decision making was Congress, when that body passed the National Health Planning and Resources Development Act of 1974.[8] This legislation, combining three previously existing health planning programs, emphasizes planning on the national, state, and local levels.[9] Approval of the limitation or expansion of health care facilities and services is the responsibility of the appropriate planning agency. Clients of health care providers are represented in these agencies, and, thus, are assured of an equal voice in the decision making process.

Kinlein, an independent generalist nurse,[10] addressed the concept of the client/clinician relationship by delineating five areas of professional responsibility: availability, accessibility, accuracy, accountability, and autonomy. On reviewing Kinlein's categories, the clinician may want to add confidentiality.

In addressing some "realistic expectations" of the role of clinical dietitians, we may conclude that there is a need for the practitioner, in collaboration with other health care providers, to clearly enunciate the criteria by which the client is the recipient of quality nutritional care. After all the client *is* the reason for our existence.

RESPONSIBILITIES TO COLLEAGUES

Again we wish to state clearly that the clinical dietitian does not perform his role in isolation. If the concept of client-centered care is to be realized, the practitioner must contribute the component of nutritional care in collaboration with other health care providers *and* the client.

With whom does the clinical dietitian collaborate? How many health care personnel are actually in practice? What and where is the site of the practice? These are questions practitioners must address while clarifying their role in relation to the role of others.

In response to the second question, Torrens and Lewis have reported that:

> *The most important trend in health care personnel during the last twenty five years has been the extraordinary growth in the number of individuals working in the health sector.*[11] *(p. 257)*

In that time, there has been a gain of 44 percent in the total U.S. work force, but a gain of 215 percent in the health care sector.[11] Of even greater significance is the number of men versus women in the health care sector. Ninety seven percent of practicing dietitians are female,[12] whereas approximately 70 percent of the workers in the remainder of the health care industry are women.[11] Nutritional care services retained their importance in the past quarter century as the number of persons employed in that sector gained by 227 percent for the years 1950 to 1975, in contrast to an overall gain of 215 percent.[11]

The site of practice presents serious implications for the future of acute care facilities. Goldsmith[13] asks the very cogent question: Can hospitals survive? Some of the societal changes identified by Goldsmith as affecting hospitals include increasing economic power of physicians, new forms of health care delivery, prepaid health plans, a changing regulatory environment, and diversification into new services such as ambulatory care, including surgery, freestanding emergency rooms, health maintenance organizations, and screening programs. A recent survey of dietitians[12] reports that 44 percent of employed dietitians are practicing in hospitals, closely coinciding with the 47 percent who reported their specialization as clinical dietetics.

In the milieu of health care, how does the clinical dietitian initiate role identification, role negotiation, and/or role clarification? In the discussion of teams in Chapter 2, Dr. Schmitt identified teamwork as having three major aspects: shared goals, individuals acting in roles that encompass a diversity of skills and experiences, and a plan for coordinated effort. Thus, the clinical dietitian must ensure that her role in providing nutritional care to clients is clearly articulated to all other team members. The corollary is clear: Clinical dietitians must have a clear understanding of the roles of the other professionals who are collaborating on providing client care. Role identification, negotiation, and/or clarification naturally follow when team members understand and appreciate the uniqueness of one another.

LEGAL RESPONSIBILITIES

According to Ducanis and Golin,[1] the legal responsibilities category of professional codes relate to the legal constraints that regulate the professional's activities.

By what criteria can society recognize that the dietitian is qualified to practice? What agencies, boards, and/or commissions exist on which society relies to determine whether a dietitian will meet their expectations in providing care? An analogy could be the pianist who emerges from an accident with a fractured right arm. He wants to be certain that the physician who performs the orthopedic surgery is not only qualified to treat his arm, but he wants assurance he can continue his career as a pianist.

Credentialing is the general process available to society to determine qualifications of professionals who serve their needs. In simple terms, credentialing is the testimonial showing that a person is entitled to credit or has a right to exercise official power.[14] Credentialing in the health professions is an umbrella term for discussions of registration, certification, and/or licensure of health professionals.

In 1971, an invitational conference on Certification of Allied Health Professions was held for the purpose of clarifying manpower certification issues. Primary among those issues were the seemingly limitless definitions in current use, and the need for establishing some commonalities of nomenclature. As an outcome of the conference, one form of credentialing, certification, was defined as:

> . . . the process by which a non-governmental agency or an association grants recognition to an individual who has met certain predetermined qualifications specified by that agency or association.[15] (p. 82)

Expanding on the definition of certification as it related to the dietitian, Hart and Sharp[16] proposed clarification of the phrase, "predetermined qualifications." They suggested that the qualifications could include graduation from an accredited or approved program, acceptable performance on a qualifying examination, or completion of a specified work experience.

Currently, society can recognize clinicians who meet these "predetermined qualifications" because they hold the designation, Registered Dietitian (R.D.). The Commission on Dietetic Registration is empowered to set standards, review qualifications of candidates, and confer the R.D. status on those who meet the standards.

Some confusion may arise from the terms certification and registration. The Study Commission on Dietetics attempted to clarify the terms by noting that registration is a listing of professionals who have met requirements and had their names placed on a registry, whereas certification is a process whereby a voluntary association warrants a person's competence by certifying that he has met certain prescribed criteria of education and/or has passed an examination. Although it has been recognized[16,18] that there are differences in the terms, it is generally concluded that society's criterion for recognizing the certification of those qualified is met by the term, Registered Dietitian (R.D.).

In contrast to certification, which is the responsibility of a nongovernmental agency, licensure is an activity regulated by government. In health science manpower nomenclature, the accepted definition for licensure is:

> . . . the process by which an agency of government grants permission to persons meeting predetermined qualifications to engage in a given occupation and/or to use a particular title or grants permission to institutions to perform specified functions.[15] (p. 82)

Licensing status has been further clarified by distinguishing between "mandatory" and "voluntary" status.[16] *Mandatory licensure* permits only those persons who have been issued licenses to practice the occupation. *Voluntary licensure* allows only persons holding licenses to use a particular title or official designation; unlicensed persons are permitted to practice but cannot use the designation accorded to licensed practitioners. The trend in the health sciences has been toward mandatory licensure.

Licensure as implemented in the United States is the province of state governments. An individual who is licensed to practice his profession in one state may or may not be able to practice in another state. Depending on the state and on the profession, reciprocity with some or all of the other states may be incorporated into the licensure law.

With the possibility of national health insurance and concurrent federal legislation, which affect third party reimbursement for professional services, the issue of licensure for dietitians emerges. A number of publications[21-23] address the issue and will no doubt serve as initial points of activity in the event licensure is undertaken by the practitioners in one or more states.

RESPONSIBILITIES TO SOCIETY

In their review of the professional code statements related to society, Ducanis and Golin[1] concluded that the statements exhibited both the professional's relationship with the public at large, and the manner in which the profession itself is presented to the public. The professional's responsibility to society and his legal responsibility are closely interwoven. The question, "Who should control the health professions: The professionals or the public?"[11] (p. 282) is one that has not yet been publicly posed, but is, in many quarters, privately discussed.

Currently, health care professionals seek a hearing of the particular contributions that they can make to overall health care. For example, the professional society of dietitians has formulated a statement for the Institute of Medicine, National Academy of Sciences, which enunciates both societal and professional barriers to delivery of the full potential of nutritional care.[24] The seven barriers are:

1. *Public recognition of the essential nature of nutrition education in the promotion of health and of nutritional care in health care programs is limited or lacking.*

2. *Adequate funding for nutritional services and the organizational structure within which dietitians can work in teams with other health professionals are lacking or deficient. Mechanisms for providing nutritional care and dietary counseling to ambulatory patients are very limited.*

3. *Public recognition of the need for on-going support for research in the basic science of nutrition and insistence on nutritional care delivery are lacking.*

4. *Basic and continuing education in nutrition is frequently not included in the curricula for medical and dental and other professional staff.*

5. *Expansion of the role of the dietitian as a primary caretaker and as a physician-extender in planning and implementing continuing care outside the acute care facility needs to be accelerated or emphasized.*

6. *Indexes of nutritional status in physical examinations and laboratory data and dietary history and assessments are not always included in routine screening.*

   a. *Even when such data are available, nutritional referral is not always triggered when it would seem appropriate.*

   b. *Dietary counseling, initial and continuing, is seldom a reimbursable service in health insurance plans.*

7. *Nutritional services tend to be more accessible to the affluent (who can afford services at a fee) and to the indigent (who are eligible for a variety of public health programs). The working poor and middle-income persons perhaps have the least access to the services of registered dietitians except during hospitalization for crisis care.*[24] *(p. 589)*

Each statement demonstrates a relationship of nutritional care to society, and the noted barrier that precludes delivery of that care. Clinical dietitians clearly must identify nutritional care as one component of health care.

SUMMARY

Professional competence, achieved through both entry-level preparation and continuing learning, ensures that clients, colleagues, and society are well served. The legality of practice reinforces the concept of professional competence through some form of credentialing.

What does the future hold for the practice of clinical dietetics? If practitioners are willing to assume the responsibilities for which they are prepared, we may sum up the answer in one word: Promise.

CITED REFERENCES

1. Ducanis, A. J., and Golin, A. K. *The Interdisciplinary Health Care Team.* Germantown, MD: Aspen Systems Corp., 1979.

2. Report of the Task Force on Competencies, Council on Educational Preparation, The American Dietetic Association. *J. Am. Dietet. A.* 73:281, 1978.

3. National Commission on Allied Health Education. *The Future of Allied Health Education.* San Francisco: Jossey-Bass Inc., Publ., 1980.

4. Baird, S. C., and Armstrong, R. V. Role Delineation for the Field of Clinical Dietetics. Technical Report Series. #1—*Literature Review and Annotated Bibliography.* #3—*Survey Design and Sampling Procedure.* #4—*Drafting "Appropriate" Responsibilities, Skill/Knowledge Statements.* #5—*Devel-*

oping *"Appropriate" Role Documents. #6—Policy and Planning Implications.* December, 1980. (Unnumbered in the series), *Role Delineation for Entry-Level Clinical Dietetic Personnel: Actual Role and Responsibilities.* June, 1980. Chicago: The American Dietetic Association.

5. Houle, C. O. *Continuing Learning in the Professions.* San Francisco: Jossey-Bass Inc., Publ., 1980.

6. Committee on Goals of Education for Dietetics, Dietetic Internship Council, The American Dietetic Association. Goals of the lifetime education of the dietitian. *J. Am. Dietet. A.* 54:91, 1969.

7. Pennington, F. C., Ed. *Assessing Educational Needs of Adults. New Directions for Continuing Education, No. 7.* San Francisco: Jossey-Bass Inc., Publ., 1980.

8. Public Law 93-641. National Health Planning and Resources Development, 1974.

9. Anderson, N. N., and Robins, L. Observations on potential contributions of health planning. *In* Williams, S. J., Ed. *Issues in Health Services.* New York: John Wiley & Sons, Inc., 1980.

10. Kinlein, M. L. *Independent Nursing Practice with Clients.* Philadelphia: J. B. Lippincott Co., 1977.

11. Torrens, P. R., and Lewis, C. E. Health care personnel. *In* Williams, S. J. and Torrens, P. R., Eds. *Introduction to Health Services.* New York: John Wiley & Sons, Inc., 1980.

12. Policy Research Corporation. *The Profession of Dietetics: Present and Future.* Chicago: The American Dietetic Association, 1980.

13. Goldsmith, J. C. The health care market: Can hospitals survive? *Harvard Bus. Rev.,* Sept.–Oct., 1980.

14. *Webster's Seventh New Collegiate Dictionary.* Springfield, MA: G. & C. Merriam Co., 1967.

15. *Certification in Allied Health Professions.* 1971 Conference Proceedings. DHEW Publ. No. (NIH) 73-246. Washington: U.S. Dept. Health, Educ., and Welfare, 1971.

16. Hart, M. E., and Sharp, J. L. The dietitian and credentialing. *J. Am. Dietet. A.* 66:455, 1975.

17. News Flash. *ADA Courier.* XV:2:1, 1976.

18. Bogle, M. L. Registration—the *sine qua non* of a competent dietitian. *J. Am. Dietet. A.* 64:616, 1974.

19. Asher, K. C., and Cioch, J. Disposition of appeals to Panel V—Commission on Dietetic Registration. *J. Am. Dietet. A.* 77:470, 1980.

20. Knotts, V. B., Hayman, J., and Lee, E. Registration examination: Content validity study. *J. Am. Dietet. A.* 78:74, 1981.

21. Grad, F. P. *Consideration of Legal Definition of the Dietitian.* Chicago: The American Dietetic Association, 1975.

22. Committee to Develop a Model Licensure Law. *Model Dietetics Practice Act*. Chicago: The American Dietetic Association, 1976.
23. Licensure activities in states. *Annual Reports and Proceedings, 1978–79*. Chicago: The American Dietetic Association, 1979.
24. The dietitian in primary health care. *J. Am. Dietet. A.* 70:587, 1977.

SUGGESTED REFERENCES

A Report on Education and Utilization of Allied Health Manpower. Chicago: American Medical Association, 1972.

Hesburgh, T. M., Miller, P., and Wharton, C. R. *Patterns for Lifelong Learning*. San Francisco: Jossey-Bass Inc., Publ., 1974.

Knowles, J. H. *Doing Better and Feeling Worse: Health in the United States*. New York: W. W. Norton & Co., 1977.

Kramer, M. *Reality Shock: Why Nurses Leave Nursing*. St. Louis: C. V. Mosby Co., 1974.

Ladimer, I., Solomon, J. C., and House, S. G. *Democratic Processes for Modern Health Agencies*. New York: S. P. Medical & Scientific Books, 1979.

Pennell, M. Y., Profitt, J. R., and Hatch, T. D. *Accreditation and Certification in Relation to Allied Health Manpower*. DHEW Publ. No. (NIH) 71-192. Washington: U.S. Dept. Health, Educ., and Welfare, 1971.

Report on Licensure and Related Health Personnel Credentialing. DHEW Publ. No. (HSM) 72-11. Washington: U.S. Dept. Health, Educ., and Welfare, 1971.

Schmalenberg, C., and Kramer, M. *Coping with Reality Shock*. Wakefield, MA: Nursing Resources, Inc., 1979.

Shimberg, B., Esser, B. F., and Kruger, D. H. *Occupational Licensing: Practices and Policies*. Washington: Public Affairs Press, 1973.

Standards of Nursing Practice. Kansas City, MO: Amer. Nurs. Assoc., 1973.

Survey of Selected Hospital Manpower. Preliminary Report. DHEW Publ. No. (HRA) 74-26. Washington: U.S. Dept. Health, Educ., and Welfare, 1973.

The Supply of Health Manpower, 1970 Profiles and Projections to 1990. DHEW Publ. No. (HRA) 75-38. Washington: U.S. Dept. Health, Educ., and Welfare, 1974.

APPENDIX A

Partial Listing of Medical Record Abbreviations

A	assessment
abd	abdomen
abort	abortion
ac	(Latin: ante cibum) before meals
ADL	activities of daily living
ad lib	(Latin: ad libitum) as needed or desired
adm	admission
AF	atrial fibrillation
A/G ratio	albumin/globulin ratio
alb	albumin
AODM	adult-onset Diabetes Mellitus
AS	aortic stenosis
ASHD	arteriosclerotic heart disease
as tol	as tolerated
A&W	alive and well
Ba	barium
bid	(Latin: bis in die) twice a day
Bl Cult	blood culture
BM	bowel movement
BP	blood pressure
BR	bed rest
BRP	bathroom privileges
BS	blood sugar; bowel sounds; breath sounds
BSP	bromosulphalein
BTL	bilateral tubal ligation
BUN	blood urea nitrogen
BV	blood volume
BW	body weight
Bx	biopsy
$\bar{c}$	(Latin: cum) with
C	centigrade or Celsius
Ca^{++}	calcium ion

CA	cancer
CAD	coronary artery disease
Cath	catheter; catheterize
CBC	complete blood count
cc	cubic centimeter; chief complaint
CCU	coronary care unit
CD	continuous drainage
CHD	coronary heart disease
CHF	congestive heart failure
Chol	Cholesterol
chr	chronic
Cl	chloride ion
cl	cloudy
cm	centimeter
CNM	certified nurse midwife
CNS	central nervous system
c/o	complains of
CO_2	carbon dioxide
COLD	chronic obstructive lung disease
conc	concentration
cont	continued
COPD	chronic obstructive pulmonary disease
CPC	clinicopathologic conference
CRF	chronic renal failure
Creat	creatinine
C/S	cesarean section
CSF	cerebrospinal fluid
CVA	cerebral vascular accident
CVP	central venous pressure
Cx	cervix
D&C	dilation and curettage
D/C	discontinue
disch	discharge
dl	deciliter
DL	danger list
DM	Diabetes Mellitus
DOA	dead on arrival
DOE	dyspnea on exertion
dr	dram
D/S	dextrose and saline
d/t	due to

DT	delirium tremens
D/W	dextrose and water
Dx	diagnosis or diagnostic
EDC	estimated date of confinement
EEG	electroencephalogram
EKG, ECG	electrocardiogram
ENT	ear, nose, throat
ESR	erythrocyte sedimentation rate
EtOH	ethanol
EW, ED, ER	emergency ward, department, room
exam	examination
expir	expiration or expiratory
F	Fahrenheit
FB	foreign body
FBS	fasting blood sugar
FeSO₄	ferrous sulfate
FFA	free fatty acid
FH	family history; fetal heart
Fl	fluid
FTT	failure to thrive
FUO	fever of unknown origin
Fx	fracture
GAS	generalized arteriosclerosis
GB	gallbladder
GE	gastroenteritis; gastroenterology
GI	gastrointestinal
Gm, gm, g	gram
Gm%	gram/dl
gr	grain
GTT	glucose tolerance test
GU	genitourinary
GYN	gynecology
h	hour
HBP	high blood pressure
Hct	hematocrit
HCVD	hypertensive cardiovascular disease
HEENT	head, eyes, ears, nose, and throat

Hgb	hemoglobin
HHNK	hyperosmolar hyperglycemic nonketotic coma
hs	hour of sleep
ht	height
Hx	history
I&D	incision and drainage
ICU	intensive care unit
IM, IM	intramuscular
imp	impression
incr	increasing
inspir	inspiration or inspiratory
int	internal
I&O	intake and output
IQ	intelligence quotient
IU	international unit
IV, IV	intravenously
IVP	intravenous pyelogram
J	Joule
K$^+$	potassium ion
kcal	kilocalorie
kg	kilogram
KJ	kilojoule
l	liter
L	left
lab	laboratory
lat	lateral
lb	pound
LLL	left lower lobe—lung
LLQ	left lower quadrant—abdomen
LMD	local medical doctor
LMP	last menstrual period
LP	lumbar puncture
LR	labor room
LUL	left upper lobe—lung
LUQ	left upper quadrant—abdomen
l&w	living and well
lytes	electrolytes

mcg, μg	microgram
MCT	medium chain triglyceride
med	medicine
mEq	milliequivalent
Mg^{++}	magnesium ion
mg	milligram
mg%	milligram/dl
MI	myocardial infarction; mitral insufficiency
ml	milliliter
MOM	milk of magnesia
MS	multiple sclerosis; mitral stenosis; morphine sulfate
Na^+	sodium ion
neg	negative
ng	nanogram
N/G	nasogastric
noct	nocturnal
NPN	nonprotein nitrogen
NPO	(Latin: nil per os) nothing by mouth
NS	normal saline
N&V	nausea and vomiting
O	objective
O_2	oxygen
OBS	obstetrics; organic brain syndrome
OGTT	oral glucose tolerance test
OOB	out of bed
OPD	outpatient department
OR	operating room
orth	orthopedics
OT	occupational therapy
oz	ounce
P	plan
PA	pernicious anemia
PAT	pregnancy at term; paroxysmal atrial tachycardia
path	pathology
PBI	protein-bound iodine
pc	(Latin: post cibum) after meals
PCM	protein calorie malnutrition

PE	physical examination
Ped	pediatrics
pg	picogram
pH	hydrogen ion concentration
PH	past history
PI	present illness
PID	pelvic inflammatory disease
PKU	phenylketonuria
po	(Latin: per os) by mouth
post op	postoperative
PP	postpartum; postprandial
pr	per rectum
prep	prepare for
prn	(Latin: pro res nata) as often as necessary
prog	prognosis
P/S ratio	polyunsaturated : saturated fatty acid ratio
pt	patient
PT	physical therapy
PTA	prior to admission
PU	peptic ulcer
q	(Latin: quaque) every
qd	(Latin: quaque die) every day
qid	(Latin: quater in die) four times daily
qn	(Latin: quaque nox) every night
qns	(Latin: quantum non sufficit) quantity not sufficient
q2h	(Latin: quaque duo hora) every 2 hours
q3h	(Latin: quaque tres hora) every 3 hours
R	right
RAI	radioactive iodine
rbc	red blood cells
RBC	red blood count
Rh	Rhesus blood factor
RHD	rheumatic heart disease
RLL	right lower lobe—lung
RLQ	right lower quadrant—abdomen
r/o	rule out
ROM	range of motion
ROS	review of systems
RTC	return to clinic

RUL	right upper lobe—lung
RUQ	right upper quadrant—abdomen
Rx	therapy, treatment, therapeutic, prescription
S	subjective
s̄	(Latin: sine) without
sc	subcutaneous
SGOT	serum glutamic oxaloacetic transaminase
SGPT	serum glutamic pyruvic transaminase
SH	social history
SOB	shortness of breath
spec	specimen
sp gr	specific gravity
SSE	soap suds enema
staph	*Staphylococcus*
stat	(Latin: statin) immediately and once only
surg	surgery
Sx	symptoms
T&A	tonsillectomy and adenoidectomy
tab	tablet
TBC	tuberculosis
temp	temperature
TG	triglyceride
tid	(Latin: ter in die) three times a day
TLC	total lung capacity; tender loving care
TP	total protein
TPR	temperature, pulse, respiration
trach	trachea; tracheostomy
UCHD	usual childhood diseases
URI	upper respiratory infection
Urol	urology
USP	United States Pharmacopoeia
UTI	urinary tract infection
vag	vaginal
VC	vital capacity
VD	venereal disease
vol	volume
VS	vital signs

wbc	white blood cells
WBC	white blood count
wdwn	well developed, well nourished
WNL	within normal limits
wt	weight

Symbols

♀	female
♂	male
>	greater than
<	less than
+	positive
−	negative

APPENDIX B

Guide to Nutrient Evaluation in Biologic Fluids

| Nutrient and Units | Age of Subject (years) | Criteria of Status | | |
		Deficient	Marginal	Acceptable
Hemoglobin[a]	6–23 mo	Up to 9.0	9.0–9.9	10.0+
(gm/100 ml)	2–5	Up to 10.0	10.0–10.9	11.0+
	6–12	Up to 10.0	10.0–11.4	11.5+
	13–16 M	Up to 12.0	12.0–12.9	13.0+
	13–16 F	Up to 10.0	10.0–11.4	11.5+
	16+ M	Up to 12.0	12.0–13.9	14.0+
	16+ F	Up to 10.0	10.0–11.9	12.0+
	Pregnant (after 6+ mo.)	Up to 9.5	9.5–10.9	11.0+
Hematocrit[a]	Up to 2	Up to 28	28–30	31+
(Packed cell	2–5	Up to 30	30–33	34+
volume in	6–12	Up to 30	30–35	36+
percent)	13–16 M	Up to 37	37–39	40+
	13–16 F	Up to 31	31–35	36+
	16+ M	Up to 37	37–43	44+
	16+ F	Up to 31	31–37	33+
	Pregnant	Up to 30	30–32	33+
Serum Albumin[a]	Up to 1		Up to 2.5	2.5+
(gm/100 ml)	1–5		Up to 3.0	3.0+
	6–16		Up to 3.5	3.5+
	16+	Up to 2.8	2.8–3.4	3.5+
	Pregnant	Up to 3.0	3.0–3.4	3.5+
Serum Protein[a]	Up to 1		Up to 5.0	5.0+
(gm/100 ml)	1–5		Up to 5.5	5.5+
	6–16		Up to 6.0	6.0+
	16+	Up to 6.0	6.0–6.4	6.5+
	Pregnant	Up to 5.5	5.5–5.9	6.0+
Serum Ascorbic Acid[a] (mg/100 ml)	All ages	Up to 0.1	0.1–0.19	0.2+
Plasma vitamin A[a] (mcg/100 ml)	All ages	Up to 10	10–19	20+
Plasma Carotene[a] (mcg/100 ml)	All ages	Up to 20	20–39	40+
	Pregnant		40–79	80+
Serum Iron[a] (mcg/100 ml)	Up to 2	Up to 30		30+
	2–5	Up to 40		40+
	6–12	Up to 50		50+

NOTE: Reprinted by permission of the publisher from "Nutritional assessment in health programs," ed. G. Christakis (*Am. J. Public Health* 63 Supp. [Nov.]: 34, 1973).

Nutrient and Units	Age of Subject (years)	Criteria of Status		
		Deficient	Marginal	Acceptable
	12+ M	Up to 60		60+
	12+ F	Up to 40		40+
Transferrin	Up to 2	Up to 15.0		15.0+
Saturation[a]	2–12	Up to 20.0		20.0+
(percent)	12+ M	Up to 20.0		20.0+
	12+ F	Up to 15.0		15.0+
Serum Folacin[b] (ng/ml)	All ages	Up to 2.0	2.1–5.9	6.0+
Serum vitamin B_{12}[b] (pg/ml)	All ages	Up to 100		100+
Thiamine in Urine[a]	1–3	Up to 120	120–175	175+
(mcg/g creatinine)	4–5	Up to 85	85–120	120+
	6–9	Up to 70	70–180	180+
	10–15	Up to 55	55–150	150+
	16+	Up to 27	27–65	65+
	Pregnant	Up to 21	21–49	50+
Riboflavin in Urine[a]	1–3	Up to 150	150–499	500+
(mcg/g creatinine)	4–5	Up to 100	100–299	300+
	6–9	Up to 85	85–269	270+
	10–16	Up to 70	70–199	200+
	16+	Up to 27	27–79	80+
	Pregnant	Up to 30	30–89	90+
RBC Transketolase-TPP-effect (ratio)[b]	All ages	25+	15–25	Up to 15
RBC Glutathione Reductase-FAD-effect (ratio)[b]	All ages	1.2+		Up to 1.2
Tryptophan Load	Adults	25+ (6hrs)		Up to 25
(mg Xanthurenic	(Dose: 100 mg/kg	75+ (24 hrs)		Up to 75
acid excreted)[b]	body weight)			
Urinary Pyridoxine	1–3	Up to 90		90+
(mcg/g creatinine)[b]	4–6	Up to 80		80+
	7–9	Up to 60		60+
	10–12	Up to 40		40+
	13–15	Up to 30		30+
	16+	Up to 20		20+
Urinary N´ methyl	All ages	Up to 0.2	0.2–0.59	0.6+
nicotinamide	Pregnant	Up to 0.8	0.8–2.49	2.5+
(mg/g creatinine)[a]				
Urinary Pantothenic Acid (mcg)[b]	All ages	Up to 200		200+
Plasma vitamin E (mg/100 ml)[b]	All ages	Up to 0.2	0.2–0.6	0.6+
Transaminase Index (ratio)[b]				
EGOT[c]	Adult	2.0+		Up to 2.0
EGPT[d]	Adult	1.25+		Up to 1.25

[a] Adapted from the Ten State Nutrition Survey
[b] Criteria may vary with different methodology
[c] Erythrocyte Glutamic Oxaloacetic Transaminase
[d] Erythrocyte Glutamic Pyruvic Transaminase

APPENDIX C

Guide to Determining Obesity from Skinfold Measurements

Age (Years)	Minimum Triceps Skinfold Thickness Indicating Obesity (Millimeters)	
	Males	Females
5	12	14
6	12	15
7	13	16
8	14	17
9	15	18
10	16	20
11	17	21
12	18	22
13	18	23
14	17	23
15	16	24
16	15	25
17	14	26
18	15	27
19	15	27
20	16	28
21	17	28
22	18	28
23	18	28
24	19	28
25	20	29
26	20	29
27	21	29
28	22	29
29	22	29
30–50	23	30

NOTE: Reprinted by permission of the publisher from "A simple criterion of obesity," by C. C. Seltzer and J. Mayer (*Postgrad. Med.* 38:A-101, 1965), © 1965 by McGraw-Hill.

APPENDIX
D
Approximate Calculation
of Ideal Body Weight

Women: For first 5 feet of height: 100–105 lbs
For each additional inch: Add 5 lbs
(e.g., female, 5′3″: ideal body weight = 115–120 lbs)

Men: For first 5 feet of height: 105–110 lbs
For each additional inch: Add 5 lbs
(e.g., male, 5′10″: ideal body weight = 155–160 lbs)

Optional: Add 5 lbs for medium frame
Add 10 lbs for large frame

APPENDIX
E
Food Frequency Schedule*

Name: _____

Date: _____

Instructions:

Indicate that you *do not eat* a food by making a check in the column labeled "Don't Eat." For each food that you *do eat,* write the number of times in a day, week, or month in the appropriate box.

In some cases more than one food has been listed on a line. If you do not eat all of these foods, underline the specific food(s) you eat. A space has been provided at the end for you to write in foods not listed which you regularly eat.

Food	Don't Eat	Do Eat Times/ Day	Do Eat Times/ Week	Do Eat Times/ Month
I. Chicken				
Beef, hamburger, veal				
Liver, kidney, tongue, etc.				
Lamb				
Coldcuts, hot dogs				
Pork, ham, sausage				
Bacon				
Fish				
Kidney beans, pinto beans, lentils (all legumes)				
Soybeans				
Eggs				
Nuts or seeds				
Peanut butter				
Tofu				
II. Milk (fluid, dry, evaporated)				

* Modified from *Nutrition During Pregnancy and Lactation* (1975 Edition). Maternal and Child Health Branch, California Department of Health. Reprinted by permission.

Food	Don't Eat	Do Eat		
		Times/ Day	Times/ Week	Times/ Month
Cottage cheese				
Cheese (all kinds other than cottage)				
Condensed milk				
Ice cream				
Yogurt				
Pudding and custard				
Milk shake				
Sherbet				
Ice milk				
III. Whole grain bread				
White bread				
Rolls, biscuits, muffins				
Bagel				
Crackers, pretzels				
Pancakes, waffles				
Cereals				
White rice				
Brown rice				
Noodles, macaroni, grits				
Tortillas (flour)				
Tortillas (corn)				
IV. Tomato, tomato sauce, or tomato juice				
Orange or orange juice				
Tangerine				
Grapefruit or grapefruit juice				
Papaya, mango				
Lemonade				
White potato				
Turnip				
Peppers (green, red, chili)				
Strawberries, cantaloupe				
V. Dark green or red lettuce				
Asparagus				
Swiss chard				
Bok choy				

			Do Eat	
Food	Don't Eat	Times/ Day	Times/ Week	Times/ Month
Cabbage				
Broccoli				
Brussels sprouts				
Scallions				
Spinach				
Greens (beet, collard, kale, turnip, mustard)				
VI. Carrots				
Artichoke				
Corn				
Sweet potato or yam				
Zucchini				
Summer squash				
Winter squash				
Green peas				
Green and yellow beans				
Hominy				
Beets				
Cucumbers or celery				
Peach				
Apricot				
Apple				
Banana				
Pineapple				
Cherries				
VII. Cakes, pies, cookies				
Sweet roll, doughnuts				
Candy				
Sugar or honey				
Carbonated beverages (sodas)				
Coffee or tea				
Cocoa				
Wine, beer, cocktails				
Fruit drink				
VIII. Other foods not listed which you regularly eat				

F

Food Practices Schedule*

FOOD PRACTICES QUESTIONNAIRE

The following questions are presented in order to obtain a picture of you from your childhood to the present. Please answer the questions to the best of your knowledge to help the dietitian understand you and your nutritional health needs.

Name _____ Date_____

Address _____ Age_____M____F____

CIRCLE THE LETTER OF THE CORRECT ANSWERS

1. Which of the following problems are in your parents' families?
   a. diabetes   c. high blood pressure   e. other _____
   b. ulcer   d. allergy   f. none

2. Which member(s), if any, of your family was obese?
   a. mother   c. brother(s)   e. none
   b. father   d. sister(s)

3. In your childhood family life, your parents:
   a. thought food   c. thought food was   e. forced children to
      was not   very important   eat whether hungry
      important.   or not.
   b. thought food   d. loved to eat.   f. other _____
      was sort of
      important

4. When you were a baby, you were:
   a. thin.   b. average.   c. chubby.   d. don't know.

5. During the ages between 5 and 10 years old, you were:
   a. thin.   b. average.   c. chubby.   d. don't know.

___

* Contributed by Beila S. Kunis, R.D., M.S., Community Dietitian, Illinois Family Health Centers, Inc., Chicago.

6. During the ages between 13 and 18 years old, you were:
   a. thin.   b. average.   c. chubby.   d. don't remember.

QUESTIONS 7, 8, & 9 FOR WOMEN ONLY—
PLEASE FILL IN BLANKS

7. Age at marriage _____   Weight _____

8. Age at first pregnancy _____   Weight before delivery _____
                                       after delivery _____
9. After final pregnancy, what was your weight? _____

---

10. Possible reasons for weight gain:
    a. home alone   d. stopped smoking   g. death in family
    b. tension   e. marital problems   h. loved to eat
    c. stopped working f. divorce   i. other_____

11. During which period did body size and/or weight begin to bother you?
    a. childhood   c. adult life   e. after children grown
    b. youth   d. married life   f. never had problems

12. Do you eat when you are:
    a. hungry?   e. served food?   i. enjoying company?
    b. alone?   f. angry?   j. tired?
    c. bored?   g. happy?   k. relaxing in front of TV?
    d. depressed?   h. in need of a reward? l. other? _____

13. Do you usually:
    a. eat alone?   f. like to eat?   j. eat all you would
    b. eat with others? g. prefer not to eat?   like?
    c. eat in restaurants? h. lose appetite when k. eat more than you
    d. eat in a hurry?   upset?   need to?
    e. eat at regular   i. lose weight when   l. eat in order to
       hours?   upset?   satisfy hunger?

14. Which of the following classifications of food do you prefer?
    a. bland flavors   d. sweet desserts   g. none of these
    b. salty flavors   e. fried foods   h. other _____
    c. spicy flavors   f. butter flavors

15. Which of the following problems have been with you over the last few years?
    a. weight gain   d. diarrhea   g. nausea
    b. weight loss   e. heartburn   h. pressure
    c. constipation   f. gas

16. Have you ever been on a modified diet before? Yes_____
No_____
If yes, what was the diet for?
a. digestive problems   d. diabetes   g. ulcer
b. heart condition   e. allergy   h. other _____
c. gallbladder   f. weight control

17. You felt that a modified diet was:
a. too difficult.   d. worth following as long as
b. not worth the effort.   necessary.
c. okay for a short period   e. too difficult to follow at work.
of time   f. too confusing.

18. Do you live:
a. alone?   d. in rented room?   g. in hotel?
b. with own family?   e. in apartment?   h. in store?
c. with other people?   f. own house?

19. Do you have:
a. cooking facilities in a   e. toaster?
kitchen?   f. broiler (stove or table model)?
b. hot plate?   g. pots and pans for cooking?
c. dry storage space?   h. a place to wash dishes?
d. refrigerator?

20. Shopping for food is done:
a. by you.   d. in small neighborhood
b. by other member(s) of   grocery.
family   e. daily.
c. in supermarket.   f. weekly.

21. What type of food do you eat as the main meal of the day most of
the time?
a. sandwich   d. spaghetti/noodles   g. pizza
b. roast meats ,   e. rice and beans   h. other _____
c. frozen dinners   f. casseroles

22. Do you have any of the following physical handicaps that limit your
ability to shop for food or prepare your meals?   Yes____ No_____
If yes, circle reason.
a. arthritis of fingers or   e. limited vision
wrists   f. limited strength to carry
b. difficulty walking   packages

c. back problems that
prevent bending
d. limit in extension of arms

g. amputation of fingers or
_____

23. Do you get regular exercise? Yes_____ No_____
If yes, circle type.
a. walking daily or as often
as possible
b. swimming or other physical sports activity

c. bicycle riding
d. housecleaning and/or iron-
ing on regular basis
e. other _____

24. At which hour would you be able to attend small group discussions
with others who have the same diet problems and concerns?
a. morning hours _____
b. afternoon hours _____
c. evening hours _____
d. not interested

APPENDIX
G
Abstracting Services

Abstracts of Hospital Management Studies. Cooperative Information Center for Hospital Management Studies, University of Michigan, Ann Arbor, Mich. Published quarterly, annual cumulative author and subject index.

Biological Abstracts. Biosciences Information Service of Biological Abstracts, Philadelphia, Pa. Published on the first and fifteenth of every month; semi-annual cumulative author and subject index.

Chemical Abstracts. American Chemical Society, Chemical Abstracts Service, Columbus, Ohio. Published weekly, annual cumulative author and subject index.

Excerpta Medica. Excerpta Medica, Amsterdam, The Netherlands. There are 41 abstract journals in the series; published at least ten times yearly; at least one issue is cumulative index of subjects.

Medical Care Reviews. Bureau of Public Health Economics, University of Michigan, Ann Arbor, Mich. Reviews and abstracts published monthly except September.

_____. New in Print. *J. Am. Dietet. A.,* Chicago, Ill. Reviews (abstracts) of selected articles in over 90 journals; published monthly as a service to readers; index issues (June and December) list titles of journals abstracted and cumulative subject index.

Psychological Abstracts. The American Psychological Association, Inc. Washington, D.C. Published monthly; semi-annual cumulative author and subject index.

Sociological Abstracts. Sociological Abstracts, Inc., San Diego, Calif. Published five times during the year.

APPENDIX
H
Current Awareness
Sources and Indexing Services

Current Contents. Institute for Scientific Information, Inc., Philadelphia, Pa. Published weekly; Reproduction of tables of content of journals; includes six editions:
CC/Agriculture, Biology, & Environmental Sciences
CC/Clinical Practice
CC/Engineering, Technology, & Applied Sciences
CC/Life Sciences
CC/Physical and Chemical Sciences
CC/Social & Behavioral Sciences

Hospital Literature Index. American Hospital Association, Chicago, Ill. Published quarterly; indexed according to subject and author. Annual cumulative index of subject and authors.

Index Medicus. National Library of Medicine, Washington, D.C. Published monthly; indexed according to subject and author.

Cumulated Index Medicus. National Library of Medicine, Washington, D.C. Annual cumulative index of authors and subjects; includes *Bibliography of Medical Reviews, Medical Subject Headings,* and *List of Journals Indexed.*

Science Citation Index. Institute for Scientific Information, Inc., Philadelphia, Pa. Published quarterly in three sections—Sources: journal lists and corporate index (listing of authors according to affiliated institutions); Subject: cross-referencing of authors and subject; and Permuterm Subject Index (PSI): indexing of all significant words within each sentence of title and subtitle of articles. Annual cumulative index of all three sections.

APPENDIX
I
Regional Medical Libraries of the National Library of Medicine

Region I: New England Regional Medical Library Service
(Connecticut, Massachusetts, Maine, New Hampshire, Rhode Island, and Vermont)
Francis A. Countway Library of Medicine
Harvard University
10 Shattuck St.
Boston, MA 02115

Region II: New York and New Jersey Regional Medical Library
New York Academy of Medicine Library
2 E 103 St.
New York, NY 10029

Region III: Mideastern Regional Medical Library Service
(Delaware and Pennsylvania)
Library of the College of Physicians
19 S 22 St.
Philadelphia, PA 19103

Region IV: Mid-Atlantic Regional Medical Library (District
of Columbia, Maryland, North Carolina, Virginia,
and West Virginia)
National Library of Medicine
8600 Rockville Pike
Bethesda, MD 20209

Region V: Kentucky-Ohio-Michigan Regional Medical Library
Program
Wayne State University
Shiffman Medical Library
4325 Brush St.
Detroit, MI 48201

Region VI: Southeastern Regional Medical Library Program
(Alabama, Florida, Georgia, Mississippi,
South Carolina, Tennessee, and Puerto Rico)
AW Calhoun Medical Library
Emory University
Atlanta, GA 30322

Region VII: Midwest Regional Medical Library (Illinois, Indiana, Iowa, Minnesota, North Dakota, Wisconsin)
Library of the Health Sciences
University of Illinois at the Medical Center
1750 West Polk St.
Chicago, IL 60612

Region VIII: Midcontinental Regional Medical Library Program (Colorado, Kansas, Missouri, Nebraska, South Dakota, Utah, and Wyoming)
Library of Medicine
University of Nebraska Medical Center
Omaha, NB 68105

Region IX: South Central Regional Medical Library Program (Arkansas, Louisiana, New Mexico, Oklahoma, and Texas)
University of Texas Health Science Center
5323 Harry Hines Blvd.
Dallas, TX 75235

Region X: Pacific Northwest Regional Health Sciences Library (Alaska, Idaho, Montana, Oregon, and Washington)
University of Washington Health Services Library
Seattle, WA 98195

Region XI: Pacific Southwest Regional Medical Library Service (Arizona, California, Hawaii, and Nevada)
Biomedical Library
Center for the Health Sciences
University of California at Los Angeles
Los Angeles, CA 90024

APPENDIX

J

Preliminary Data Schedule

To the client: This questionnaire is designed to help the dietitian provide you with the best nutritional care possible. Often this information is of real value in planning that care. If you are reluctant to fill out this form, please feel free to discuss your reluctance with the dietitian. The information is available only to the dietitian and the other health professionals assigned to your care.

1. Full Name_____ Age_____
2. Address _____
3. Previous address, if less than 2 years at above:

   _____

4. Marital status (circle)   S   M   D   W
5. Spouse's name_____ age_____ (D if deceased)
6. Children (name)_____ age_____ (D if deceased)

   _____ age_____

   _____ age_____

   _____ age_____
7. Parents (name)_____ age_____ (D if deceased)

   _____ age_____
8. Other people living at your residence: Relation, if any:

   _____ age_____

   _____ age_____
9. Occupation_____ Employer_____

   How many years?_____
10. Previous occupation_____ Employer_____

    How many years?_____
11. Spouse's occupation_____ Employer_____

    How many years?_____
12. Spouse's previous occupation:

    _____ Employer_____

    How many years?_____
13. Education (circle highest level):   G.S.   J.H.S.

    H.S.:   1   2   3   4

    College: 1   2   3   4

    Grad. degree

340

14. Spouse's education (circle highest level):
    G.S.   J.H.S.
    H.S.:   1   2   3   4
    College: 1   2   3   4
    Grad. degree
15. Ethnic group_____
16. Place of birth_____
17. Country of citizenship_____
18. Residency in other countries_____
19. Religious affiliation_____
20. Childhood illnesses_____
21. Serious illnesses (check those that are applicable):
    Emotional   Heart disease   Thyroid disease
    Diabetes Mellitus   Strokes   Gastrointestinal disease
                         Anemia   Other_____
22. Surgery_____
23. Past hospitalizations_____
24. Present physical handicaps_____
25. Present health concerns_____
26. Ht._____ Weight_____
27. Diet prescription_____
28. Food related concerns/needs:
    _____
    _____
    _____

29. Hobbies and recreation_____
30. Social preferences (check those that are applicable):
    Activities: Large group (50 +)_____ Small group (7–15)_____
    Moderate group (15–50)_____ Intimate (2–6)_____
    Frequency of participation: Often_____ Occasionally_____
                                 Seldom_____
    Nature: Party_____   Educational_____
             Sport_____   Entertainment_____
             Charity/service_____
             Other_____
31. Primary care provider_____

APPENDIX
K
Self-Evaluation Guide for Clinical Dietitians*

Below are listed tasks that clinical dietitians may perform; you may be doing many of these tasks now. The rating scales printed to the left and right of each task can help you decide whether you would like to change your job and what you would like to change. On the left, circle the number representing how often you perform each task in your present job; on the right, circle the number showing how often you think you should or would like to do that task. Only individual preference is important; there are no right or wrong answers. Rate each task on a scale of 1 to 5:

1 = Never 2 = Rarely 3 = Occasionally 4 = Usually 5 = Always

Present Frequency	Task	Desired Frequency
1 2 3 4 5	Gather and record dietary status information for each client	1 2 3 4 5
1 2 3 4 5	Evaluate nutritional risk of each client based on nutritional status information	1 2 3 4 5
1 2 3 4 5	Evaluate client's desire and ability to learn about modifications in food intake	1 2 3 4 5
1 2 3 4 5	Record interpretation of assessment information in dietetic cardex and on medical record	1 2 3 4 5
1 2 3 4 5	Verify primary care provider's nutritional care prescription	1 2 3 4 5
1 2 3 4 5	Establish priorities each day	1 2 3 4 5
1 2 3 4 5	Define criteria for evaluating the quality of nutritional care	1 2 3 4 5
1 2 3 4 5	Establish objectives of nutritional care for each client	1 2 3 4 5

* Adapted with permission from Schiller R.M. *Improving nutritional care: Readers respond* (*Dietetic Currents* 7:25–28, 1980; published by Ross Laboratories, Columbus, Ohio).

Present Frequency	Task	Desired Frequency
1 2 3 4 5	Guide clients' setting of their own learning objectives	1 2 3 4 5
1 2 3 4 5	Prepare learning materials for client use	1 2 3 4 5
1 2 3 4 5	Supervise meal service	1 2 3 4 5
1 2 3 4 5	Select modified menus for clients	1 2 3 4 5
1 2 3 4 5	Adjust clients' menus to accommodate changes in nutritional care prescriptions	1 2 3 4 5
1 2 3 4 5	Assist clients in menu planning of food selection for home use	1 2 3 4 5
1 2 3 4 5	Instruct clients about nutrition and necessary modifications	1 2 3 4 5
1 2 3 4 5	Make provisions for continuity of care	1 2 3 4 5
1 2 3 4 5	Gather, record, and interpret information on clients' progress toward achieving nutritional care objectives	1 2 3 4 5
1 2 3 4 5	Monitor, record, and report client response to intervention	1 2 3 4 5
1 2 3 4 5	Contribute to intradepartmental and/ or interdepartmental care audits	1 2 3 4 5
1 2 3 4 5	Present at or otherwise contribute to medical rounds and case conferences	1 2 3 4 5
1 2 3 4 5	Delegate technical duties	1 2 3 4 5
1 2 3 4 5	Develop recipes using special dietary products	1 2 3 4 5

Note the tasks that you have given very different ratings on the right and left. For example, you may have given "Select modified menus for clients" a present rating of 5 (always), but you feel confident that other personnel could assume much of this task; therefore, you may have selected 2 (rarely) or 3 (occasionally) as the desired frequency.

Choose one or two of the tasks with disparate ratings that you are keenly interested in changing soon. Your answers to the following questions will help you map out a plan of action to achieve these changes:

• To make this change, do I need new knowledge and/or skills?
• Which of my present duties can I delegate to others to make room for new ones? To whom will I delegate? Are there tasks that need not be done by anyone?
• Do I need new forms or procedural guidelines for the new duties? If so, who should develop them?

- How will I get the cooperation I need?
- Who will support me in making the changes and in my new role?

After you have answered these and any other questions of your own, you can plan the attainment of your goal(s) in manageable steps, establish deadlines for each step, recruit the help you need, and proceed with your plans. Thereafter, you can evaluate your progress periodically, celebrate your successes, and, if you wish, return to this form to identify new areas for change, adding tasks not listed above.

Glossary

Assessment   the gathering and analysis of data related to the status of the client at the point of his entry into the nutritional care process

Baseline Data   the factors or criteria identified from among the total assessment data that are to be the focus of intervention and change

Clinical Dietetics   nutritional care, offered in an environment where clients and their needs, physical, socioemotional, and intellectual, are the primary foci of professional effort

Diet History   the *tool* by which data describing a client's past and/or current food intake and food behaviors are collected. The food intake description should provide a quantitative and qualitative estimation of typical consumption. The food behaviors are characterized by usual pattern of food and nutrient consumption, variations of that intake, the impact of other significant variables, and the *process* that represents the procedure for collecting the data

Dietary Status   a statement describing what an individual has been eating which gives no direct indication of nutritional status (C. M. Young)

Dietetics   a profession concerned with the science and art of human nutrition care, an essential component of the health sciences. It includes the extending and imparting of knowledge concerning foods that will provide nutrients sufficient for health and during disease throughout the life cycle and the management of group feeding for these puposes (American Dietetic Association)

Evaluation   the process of gathering information about the effectiveness of intervention in producing the desired changes in the baseline data factors. It also includes an examination of the positive and negative influences on the change, or lack of it

Goal   an end toward which effort is directed

Health Team   a group of health professionals with a variety of skills, knowledge, values, and attitudes who work together to solve health problems (B. Siegel)

Implementation   the process of putting into action the plan for nutritional care that includes the long term goals, short term objectives, and intervention strategies

Nutrition   the science of food, the nutrients and other substances therein, their action, interaction and balance in relation to health and disease, and the processes by which the organism ingests, digests, absorbs, transports, utilizes and excretes food substances. In addition nutrition must be concerned with certain social, economic, cultural and psychological implications of food and eating (Council on Foods and Nutrition, American Medical Association)

Nutrition Education   a multidisciplinary process that involves the transfer of information, the development of motivation, and the modification of food habits where needed. . . . the bridge that carries appropriate information from the research and development laboratories to the public, the ultimate user (R. L. Leverton)
. . . the means to develop each individual's nutritional knowledge in such a way that he will be motivated to choose a nutritionally adequate diet (Society for Nutrition Education)

Nutritional Assessment   the process of describing the nutritional status of individuals or groups. The process involves the evaluation of subjective and objective data, utilizing a variety of measurement tools including the diet history, anthropometric measures, and laboratory determinations

Nutritional Care   the creative act of translating the bodies of knowledge of nutrition and other scientific disciplines to resolve the food problems and concerns of humans, through the provision of nutritional counseling and the provision of nutrient sources

Nutritional Care Plan   the tool that is the documentation communicating the management strategies devised in nutritional care planning

Nutritional Care Planning   the process that follows assessment and incorporates a series of management strategies designed to facilitate controlled change on the part of the client to realize optimal nutritional status

Nutritional Counseling   the total process of providing clients with the ability to self manage their own nutritional care

Nutritional Status   actual nutritional condition . . . as measured by physical examination, laboratory determinations, pathologic morphology, and therapeutic response under controlled conditions . . . [and] influenced not only by dietary intake but also conditioning factors, such as increase in nutrient requirements, excretions, or destruction and interferences with nutrient intake, absorption, or utilization which may be operating either currently or in the past (C. M. Young)

Objective   an observable, verifiable step toward attainment of goals

Planning   the process of identifying needs that are translated into long term goals, short term objectives, intervention strategies, and evaluation tools and strategies

Preliminary Data   the information compiled, usually before encountering the client, for the purpose of developing a profile

Process   a sequence of activities or events designed to produce a determined goal or outcome

Profession   a body of persons engaged in (a) . . . common mission . . . bound together by a common discipline in a spirit of fraternity, learning, and public service. The profession is synonymous with its membership (American Dietetic Association)

System   interacting, interdependent parts composing a viable, unified whole. An open system is in contact with the environment and is subject to change. A change in any subsystem impacts on the total system

Tool   a means to an end, as an instrument or implement used to accomplish a purpose

Index